CONTEMPORARY CATHOLIC
HEALTH CARE ETHICS

CONTEMPORARY CATHOLIC HEALTH CARE ETHICS

Second Edition

David F. Kelly
Gerard Magill
Henk ten Have

GEORGETOWN UNIVERSITY PRESS
Washington, DC

Library of Congress Cataloging-in-Publication Data

Kelly, David F.
    Contemporary Catholic health care ethics / David F. Kelly, Gerard Magill, Henk ten Have.—2nd ed.
        p.   cm.
    Includes bibliographical references (p.   ) and index.
    ISBN 978-1-58901-960-7 (pbk. : alk. paper)
    1. Medical ethics—Religious aspects—Catholic Church.   2. Medical care—Religious aspects—Catholic Church.   3. Medicine—Religious aspects—Catholic Church.   I. Magill, Gerard, 1951–
II. Have, H. ten.   III. Title.
R725.56.K438   2013
174.2—dc23

                                                                                    2012023873

20   19   18   17   16   15   14   13   9 8 7 6 5 4 3 2
First printing

To the students of the Duquesne University
Center for Healthcare Ethics,
past, present, and future

Contents

Acknowledgments

THE REVISED VERSION of this book is dedicated to the students—past, present, and future—of the Duquesne University Center for Healthcare Ethics. All three authors are on its faculty. What we present here has been explored with our students in the classroom and in the clinical context. We are grateful to Georgetown University Press for its editorial support. We thank Duquesne University and the Center for Healthcare Ethics for personnel and technical support. In particular we wish to thank Aimee Zellers, a graduate assistant at the Center, for her assistance in finalizing the manuscript for this second edition.

Introduction

THE FIRST EDITION OF THIS WORK, which is here revised, is Kelly's third book. His first is his published dissertation, which is still in print, *The Emergence of Roman Catholic Medical Ethics in North America* (Kelly 1979). That work, like most dissertations, is almost entirely theoretical. It has become a good source for scholars who want to understand Catholic medical ethics. In 1990, after a sabbatical year taken at St. Francis Medical Center in Pittsburgh, he wrote *Critical Care Ethics* (Kelly 1991). That work is largely practical, intended to serve as a guide on practical issues in hospital ethics. All of its chapters except one were originally talks given to health care professionals.

In the present book, the authors draw both from theory and from practice with the hope that this book might serve as a textbook for students and a resource for practitioners. This single volume in Catholic health care ethics includes its theological basis, its methodology, and its application. Part I, on theology, is a revision and expansion of a long article/small book Kelly wrote for the National Association of Catholic Chaplains in 1985. Part II, on method, was largely new to the first edition, and draws mainly on Kelly's first book and on research done and notes written for a graduate course now available online from Duquesne University. Much of part III, on application, is a development and expansion of chapters in *Critical Care Ethics* and draws also from course preparation. Some chapters are newly written for this book. It is mostly in part III that the second edition is revised, expanded, and updated. Here important additions have been made by Magill and ten Have.

Part I offers a theological basis for health care and health care ethics. It speaks to theological anthropology and proposes a Catholic Christian approach to the meaning of human life as that applies specifically to health care. It includes a brief history of the relationship of religion and medicine and makes claims about how theology ought and ought not to be applied to health care ethics.

Part II introduces the reader first to the terminology and approaches used by philosophical secular bioethics, including normative ethics and metaethics, and then to the methodological approaches of Catholic bioethics. It draws these two together, showing how the same questions are variously answered and suggesting how Catholic methodologies might be categorized in general philosophical language. The section on Catholic method includes a detailed analysis of the principle of double effect and its applications, thus presenting the official teaching of the Catholic magisterium (pope and bishops) on many specific bioethical issues. In particular, the issue of birth control is examined in its historical and contemporary forms. Thus, part II includes some application along with method.

Part III deals with many important issues in contemporary health care ethics. There is an especially strong emphasis on end-of-life issues because this is the area where ethics comes into play most visibly in hospitals and nursing homes. Eight chapters, chapters 13 through 20, offer considerable detail about the real questions that constantly trouble patients and their families as well as health care practitioners. Though there are some references in this section to theological and methodological issues developed earlier, this section is designed so that it can stand on its own and be relatively complete for those whose interest may be limited to this area. These chapters describe in detail American ethics and law about forgoing treatment, and are not specifically Catholic, though they do point out that much of what has become American policy in the area was taken from Catholic medical ethics. Chapters on pain and pain management and on ethics committees are also of immediate practical importance to health care practitioners.

Following the section on forgoing treatment and end-of-life care come chapters on other essential issues in health care ethics. It is here that the book's expansion is most apparent. Chapters 23 and 24 concern research ethics and organizational ethics, important areas not covered in the first edition. Chapter 25 deals with stem cell research, and is followed by two chapters on genetics that provide greater breadth and depth of this essential area than was given in the first edition. Next are two chapters on the just allocation of health care resources. The final chapter, newly added, is on global bioethics, providing insight into how this field of study can no longer be seen from a purely parochial perspective. After the text is a glossary defining some important terms.

There are a number of books about various aspects of health care ethics written by Catholic scholars. The one most commonly cited is by Benedict Ashley and Kevin O'Rourke, the latest edition of which adds Jean deBlois to its authors. In longer and shorter versions, this excellent work presents and defends the official teaching of the Catholic Church on medical ethical issues (Ashley and O'Rourke 1997, 2002; Ashley, deBlois, and O'Rourke 2006). We use this text in our courses and will continue to use it. But this is not the only approach one can take to Catholic health care ethics. A significant number of Catholic scholars are critical of some aspects of the received tradition, and we are among them. We are convinced that there are problems with the method usually used in traditional Catholic medical ethics and with some, though by no means all, of the conclusions reached by that method. And we think that this approach has been untrue to the Catholic theology that ought to serve as the basis for health care and health care ethics. This book is our attempt to present an alternative approach. Many of the practical judgments reached here are in fact the same as those reached by the received tradition. This is especially true in the crucial issues concerning ethics at the end of life. But in some areas there are differences. Catholic moral theology has not been completely constant over the centuries; it has learned and developed. The contemporary dialogue and debate contributes to that development.

When this work is used as a class text, it may be better to read the book as it is written (rather than turning directly to the chapters on application). In our experience, students need more help in working through the methodological issues than they do in grasping the more specific applications. If the practical questions are treated first, it is all too easy to ignore method completely. That does not mean that all readers will find this the best way to use this book. Some will be interested only in certain of the applications, and others may prefer to start there and then return to the theory section to follow up on methodological issues implied or referred to in the later chapters. But to look only to the applications without a grasp of the method risks the result of a superficial understanding of the discipline. Though we do describe alternative approaches to ethical, moral-theological, and bioethical method, the book intends to present a unified approach, and it is in parts I and II that we develop the foundation for that approach. It may well be that readers who find themselves disagreeing with conclusions drawn in the application chapters would better understand those issues after reading the earlier sections. Medical ethics should not be haphazard; parts I and II offer the chance to analyze, deepen, and increase the coherence of one's approach to bioethics.

Health is clearly a human good. It is connected to human wholeness, to human well-being. Yet is hard to define precisely. On the one hand, health cannot be limited to physical or bodily health, since we rightly speak of mental health, moral health, spiritual health, economic health, and so on. Holistically, health is "optimal functioning of the human organism to meet biological, psychological, social, and spiritual needs" (Ashley and O'Rourke 1997, 25). The World Health Organization (WHO) defined it in 1958 as "a state of complete physical, mental, and social well-being and not merely the absence of disease and infirmity" (Ashley, deBlois, and O'Rourke 2006, 35). On the other hand, the ethics of health care deals with a limited aspect of this wider sense of human well-being. Although health is jeopardized by any number of things, from poverty and war to earthquakes and famine, health care ethics is not ecological ethics or the ethics of war or of international monetary policy. Health care ethics cannot be all of ethics (Kelly 1979, 408–16). Health care ethics is interested in the procedures and the systems of "health care"—that is, those that are designed to restore us to physical and psychological health when this has been diminished by disease. It is thus concerned primarily, though not solely, with "health in the narrower sense of optimal functioning at the biological and psychological levels" (Ashley and O'Rourke 1997, 25). This book concentrates on the issues of physical health care not because mental health care is unimportant but because many of the ethical issues connected with it are too complex for an adequate treatment here. Much of what is treated in the book, however, can be applied to both physical and mental health care.

Abbreviations

AID	artificial insemination by donor
AIDS	acquired immunodeficiency syndrome
AIH	artificial insemination by husband
ANT	altered nuclear transfer
ANT-OAR	altered nuclear transfer-oocyte assisted reprogramming
ASBH	American Society for Bioethics and Humanities
AU	act utilitarianism
CDF	Congregation for the Doctrine of the Faith
CHA	Catholic Health Association
CPR	cardiopulmonary resuscitation
CRO	contract research organization
CT	computed tomography
DCD	donation after cardiac death
DMD	Duchenne muscular dystrophy
DNA	deoxyribonucleic acid
DNR	do not resuscitate
DPA	durable power of attorney
DRG	diagnosis-related group
EMTALA	Emergency Medical Treatment and Labor Act
ER	emergency room
fMRI	functional magnetic resonance imaging
GIFT	gamete intrafallopian transfer
GNP	gross national product
HEC	hospital ethics committee
HFEA	Human Fertilisation and Embryology Authority, Great Britain
HHS	US Department of Health and Human Services
HIPAA	Health Insurance Portability and Accountability Act
HIV	human immunodeficiency virus
HMO	health maintenance organization
ICU	intensive care unit
IEC	institutional ethics committee
IOM	Institute of Medicine
iPS	induced pluripotent stem (cells)
IRB	Institutional Review Board
IVF	in vitro fertilization

MANH   medically assisted nutrition and hydration
MCAD   medium-chain acyl-CoA dehydrogenase deficiency
MCO   managed care organization
MCS   minimally conscious state
MRI   magnetic resonance imaging
NBAC   National Bioethics Advisory Commission
NICE   National Institute for Clinical Excellence
NFP   natural family planning
PAS   physician-assisted suicide
PDE   principle of double effect
PET   positron emission tomography
PKU   phenylketonuria
PPACA   Patient Protection and Affordable Care Act
PSDA   Patient Self-Determination Act
PVS   persistent vegetative state
RAC   Recombinant DNA Advisory Committee
rDNA   recombinant DNA
RNA   ribonucleic acid
RU   rule utilitarianism
SCNT   somatic cell nuclear transfer
TOTS   tubal ovarian transfer with sperm
UDDA   Uniform Definition of Death Act
UNESCO   United Nations Educational Scientific and Cultural Organization
USCC   United States Catholic Conference
WHO   World Health Organization
WMA   World Medical Association

PART I

Theological Basis

CHAPTER 1

RELIGION AND HEALTH CARE

Introduction

IN THE UNITED STATES in the late 1960s a new development occurred in a long-standing area of inquiry. What had been the largely intrareligious study of the morality or ethics of medical practice became "bioethics."[1] Displaying perhaps a combination of arrogance and ignorance, American bioethicists often claim, or at least imply, that this field of study was created brand new by the philosophers who coined the term. Without question what happened in the last four decades of the twentieth century was a major development, essential to the emergence of what the discipline has become. Secular philosophers (those who speak from no religious tradition) began in the 1960s to show interest in a field they had for a long time ignored, and this interest and excitement made bioethics a far more influential endeavor than it had previously been. New research centers and professional groups were established. Governmental oversight bodies were appointed. Scores of new journals appeared. And the religion-based approaches that had preceded this new development have been influenced and to some extent eclipsed by it.

It is nonetheless entirely inaccurate to suggest that the new American bioethics of the late twentieth century owes little to its religious forebears. As the second and third parts of this book make clear, much of what bioethicists claim, many of the judgments they make, are based on conclusions reached by religion-based approaches to medical ethics.[2]

From the American perspective—indeed, from the perspective of the West in general—the Roman Catholic tradition has been most influential. Catholics developed over many centuries a highly specified approach to medical ethics. The Jewish tradition also created a detailed and centuries-long tradition of medical ethics, but it had less influence largely because Catholic immigrants to the United States outnumbered Jews and because, as discussed in detail in part II, Catholics adopted a natural law approach to morality, claiming that moral judgments were based on reason and, hence, applicable to all humans, whereas Jewish scholars were less apt to insist on this, basing moral claims at least in significant measure on rabbinic interpretations of scripture (Mackler 2000, 2–12).

In any case, religion has been of major significance in shaping health care ethics as we know it today. Religion develops an understanding of the human person on which an ethic of health care can be based. Thus, the first part of this book is directly theological. Readers who work on health care ethics from a religious perspective will find this part especially useful and perhaps in some sense normative. But even readers who do not find religious anthropology persuasive may want to discover what Christianity has to say on these issues. Bioethics, after all, even in its secular garb, deals with patients and health care providers who are religious and whose faith affects their approach to health care. It is clear that American bioethicists need at least a decent knowledge of the Catholic and Jewish traditions if they are to practice well. Bioethics has emerged from religious roots and cannot be understood apart from them.

Nor is it true, as is often stated by those who reject the role of religion in public bioethics discourse, that religions are not helpful because they disagree with one another. It is true that they do often disagree. But so do secular thinkers and secular approaches. Somehow it is thought valid to ask both liberals and conservatives about stem cell research despite the fact that they usually disagree, but it is invalid to ask both Catholics and Jews because they may also disagree. The richness of religious language often adds an essential dimension otherwise missing from the discussion.

Religion is concerned with the meaning of human life in its ultimate dimensions. Religious faith is the human person's response to God's revelation as God discloses to us who we are in the divine plan. Theology is our search for a greater understanding of this revelation and of our response to it. Thus, religion, revelation, faith, and theology are all centrally interested in the meaning of human life. Why do we exist? When and how do we live at our human best? What kind of respect do we owe our own human lives and those of others?

Sometimes religion has tended to understand human life from an overly spiritualized or angelicized perspective. This has occurred from time to time in certain movements in Christian and Catholic theology. When this occurs, religion tends to reject the importance of the body, of human health, and of the processes of health care. These aspects of human life are then considered irrelevant to spiritual growth or are even seen as hindrances to it. The human person is turned into a kind of inferior angel whose true home is the world of the spirit. Religion is reduced to the otherworldly.

More often religion has included in its searching and its theologizing these essential aspects of human living. Human health and health care have been of central importance to much of Christian theology and Christian practice. Religious women and men, clergy and laity alike, have dedicated their lives to human healing, both of the body and of the spirit. Theologians and health care professionals have worked together in developing theologies and anthropologies of health care and of health care ethics. Health care and religion have something to offer one another.

The aim of part I is to explore the idea of a theological basis for health care and health care ethics. What can Christian theology bring to our understanding of human health, of human health care, and of bioethics? We explore the topic in several stages. The first chapter is an overview of the history of the relationship of religion and medicine, suggesting some of the main lines in the Christian theology of health care. The second and longest chapter develops the theological basis for human dignity, exploring the theological themes that serve as the fundamental basis for health care. The third chapter speaks of the integrity of the human person and explores both dualistic and holistic approaches to Christian anthropology. Here we also try to deepen our understanding of how God works through human actions, of the relationship of divine and human (natural) causality in health care. Chapter 4 speaks of the sanctity and quality of life, two concepts often seen in opposition to one another as principles for health care ethics, and also discusses the problems of individualism and corporatism in health care. Finally, chapter 5 is a methodological analysis of how theological principles have worked and ought to work in the actual practice of health care ethics. It deals especially with divine sovereignty over human life and with the meaning of human suffering as principles in medical ethics.

The scope of these first five chapters includes themes common to all religions, but the focus is on Christian theology generally and on the Roman Catholic tradition specifically. This focus reflects the historical influence of Catholic medical ethics.

Religion and Health Care

Until the last forty years or so, Roman Catholic theologians and philosophers, together with Jewish scholars, were virtually alone in the field of medical ethics. Although other philosophers and theologians studied ethics and moral theology in general, and although they applied moral principles to sexual and social issues, they never developed in depth the science and art of health care ethics. Professional associations of physicians such as the American Medical Association did promulgate and interpret codes of medical ethics, but these were more likely to be codes of etiquette for members of the profession intended to enhance the prestige of physicians than they were actual moral analysis of health care procedures and structures. As has already been noted, this situation has changed radically in recent decades as bioethics has become a rapidly growing field of study for philosophers, health care professionals, lawyers, historians, sociologists, theologians, and religionists of various backgrounds and religious affiliations.[3]

The fact that, until recently, only Catholics and Jews developed detailed studies of health care ethics does not mean that only they were interested in the larger relationships of religion and medicine. Even though the Roman Catholic tradition was the most detailed and the most influential, and even though only this tradition produced a truly systematic and extensive literature in health care ethics, the relationship of medicine and religion is significant within the larger Christian tradition and generally in the religions of our world. Religion deals with the core questions of human existence and is thus interested in issues of healing. The human person is an embodied spirit, an animated body, and so human health involves spiritual and physical aspects in inseparable interaction. Although one or the other of these may rightly be emphasized for certain purposes, the complete separation of the human person into spiritual and physical parts is detrimental. Until the Enlightenment of the eighteenth century, the radical separation of medicine from religion was not attempted, and religions generally included physical healing in their ministry to whole people.

A number of world cultures have combined the two arts of healing in the same person. Egyptians and other Near Eastern peoples, Asians, and some of the Celtic and Germanic tribes did this. The "holy man" was the physical healer as well as the religious leader. What we know today as modern medicine, of course, was not available, and these healers combined a trial-and-error approach (empirical medicine) with religious practices of a supernatural or magical kind. Westerners are starting to find out that, although some of what "primitive" peoples do and did to heal themselves is ineffective, many of their techniques do work, and we are adding this "alternative and complementary medicine" to our own medical repertory (Callahan 1999). Perhaps more important, we are discovering anew what "primitives" were never tempted to forget, that healing concerns whole people and is most effective and most ethical when it addresses the needs of whole people. Physicians who forget this and see only parts of a body, and clergy who forget it and see only angels or souls, run the risk of doing a great deal of harm (Kelly 1979, 47; Agnew 1967, 581–82; Pompey 1968, 14).

Historians often refer to the Greek physician Hippocrates of the fifth century BC as the founder of scientific or rational medicine. He introduced a rational approach to medicine, insisting on the process of diagnostic analysis. For Greek medicine—and for Roman medicine, which followed it—this replaced the previous combination of "empiricism" (trial and error) and magic (Kelly 1979, 47; Entralgo 1969, 15; Agnew 1967, 582; Pompey 1968, 15). But it did not separate religion and medicine. Hippocrates saw medicine not as something secular but as a part of his religion. The changes he introduced were as much religious as medical. Nature was sacred, not secular, and to study it and heal it was to act religiously. For Hippocrates, disease and health followed laws of "natural" causality, but these laws were nonetheless sacred, not secular (Kelly 1979, 48; Entralgo 1969, 42–44).

Following the time of Hippocrates, most Greek and Roman doctors were not official religious leaders, and this practice continued during the first centuries of Christian Rome. Physicians of the time recognized, however, that their vocation was of religious significance. They were to serve as Christ had served, to heal as he had healed, even to save as he had saved. The Christian concept of agape (love or charity to others in imitation of Christ's love of humankind) entered their understanding of the Christian medical vocation, and with it came an insistence that doctors must treat the poor for free, must care even for incurable patients, and must consider spiritual as well as physical needs. Patients were more than objects to be treated if curable and otherwise ignored (Kelly 1979, 49; Entralgo 1969, 54).

As the structures of the Roman Empire collapsed, so did the approach to medicine the Romans had inherited from the Greeks. But in accord with the importance Christianity gave to healing and to caring for the poor and the suffering, specifically religious Christian institutions began to take up the work of the "lay" doctors. Monks in their monasteries cared for the sick, and some bishops built hospices for travelers and indigents. Thus, priests and religious women and men began to take over the work of the physician (Kelly 1979, 49–50; Entralgo 1969, 56–57, 60–62; Pompey 1968, 17–20). It is interesting to note that the results were at best mixed. At first, these monks and nuns studied and followed the medical practices of the best of the Greek and Roman doctors, and they added to this what they discovered in their missionary wanderings among the pagan tribes of Europe. Gradually this learning was rejected, and the same combination of trial-and-error with specifically religious remedies that we noted in pre-Hippocratic medicine replaced it. It seems as if there was little interest in exploring how to be a better doctor or in trying to understand disease and its cure (Kelly 1979, 50; Entralgo 1969, 65–70; Pompey 1968, 18–19). For the monks, medicine was not so much an art to be studied and wondered about as it was an added responsibility. Their primary desire was to be monks, not physicians. In this context, and in the general social disintegration of the time, medical care diminished in quality. But once again the Christian religion and its institutions had given evidence of the importance of health and health care to religion.

In the High Middle Ages of the twelfth and subsequent centuries, medicine again came alive as a discipline in its own right. Educational centers appeared in the great cities of Europe, and these universities began to teach medicine to interested students. Fewer and fewer physicians now were priests or monks (Kelly 1979, 50–51; Entralgo 1969, 62, 74). In fact, church synods and councils began to forbid the clergy to practice medicine, probably because they did not want them to earn their living at it and thus fail to carry out their religious duties, and because the primitive state of medicine at the time often meant that physicians would be involved in useless or harmful procedures that could bring notoriety and even criminal charges (Kelly 1979, 51; Pompey 1968, 23, 25–26). Of more lasting importance in the reemergence of medicine was scholastic theology, especially that of Thomas Aquinas and his followers, which rediscovered the philosophy of Aristotle with its insistence on nature and on natural laws. Medicine could emerge again as an art to be studied and explored. But in this revival medicine was still religious. The intellectual context of the time was theocentric, and the study of medicine was perceived to be a part of the study of God's creation as God willed it to be (Entralgo 1969, 78–79, 83–90). For many of the lay doctors of the Middle Ages, and of the Renaissance and Baroque eras that followed, the care of the sick was a specifically Christian vocation (Entralgo 1969, 91–100; Pompey 1968, 30). Sir Thomas Browne's 1642 book is a classic example of how one physician viewed his vocation (Browne [1642] 1963).

This started to change in the eighteenth century, when European intellectual patterns came to be dominated more and more by the Enlightenment. Enlightenment philosophers such as Voltaire, Kant, Newton, Locke, and Hume began to stress the importance of human reason and of scientific analysis for human progress in isolation from and even in opposition to religion (Kelly 1979, 61–62). They saw that the preceding centuries had often been engulfed in interreligious disputes that had caused turmoil and considerable suffering for the people. They thought that a freedom from this kind of darkness would release humanity from the shackles that kept it bound to reactionary authoritarianism. They thus rejected much of religious authority, especially when they perceived it as hindering human development, which they tended to identify with scientific and technological progress. Human reason could achieve a better society. Religion was accepted only, or at least primarily, for its utilitarian function of teaching people how to behave morally for the establishment of a better society.

In this intellectual environment, medicine tended for the first time to separate itself ideologically from religion. In the previous centuries, most doctors had been lay Christians, not priests and religious. But they had seen their vocation as quite clearly a part of their Christian religion and of its worldview. Now medicine was to become secular, unreligious, and sometimes even antireligious (Pompey 1968, 8–11).

It was in the eighteenth century that Christian theologians began to develop a specific field of study and body of literature to explore the interface of religion and medicine. What had previously been sporadic or had been incorporated into larger treatises of systematic or moral theology now found its own expression and a beginning of cohesion in a subdiscipline of pastoral theology known as pastoral medicine. Theologians and some Christian physicians recognized that the complete separation of medicine from religion was harmful to both disciplines, and pastoral medicine emerged as an attempt to correct this. The term "pastoral medicine" is generally unfamiliar today, especially in the United States, but it was the primary prediscipline to the Catholic medical ethics of the twentieth century. As pastoral medicine arose in the eighteenth century, and as it continued into the nineteenth and twentieth centuries, it tried to bridge the gap between religion and secularized medicine by including all aspects of the interface of these two disciplines (Kelly 1979, 62; Fleckenstein 1963, 160).

Pastoral medicine thus developed two emphases, one medical and the other theological. The first emphasis was to teach the theologians and the parish clergy what they needed to know about medicine. Theologians would need this knowledge in their study of Christian anthropology in order to understand better the meaning of human persons as God created us and intends us to live, the way in which human beings act and react, the theological questions of body–soul interaction and of grace and human freedom, and in order to develop a moral theology of medical practice. The parish clergy would need medical knowledge in their parish ministry as counselors and confessors, and to enable them to provide first aid and basic medical advice to parishioners where doctors were lacking (the tendency of medical personnel to gravitate to the big cities is not new, and rural sections of Europe in the eighteenth century were often without physicians). The second emphasis of pastoral medicine was theological and ethical. Doctors could learn from theologians about the spiritual dimensions of the person and about the application of moral–theological principles to medical practice (Kelly 1979, 60–61).

As pastoral medicine developed, it emphasized first one, then another of the various aspects it included. During the eighteenth century, under the influence of the Enlightenment, much of it was limited to manuals of first aid for rural priests and ministers. Religion was to be useful in some measurable way, and physical healing and hygiene to prevent disease were ways to achieve this goal (Kelly 1979, 63–64; Niedermeyer 1955, 1:15–19, 53–54; Fleckenstein 1963, 160–61; Pompey 1968, 8–12, 33–117, 295–96). In fact, some of the early literature quite clearly argued that this was to be the clergy's primary task. It transformed the clergy into doctors. At the other extreme were works of pastoral medicine that altogether rejected the Enlightenment search for better medical science and argued for a supernaturalist approach that would change doctors into clergy (Niedermeyer 1955, 1:55–57). In the nineteenth and twentieth centuries pastoral medicine moved more and more in the direction of moral theology or medical ethics, and some books were really medical ethics texts. Yet despite these shifts in emphasis and tendencies to limit the field to one or another aspect, pastoral medicine maintained a dialogue between medicine and religion.

The years since the 1960s have seen a new revival of the study of medicine and religion and of medicine and ethics. Medical ethics, long a Roman Catholic discipline, is now quite ecumenical. Nurses, physicians, lawyers, and other professionals involved in health care and in health care institutions are studying with philosophers and theologians to develop better approaches to the complex individual and structural questions that beset the health care system. Medicine no longer considers itself separate from the wider concerns of the meaning of human existence, traditionally the subject matter for theologians and philosophers.

There are many reasons for this. Some are obvious to all who are involved in health care in any way: the rapid growth in medical technology with its tendency to dominate medical care to the exclusion of personal interaction and personal choice; the rise in health care costs; the availability of instant communication techniques in the media, which bring public attention to the advances and the failures of the health care delivery system; and new problems connected with transplants, allocation of resources, genetic engineering, and so on.

Beneath these readily apparent reasons are more subtle ones. Theology has long been a source of ethical reflection. As early as the fifteenth century, physicians were singled out for analysis in the moral manuals of the Catholic tradition along with judges, clergy, and politicians. Over the centuries, only health care providers have received detailed attention, an attention due to the special nature of health care itself. It is because medicine is of its very nature a relational profession that it has such an intrinsic moral component. In the practice of medicine, in the provision of health care, professionals put their knowledge and skills to use in dealing with nonprofessionals at exceptionally intimate and vulnerable moments. Patients are by definition those who undergo, those who suffer. The patient, who undergoes, is vulnerable. Thus, sociologists note that professionals have a "guilty knowledge," a knowledge of things dangerous to know. It is this combination of vulnerability and guilty knowledge in the clinical life-and-death context of medical practice that sets health care apart as a particularly moral enterprise.

There is an even deeper reason for the long relationship of medicine and religion, one especially apparent in recent decades. Medicine, particularly when it is in a period of rapid change, tests our understanding of the very meaning and importance of human life. Biotechnology, genetic engineering, and similar contemporary pursuits emphasize this. And it is a religious question. Religion and medicine are both concerned with the existential center of the human person, with sickness, sin, health, and salvation. Both deal with limit situations, with moments and events and questions in our lives that put our very selves to the test of meaning. A theological basis of health care and of health care ethics will have to deal with this, with questions of Christian anthropology, with questions about what it means to be human.

Notes

1. The term "bioethics" was coined by Van Rensselaer Potter, who wrote *Bioethics: Bridge to the Future* in 1971 (see chapter 30 in this volume). The term was then adopted by others to imply a shift in emphasis from the "medical ethics" that had preceded it, adding to the previous emphasis on the doctor-patient-treatment context an emphasis on biological research and bio-medical techniques.

2. Throughout its history, various terms have been used to designate the field. In this book we will use "bioethics," "biomedical ethics," "medical ethics," and "health care ethics" more or less interchangeably, though in some cases historical context will suggest the use of one or another of them. For a detailed analysis of the various names used, see Kelly 1979, 106–8, 219–21, 407–8.

3. The first influential modern work written by a Protestant was Joseph Fletcher's *Morals and Medicine* (1960).

CHAPTER 2

THE DIGNITY OF HUMAN LIFE

CATHOLIC MORAL THEOLOGY has traditionally argued that ethics (what we ought to do) must be based on anthropology (who we are). Contemporary theologians have drawn from both the tradition of Catholic theology and the developments of modern philosophy to explore anew the meaning of human life as God intends it. This chapter suggests a theological basis for the dignity of the human person. Health care and health care ethics presuppose at their very core that the human person is of special worth, and the Christian understanding of the human person supports this concept of human dignity.

Catholic theology has traditionally argued for the dignity of the human person from two theological bases: creation and redemption. It was God's original purpose to create the human person with a special status within creation. But sin tainted the original goodness of humankind, and, though we never entirely lost our position as specially valued images of God, we were found to need a savior, a redeemer to restore us to God's grace and favor. Thus God decided to send Jesus as savior, to return to us the capacity of life according to God's original design.

This approach to the theological foundation of human dignity is of value, and its emphases on creation and redemption are essential to the Christian story of God's loving care for human beings. But contemporary theologians are apt to point out that this approach suggests too much that Jesus Christ is an afterthought in God's plan for human destiny. The God who creates is the same God as the God who saves from sin, say such theologians as Karl Rahner and Edward Schillebeeckx, and it was God's will from the beginning that all of humankind should share in the divine life in and through Jesus Christ. God did not "decide to send Jesus" only as an answer to sin. The tradition of the felix culpa ("happy fault"), for all its beauty, is inadequate. It was not sin that caused the incarnation of God in Jesus Christ; it was God's original creation of human dignity and destiny that laid the basis for the divine communication of God's self to humankind in the God-Man Jesus Christ. For Schillebeeckx, "'Christology' is concentrated creation: belief in creation as God wills it to be. It is not a new divine plan for a creation which has gone wrong. . . . Belief in creation is essentially bound up with belief in the person of Jesus as God's definitive salvation for men and women" (Schillebeeckx 1982, 118). Human dignity, created by God and revealed in Jesus, the human face of God, is at the center of the Christian message. It serves as a basis for the theological anthropology that grounds health care and health care ethics.

Christian theology has often referred to our human dignity as an "alien dignity" (Thielicke 1975, 231). Sometimes this implies that it is not really we who are special but rather that our dignity is only borrowed temporarily from God, as if God might at any moment decide to eliminate it. In this scenario God becomes something of an uncaring experimenter. God grants us a temporary set of attributes to see what we might do with them, to see if we will jump the hurdles. God may be intrigued but does not ultimately care. The entire Christian message of the incarnation rejects this interpretation of alien dignity. Alien dignity means something quite different. Having freely chosen to create human beings, God has also freely chosen to involve God's very self with us, with our plans and our sufferings, our virtues and our sinfulness. That is what the cross and resurrection of Jesus mean. Our dignity is indeed "alien." Properly understood, however, the alien nature of human dignity means not that human dignity is a fiction, nor that it is extrinsic to ourselves, but that it is established by God. That God keeps us in existence does not reduce who we are but ennobles us. Alien dignity means that our worth is not found in any mere usefulness granted us by other women and men. We are of worth. That worth is from God, not from the individual or social agreement of other humans. We are of more than utilitarian value. Our worth remains even when sin-filled persons or sin-filled structures ignore it. It is alien because it transcends us and our possibilities of rejecting it. It is this approach to human dignity that best serves as foundation for health care and health care ethics. The Christian message, when properly understood, adds a theological, religious dimension that reinforces the basis for health care and health care ethics. Humans are intrinsically worthy. God has said yes to human life.

The concept of human dignity as developed in Christian theology can be explored through various themes. Following the outline of John F. O'Grady, in *Christian Anthropology: A Meaning for Human Life* (1975), this chapter treats four such themes: the human person as image of God, chosen by God, ordered to God in grace, and alienated from God by sin.[1]

The Human Person as the Image of God

The Christian understanding of the human person considers men and women to be the pinnacle of God's creation. We are made in the image of God (O'Grady 1975, 10–11). The very beginning of the Bible makes this clear. The Jewish and the Christian understanding of the meaning of human personhood as created by God in the beginning is one of total goodness and of almost divine stature.

In the stylized poem of the first chapter of Genesis, the author waits until the sixth and last day of God's creative activity to create the land animals and man and woman. God has prepared for this moment. First came light; then land and water; then the plants; then the sun, moon, and stars; and, on the fifth day, the fish and the birds. These last receive a blessing to go forth and multiply. At the end of each day, "God saw that it was good" (Gn 1:1–25).

Finally, on day six, "God said 'Let us make humankind in our image and likeness.' . . . God created humankind in God's image. In the divine image God created it. Male and female God created them" (Gn 1:26–27). Men and women receive the same blessing as the other animals to go forth and multiply, but to them is also given "dominion" or authority over the rest of creation. At the end of the sixth day, God saw that what had been created was "very good."

Two of the key words here are the Hebrew words "*selem*" and "*demuth*," usually translated "image" and "likeness," respectively. The first word suggests an actual physical resemblance. People look like God. The second word corrects that impression while adding to the impact by repeating that God creates us to be of almost divine stature. We are not photocopies of God, but in a very concrete way we resemble God and are God-like (O'Grady 1975, 10–11).

Much of the tradition of Christian theology, influenced by Greek philosophy, has tended to interpret this theological theme of creation in God's image in a very spiritualized and dehumanized way. Since much of Catholic theology has depicted God as pure and perfect spirit, unchanging, and completely indivisible, theologians have tended to emphasize only the spirits, souls, or minds of women and men in the context of our created imaging of God. Only our souls are created in God's image, according to this approach, not our bodies. But a human soul is not a human person. The book of Genesis tells us that humankind is created in God's image. There is no implication in most of the Hebrew Scriptures that men and women are split into two parts. That is, there is little or no anthropological dualism. Nor is there an "original dualism" (O'Grady 1975, 11). Unlike some other religions contemporaneous to Jahwism, the Hebrews rejected the idea of two creative forces or gods—one good creating spirit and light, the other evil creating matter, darkness, and sin. It was not just a part of the human person that was created in the image of the one God. Rather, the human being, the body–soul complex, the existing person is like God.

Why? What is it about the human person that makes her or him like God? The answer is complex, but it is at least partly because humans, like God, have dominion over the rest of creation (O'Grady 1975, 11–14). We exercise authority in God's name over the earth and the animals. Adam names the animals, a sign of authority over them. Unlike the rest of creation, in the language of contemporary theology we can be said to transcend who we are. We are open to self-creation in and through history. We can hope for a future and act to bring it about. Alone in creation—at least the creation we have so far come to know—women and men can reflect on who they are, can be aware of what they are not, and can decide, within the limitations of created finitude, to change themselves and their society. The very enterprise of health care depends on this kind of understanding of the human person, even if the understanding is not explicitly theological. Scientific knowledge requires both a faith in the ongoing coherence of nature and the possibility of making leaps into the unknown, of hypothesizing about the future, and of making that future real. Thus, the biblical teaching on the human being as created in God's image, or a secular equivalent of it, is in some ways essential to the ongoing task of health care.

In biblical times, this notion that human beings were the image of God was very different from the idea of humanity prevalent in some other religions. In many of these, humans were subservient to the forces of nature. Humans were to worship these forces and in some cases actually sacrificed themselves or their conquered enemies to them. For the Hebrews, in contrast, human beings were not set below the rest of creation, but above it. Nature was not divine. It was created, like humans, by God. This was the natural order of things: God the creator in dominion over all of creation, including human beings, and humans acting for the Lord in dominion over the rest of creation, constituted the original harmony desired by God (O'Grady 1975, 12).

This emphasis on the created goodness of human persons and on our almost divine stature does not require a literalist belief in the details of the Genesis story as if this work were scientifically or historically "accurate." If time travelers could go back with video cameras, they would see something quite different from the idyllic garden pictured in the book of Genesis. The goodness of God's creation is not that of a created infinity, of a created perfection, were such a thing logically possible. We are not God. This is symbolized for us even before the fall in the fact that God gave a command that separated humanity from Godhood. Humankind was not to eat of the fruit of the tree that only God could digest.

This has important implications for an anthropology that proposes to found a health care ethic. It means, first, that human beings are created in a dignity that makes them both creatures and cocreators with God. We are not merely equal to the rest of creation. We are to some extent cocreators, or at least coagents with God in bringing God's plan for creation to fulfillment. Yet we are not God; we are creatures. Our creative powers are limited, both by our creaturely finitude and by sin. Not only can we make mistakes but we can also sinfully break up the fabric of God's creation and of our own society. I will return to the ethical implications of this theological principle of creaturely cocreator in chapter 5. The understanding that Genesis is not meant to present a historically accurate idyllic picture of a perfect garden is important for a second reason as well. It is important to know that there never was a time when creation was not finite. Sometimes we get the idea from certain interpretations of Genesis that in the beginning life was totally without struggle, without work—indeed, without growth and maturation. Education was instant, love easy, healing unnecessary. This approach can lead us to see our life and work mostly as the unfortunate consequences of that "original sin." Had there been no sin, there would have been no work, no reading, no art, no struggle to create, no medicine, no progress or regress, no tripping and falling. Admittedly, it is very difficult to distinguish, in this real world of ours, between sin, which God did not want, and human finitude, which was part of the divine plan. But a more nuanced understanding of the theology of creation at least tries to grasp more adequately the built-in finitude of our creation, understanding it not essentially as a sin-caused obstacle but as the very possibility of creation in the first place. God never intended to make us God. What God did was create a "good creation." And in that creation, the creature *ha adam*—humankind—was of very special worth.

This more nuanced approach to the notion of creation in God's image is also helpful in understanding and responding to some recent criticisms of Christian anthropology that have emphasized its potential dangers. Some have argued that it is precisely because we think we have dominion over the earth that we have caused such human and ecological havoc. Those who take this view argue for an anthropology that sees the human being as merely one more kind of animal, more complex, perhaps, but differing only in degree and not in quality from the beasts. They charge Christianity with "humanocentrism," or with "speciesism," with forgetting the rest of nature in its rush to depict men and women as God-like.

Although there is much truth to these charges, at least in their practical ethical implications, it is unhelpful to reduce the stature of the human person to that of nonhuman nature. The human person, as created by God, experiences herself or himself as transcendent. This is a phenomenon of human life. It is not evil humanocentrism to recognize and make theologically explicit the vast difference in freedom and dignity between human beings and the other creatures with which we are familiar. To fail to do so is perhaps to hate oneself by rejecting one's own nature.

But this does not give us a license to run roughshod over the rest of creation. God's universe is good in itself, even prior to the arrival of our species. God's purpose in creating cannot be restricted to what is good for humanity. The Jewish and Christian notion of human dominion over creation is not intended to be absolute. It is a created and limited dominion.

There are two reasons why this is so. The first requires no real theological sophistication and can be supported simply from human self-interest. An absolute dominion would lead to devastating results for the human species itself were we to act on it in an unlimited fashion. Human beings are part of the ecosystem and depend on it. Our self-transcendence does not change this. The second reason is theological. Humankind is called to exercise its authority in creation not as God but as cocreative creature. Though we are created with special dignity and preeminence, and with special authority and "dominion," we are nonetheless created along with the rest of God's work. God's will is not that we undo what God presents for both divine and human honor and glory but that we transform creation and ourselves as caretakers of what God has made. People are called to exercise stewardship, not total domination.

The theme of the human person as the image of God continues in a particular way when Christian theology proposes Christ as the perfect image of God. If all women and men are created in God's image, Christ is the perfect image of the Father. For the rest of us, the image is tarnished, but not for Jesus. Thus, Paul tells us that "Christ is the likeness of God" (2 Cor 4:4) and "the image of the invisible God" (Col 1:15). Jesus exercises his dominion as God does, and as God wants us to exercise it. What women and men are called to be in creation is realized in Jesus.

The Human Person Chosen by God

The theme of the human being as image of God is one of the core creational themes of Christian anthropology. As we turn now to the theme of divine election, and when we later discuss the theme of the ordering of humanity to God in grace, we should remember that these are not added to the first theme in any separable way. That is, God's election and the gift of God's grace are not decisions added later or superimposed by God as afterthoughts. Rather, they reflect from different theological perspectives the very same intrinsic dignity of human life that we have already discovered. God created human beings with a destiny to be chosen. The best of Christian theology does not see that destiny, and its actual achievement in grace, as another layer added to ungraced, undestined natural humanity. The human person is special, according to Christian theology, because we are created at the start with a graced destiny of self-transcendence.

That human beings have a destiny in God's original creating will can properly be called a kind of "predestination" (O'Grady 1975, 25). Human dignity arises in large

measure from the fact that God has created us with this predestiny to transcend ourselves, to move beyond our own horizons and that of our surroundings to share God's
life. Even those of us who do not accept this belief in its specifically Christian form
experience the phenomenon of human freedom with its call to move beyond who we
are, to seek the infinite, to share in the spirit of God.

The term "predestination" has, of course, another meaning as well—a meaning that,
in its more extreme and simplistic forms, contradicts and undermines the very possibility of true self-transcendence and thus destroys in large measure the theological basis
for human dignity. This second meaning is unfortunately the more common one. Here
predestination means not the creating will of God that all humans be ordered to God
through grace, but a kind of arbitrary divine decision whereby only some are given
the real possibility of salvation, while others, comprising most of humankind, are left
inevitably without God's power and life, condemned to endless death. God decides
ahead of time who will be saved and who will be damned. Human freedom has little or
nothing to do with it. God's grace, when it is offered, overwhelms freedom totally; the
saved have no choice, since this kind of grace cannot be rejected. Nor do the damned,
since God withholds grace from them and leaves them to the power of sin and death.

The theological problems of the relationship of grace and freedom, or of "nature
and grace," are complex, and even such theologians as Karl Rahner have not "solved"
them. The divine–human relationship is a mystery.[2] But it is at least clear that God's
creating desire and plan for human beings includes a destiny that respects the human
freedom and capacity for transcendence that God has given men and women. Thus, it
is in this more theologically precise sense that the term "predestination" is best used.
God has planned, in creation, that human persons should live full human lives with
God in Christ. God has predestined all women and men to live with God's own self
(O'Grady 1975, 24–25).

The Jewish and the Christian teachings on election make more specific certain
historical and symbolic events through which God is seen to work the divine salvific
plan. Christians specify three principal events or stages in the unfolding of God's plan
for human salvation: creation, election, and incarnation.

We have already discussed at some length the first principal stage, the creation of
men and women in the image of God with a special blessing and a special task. Humans
are to share in God's work of transforming the world and themselves in accordance
with God's plan. This creative alliance is continued in an ongoing covenant between
God and all humanity, a covenant symbolized in events that the Bible narrates as having
preceded the more important covenant with the people of Israel that would follow later.
Two examples here can give us an indication of how God continues this creating alliance with all people.

The first occurs after Cain kills Abel in the fourth chapter of Genesis. God punishes
Cain for this act of murder, but even here God agrees to give Cain a token that will be
a sign to others who might harm him that God still holds Cain in his favor and protection. This event is a symbol of God's ongoing relationship to created humanity.

The second example is better known, and it, too, symbolizes the universality of
God's covenant with the human person. The eighth and ninth chapters of Genesis
narrate the story of Noah and his family, saved by God from the flood. After the flood
ends, God repeats to Noah and his family the same blessing given to Adam and Eve at

the moment of their creation. God adds a covenant with them, an alliance with all of humanity that pledges God's fidelity and sets in the sky a token of that pledge: the rainbow, a sign that God would never again in wrath destroy the world by water. All of humankind is special to God.

The second principal stage in the unfolding of the history of salvation is, of course, the election of the chosen people of Israel. This event is seen first in the call to Abraham and is then repeated over and over again throughout the Old Testament. God calls Abraham out of his own land to a new land that God will give him. Abraham will be the father of a new and special people. God symbolizes the degree of commitment to Abraham and to the people of Israel by agreeing that if God should ever reject the people, which will never happen, it will be right for God to be destroyed. The oath ritual in Genesis 15 is a kind of early and solemn "cross my heart and hope to die." The ritual was used to solemnize treaties between persons or peoples. The parties to the treaty would kill a number of animals, cut them in half, and then walk between the pieces. The idea was that if they violated the treaty, they would deserve death and dismemberment. Here it is God (a fiery oven) who walks between the pieces of the animals. God is committed to the chosen people. "You will be my people and I will be your God."

The election enters a new and advanced stage with Moses, when God leads the people out of Egypt, symbolizing a release from bondage and oppression. God gives them the law, which they receive not as a new burden of impossible tasks but as a gift from God establishing anew the covenant God continues to make with the specially chosen people. The alliance is again renewed through the kings, who will rule the people in God's name.

The covenant does not always work out well. The prophets constantly remonstrate with the people about their failure to fulfill their responsibilities. The people are unfaithful to God. They oppress the poor and the powerless. They refuse to accept their task of transforming self and society in accordance with the divine plan for their destiny. Sin alienates them from the God who has chosen them. Yet the dignity of their lives remains. God's fidelity to the election remains. God punishes and calls them to repentance, and when they repent, God again accepts them and the alliance is renewed and repaired (O'Grady 1975, 29-31).

The third stage in the working out of God's plan for human destiny, as this is seen by Christians, is the incarnation. When the time was right, God came as a human being to reveal God's own self to women and men. The predestination of humanity is accomplished in the enfleshment of God in Jesus, and through the cross and the resurrection. Here is the new election, the new covenant, the transformation of humanity from the order of Adam to the order of Christ. God gives God's very self to created humanity in a self-communication.

The life, teaching, and death of Jesus reveal how important humans are to God. God is involved in the actual living of a human life and in the actual dying of a human death. The Christian scriptures leave no opening for an idea that has sometimes invaded our theology and our piety: that Jesus was not really human but only a kind of extraterrestrial visitor from a spiritual world. That heresy has been with Christianity throughout much of its history. Perhaps it is because we are unable to accept the idea that, for God, we are worth the incarnation, the humanization of divinity. Perhaps it is because when we reject the possibility of God's forgiveness we need some kind of excuse to distance ourselves from the challenge Jesus gives us to live life as fully and as lovingly as he did. So we say that the reason he could live that way was because he was God, and not really human. Whatever the reason, the docetic heresy, the idea that Jesus merely appeared to be human, that he was a kind of visiting deity masquerading as one of us, undermines the central Christian basis for the dignity of the human person. If God could become a human being, the dignity of humankind is indeed demonstrated in a new and exciting way.

Christians believe that Jesus establishes a covenant, a new development in the alliance of God with the chosen people. Christians are called to make this covenant manifest, to be its sacrament, to sign forth the alliance by their lives and their actions and their very beings. The first letter of Peter states: "You are a chosen race, a royal priesthood, a holy nation, a purchased people; that you may proclaim the perfections of him who has called you out of darkness into his marvelous light" (1 Pt 2:9). Christians have a task to make manifest what has been revealed to them about God's plan for humankind. They are to strive for peace and justice, for the transformation of self and world in accordance with the dignity and the cocreative challenge given them by God in creation, in election, and in incarnation. Like Israel, Christendom has failed to live up to the covenant. Christians oppress the poor. They violate their own dignity. They are unfaithful to the God who has chosen them and who has shown them the way in Jesus. Yet, as with the people of Israel, God calls them to repentance and is faithful to the alliance (O'Grady 1975, 32).

The Human Person Ordered to God by Grace

The dignity of the human person as created by God and as destined to divine life is oriented or ordered to this life through grace. We have already noted the complexities of any theological attempt to spell out the relationship of grace and human nature with any precision when treating of the two meanings of predestination. Christian theology has tried, not always successfully, to maintain a balance between the created freedom and dignity of the human person and the gratuitous grace of God. Contemporary theologians, especially Karl Rahner, have furthered this attempt in an important direction by refusing to allow any easy separations between "nature" and "grace." Though not identical, the natural and supernatural orders in the human person cannot be separated. And while the exact relationship is mysterious, the mystery reflects the complexity of the human person actually existing in the world and is not so much a problem to be solved by theological analysis as a disclosing and unfolding of what it means to be a human being (O'Grady 1975, 52–56; Rahner [1954] 1961; 1963, 3–44; [1959] 1965).

All of this, which seems sometimes so abstract, is essential to any attempt at establishing a theological basis for health care and health care ethics. Health care providers develop sensitivity to their patients. Those who approach their work from a specifically Christian perspective will find that this sensitivity is affected by their theology of the human person. In chapters 3, 4, and 5, we deal more specifically with the problems of dualism, with the relationship of divine and natural causality, and with the use of theological principles specifically in health care ethics. But all of this depends on an adequate theology of the meaning of human life. For Christians, this must of necessity include the issues of nature and grace. If these two aspects of human life are seen as antagonistic to one another, so that human "nature" is somehow unworthy of care, then health care can never be a truly Christian vocation. Only grace and the supernatural life of the soul have importance. The mystery of graced nature remains a mystery, but it is important to grasp that in humankind God's gift of grace does not mean that human "nature" is less worthy but that it is more worthy. That the human person is ordered to God by grace is one further dimension of the dignity of the totality of human life, not a reason for splitting people into matter and spirit and limiting our ministry to the spirit. It is the whole person who is graced. For Catholic theology, at least in its better moments, grace does not overwhelm human freedom, nor is the human being so radically depraved as to be without reception for, or a natural affinity to, grace. Grace reaffirms and enhances the dignity and the nobility of human life (O'Grady 1975, 58–59).

Grace is experienced. If it is true that God, in creation, has destined us to share divine life in Jesus, then that divine life ought somehow to be experienced. The actual experience of God's life through grace has been the subject of analysis by theologians and psychologists, and of poetry and expressive prayer and narration by those we call mystics. For some, the experience of grace, or the religious experience, is a feeling of total dependency on God, or a blind leap into God's void. Rudolf Otto, in his classic work *The Idea of the Holy* (Otto [1923] 1950), suggests that true religious experience is the experience in human life of the fascinating and scary mystery who is God. The mystics have tried through narration and symbol to describe their encounters with God's presence in their lives, but these attempts never capture adequately the experience itself.

The fact is that "grace," or the experience of God's life in our human lives, can never be adequately defined. There are two reasons for this. The first is the more commonly recognized. Since grace is of God, grace is of its own nature mysterious. It transcends our comprehension. The second is less obvious but perhaps of greater importance for health care. If grace is not something separable from our own humanity, if—although not identical to human nature—grace can never be separated from our humanity or analyzed apart from it, then the mystery of human nature itself, the transcendence of the human person in our actual lived experience, imposes its own mystery on the mystery of grace. Grace, in other words, is mysterious not only because it is supernatural, thus going beyond our comprehension; it is also mysterious because it is human. Human persons, in our unfathomable humanness, are the ones who are graced. Grace does not exist on its own, out there somewhere in a large reservoir waiting for people to turn on the tap. It is human beings who are graced, and grace thus shares in the human mystery.

In the scriptures, grace is really any and all gifts of God to women and men. Grace is a free gift. It is not something contractually owed. God does not owe us creation, nor does God owe us salvation or our human destiny—though having created us, God owes us the respect due to his own handiwork. Grace is any and all communication of God to us. It is the process whereby God tells us about herself, calls us closer to divine life.

Various theologians in the development of Christian theology have given different emphases to grace and have seen the relationship of grace and human nature differently (Getz 1982). For Augustine, in the fifth century, grace was primarily a medicine that healed a humanity corrupted by original sin. His purpose was to heal; Augustine was no hater of humanity. Yet there is in Augustine a kind of pessimism about human nature, especially in its bodily and sexual aspects. Augustine emphasized the power of grace, and although he usually tried to maintain the tension between this divine power and human freedom (Augustine 1887b, 5–10), there are places in his theology where he lets go of that tension and almost eliminates freedom from the balance. He sometimes argues for the more simplistic forms of predestination where humanity becomes God's plaything, and the vast majority of humankind is condemned (Augustine 1887f; 1887e; 1887b, 41–46). Nonetheless, Augustine maintains the biblical notion that God created humankind good, and that God intended men and women to share divine life in Jesus Christ. For Augustine, humankind's purpose from the very beginning was to share in God's life.

Thomas Aquinas, in the thirteenth century, was considerably more positive about the worth of human nature. Even without grace, human nature in its "pure" state and in its fallen state retains its natural tendency toward God, its desire to see God, its affinity for God's grace. If Augustine's starting point was original sin and the need for healing grace, Thomas emphasizes the goodness of human nature as created by God and sees grace as elevating that nature to a new, added, supernatural level with its own new purpose (Thomas Aquinas 1945, II, 997, *Summa theologica* Ia IIae, q. 110 in corp., also *ST*, IIa IIae, q. 171, ad 3). In this way, Thomas better expresses the continued worthiness of the human person and better maintains the dialectic between freedom and grace. Grace builds on nature; it does not oppose it. Grace opposes sin. This was true for Augustine, too, but since for him human nature had been thoroughly and radically depraved by sin, there was little or nothing good left in it for grace to build on. Thus, for Augustine, grace opposed (sinful) human nature, whereas for Thomas, human nature, in its freedom and capacity to receive grace, could work more harmoniously with it.

But Thomistic theology, especially as it developed in theologians who followed after Thomas, tended to split nature and grace too much. Grace built on nature, true. But grace was something added to nature, as if nature could exist without it. Thus the danger came of a new kind of dualism, one that split the human person into the merely natural and the newly supernatural. This distorted the mysterious interaction in human life, the dialogue of the divine and the human. In some theologies it also led to the reification of grace. If grace was separated from the human mystery, perhaps "it" could be comprehended as a thing on its own. The various distinctions among kinds of grace, and the tendency to think about amounts of grace earned and lost and kept somewhere in escrow till the next confession, came from this separation. Paradoxically, as grace became more and more supernatural, separated from the human, it became more and more definable and comprehensible. It could become a thing added to human nature, rather than an integral aspect of the alien dignity of human life in its mysterious richness.

Contemporary theologians, particularly Karl Rahner, have tried to overcome the dualism inherent in some earlier concepts of grace. Rahner's approach has been called "transcendental Thomism" because he tries to build on Thomas's notion that human nature has a built-in capacity for or affinity with grace while he changes the tendency in some older theologies to separate nature and grace. Rahner talks about a "supernatural existential" (Rahner 1963, [1954] 1961). Human beings, as we exist in this world, participate in the supernatural order and are never totally separate from it. Even those who reject God's grace are, as human beings, related toward it even in its absence. This "supernatural existential" means that saving grace is not limited to those who are explicit believers in Christ. Grace is not added to human nature as an extra. There is only one order of human existence, and it includes our supernatural destiny as God intended in our creation.

For Rahner, grace is God's self-communication to women and men. And it is we, as humans, who are the primary communicators, the sacraments of God's revelation. We humans are the symbols through whom God's revelation comes. Among us humans, Jesus Christ is the perfect symbol, the most complete communication, the definitive grace.

A definition from another time and context can summarize our brief survey of the dignity of human life as ordered to God in grace. The Council of Trent in the sixteenth century declared that grace is God's love for us as that love is in us and changes us. God's gift of grace to human persons is an integral part of the dignity of human life.

The Human Person Alienated from God by Sin

In exploring the biblical and the theological notion of the dignity of the human person, we have already mentioned the reality of sin. This final brief section on sin in the human condition comes last among the themes for good reason, because for the Christian, the dynamic of sin, important as it is, is secondary to the dynamic of creation-election-grace. God's plan from the beginning was and is for the supernatural human destiny of all men and women. Human sin opposes that plan, but in God's power and love sin never really threatens to destroy it. The supernatural existential in God's graced creation is not just an equal antagonist holding its own against the powers of sin and death. Rather, the order of grace has achieved the ultimate victory over sin. This is the good news of the gospel (O'Grady 1975, 62–92; Mahoney 2003, 724–26).

Nonetheless, sin remains an important and often devastating dynamic in human life. Those who are involved in health care know this from experience. First, and more obviously, there are the ethical issues connected with health care—the issues that comprise "medical ethics"—and these issues have to do with right and wrong, with human choice, and often with greed, sloth, deceit, lust, envy, hubris, violence, and waste—in a word, with sin. These dynamics exert their influence not only in the individual acts of sinful people, including both healers (health care providers) and patients (health care recipients), but also in the very structures of the way health care is delivered. Some of these issues are relatively simple; many more are excruciatingly complex. It is not always easy to know precisely where the "sin" is or what the morally right solution is. Yet despite this, we sense the reality of sin, of brokenness, and of the injustice and cruelty that we people do to one another.

Second, and less obviously, there is a deeper dynamism of sinfulness inherent in the human condition that can appear in times of sickness. Here distinctions between sinfulness and created human finitude blur. Not all limitations are sin or sin's results. It is sometimes hard to know what is sin or the effect of sin, what is truly evil, and what is merely part of the necessary processes of growth and decay inherent in creation. We have seen that among the species we know, humans alone are aware of their future and can hope for a true transcendence beyond their present limitations. Yet this very capacity brings with it a loneliness, an anxiety, a recognition of limits, a human confrontation with death. Sensitive health care professionals are aware that the medical enterprise, with its vulnerability and "guilty knowledge" in combination with what is often a life-and-death context, brings out these human encounters at their deepest and most significant level. This can be terrifying. It can also be faith-filled, trusting, and consoling. The Christian belief that God in Jesus Christ has triumphed over sin and death adds a hope and a faith that human life is ultimately meaningful. This does not remove the pain of confronting sin and the ultimate limits of creation. It does not easily answer the challenge that comes to us from the experienced absurdities and evils that plague human living. But it does offer a faith and a hope that God's plan will be brought to fruition despite the power of sin and alienation. God's destiny for humankind is prior to and greater than the sin and death that would deny it.

The question of how evil can exist in a world created by a good and loving God yields no easy answers. Yet some approaches are more adequate than others, especially in the context of health care and health care ethics. For some Christian theologies and pieties, all human limitation is the result of personal sin. Disease is a sign the sick person has sinned. Natural calamities like droughts and floods are signs of God's wrath on sinners. The Bible itself often connects calamity and misfortune with the sins of Israel. Often such a connection does indeed exist. Sickness can be the result of abuse or violence. "Natural" calamities can be the result of environmental exploitation or of unjust economic and political systems. But the facile identification of all limitation, of all sickness and suffering and decay, with sin and its results is inadequate and even harmful, especially in the context of health care. More adequate Christian theologies and pieties recognize that God could not create a second God. God could only create something created, and creation has within itself, seemingly of necessity, characteristics of finiteness, characteristics of limitation, characteristics of growth and decay, even characteristics of violence. The alternative to this may not be perfection; it may be nothingness.

Then, too, there is human freedom. The human person, in his or her freedom, is given the possibility of rejecting for himself or herself the realization of God's plan. Contemporary moral theology is far less apt to identify specific ways in which this is done (mortal sins) than was the moral theology of prior times. But Catholic theology has traditionally upheld the possibility of such a rejection. True freedom, of course, is not the freedom to sin; it is the freedom not to sin that comes with grace. But God gives us grace in a way consonant with our own human freedom. God does not overwhelm our freedom but invites it to an acceptance of the eternal plan for humankind. Thus, in a paradoxical way, human freedom requires the possibility of sin. If it is to have the possibility of saying yes, which is truly freeing, it must also have the possibility of saying no.

This is the heart of what many of today's Catholic moral theologians mean by the term "fundamental option." The idea is often misunderstood to mean a kind of laxism or even subjectivism. But "fundamental option" does not do away with the possibility of mortal sin, the possibility of choosing death instead of life. Nor does it imply that real sinning is only internal, that those who may cut themselves off from God and from neighbor must do so by some kind of deep introspective decision that has no direct connection with others in the real world. It is true that the Bible, and all of moral theology, is clear that sin is ultimately a violation of God's holiness. But the same Jewish and Christian tradition proclaims loudly that sins of injustice, greed, and lust against other persons are equally sins against the holiness of God, precisely because God has created humanity in God's own image and likeness, has predestined it to share divine life, and has established that destiny through grace. A fundamental option for evil, like a fundamental option for good, is symbolized, established, and confirmed through human choices and human acts.

The reality of sin in our human world is both individual and structural. There has been a direction lately in Catholic moral theology toward a reemphasis of structural and systematic sin. Structural sin was never really forgotten in the Catholic moral tradition, though it was often underemphasized. Ethicists now recognize the interdependence of structures and individual actions. When structures are unjust, and to the extent that they are sin-filled, their oppressive tyranny often surpasses the evil of individual sinful actions. And individuals who find themselves within such structures are less free to say yes to God's plan.

The reemphasis on structures and systems within Catholic moral theology in general has had important results in health care ethics. Prior to the 1960s, Catholic medical ethics was concerned almost exclusively with topics of immediate concern to medical professionals in their daily practice (Kelly 1979, 221–27). Most of the larger issues of pastoral medicine were ignored. Little attention was paid to the nature and biases of medicine itself, or to the social and economic factors so essential to health care. Topics concentrated on the individual medical actions of physician, nurse, and patient. Many concerned reproduction. The methodology of Catholic medical ethics, the way it analyzed issues of health care, was especially apt for these kinds of topics and stressed specific distinctions of actions in their precise physical or biological components. Chapters 10 through 12 examine this in detail.

This has now changed. Many Catholic moralists are interested in the more complex issues concerning structural sin in the health care system (Kelly 1979, 407–16). Unfortunately, as we will see in chapters 28 and 29, there is sometimes a tendency to think that easy answers are available, a tendency similar to the past idea that individual medical procedures were open to simple moral analysis. Some approach structural issues in medicine with the same kind of facile condemnation they now reject when it is applied to individual procedures. Despite these dangers, however, the shift in emphasis toward recognition of the importance of structural sin is beneficial to health care ethics.

The dynamic of sin is an important and fundamental dimension of human life. But more important from the Christian perspective than the order and dynamic of sin is the order and dynamic of grace. Sin is not dominant. For the Christian, sin is seen in the context of the prior and more fundamental order of graced creation with its God-given destiny. Sin is relativized by the forgiveness and reconciliation that God offers in Jesus. The alien dignity of the human person is established by God and thus worthy of human respect.

Notes

1. Jack Mahoney approaches this using the four doctrinal pillars of Christian faith: creation, sin, salvation, and fulfillment (Mahoney 2003, 721–27).

2. For a typology of the ways in which divinity and humanity are understood to interact, see Getz 1982.

CHAPTER 3

THE INTEGRITY OF THE HUMAN PERSON

T HE PURPOSE OF THIS CHAPTER is to explore, in the context of health care, two contrasting approaches to a theological understanding of the human person and of the relationship between God and humankind. These contrasting approaches are dualism and holism.

The chapter has two parts. The first will develop in general the issues involved in the problem of dualism. The second will explore how dualism and holism yield different directions in our understanding of how God works in the world of women and men. That is, the second part of this chapter discusses the theological question of the relationship of divine and human causality. Who causes what? How do God and humans interact in causing change? Does human healing contradict or cooperate with divine healing?

Dualism and Holism

We have already alluded to dualism and holism in discussing the theological basis for human dignity. For the Hebrew there was little if any idea that the human person was split into two more or less separable parts: body and soul. But this integrated view of the human person was not the only one influencing Christian theology. For many centuries a second, more dualistic understanding of the human person was dominant, and its dominance affected our understanding of ourselves as embodied creatures.

The terms "dualism" and "holism" are important ones in contemporary theological anthropology, but they are not easy to define. A number of different sorts of dualisms can be described. There is "anthropological dualism," which designates a split in the human person between bodily and spiritual aspects. Inevitably in this kind of dualism there is the judgment that the spiritual aspect, or soul, is the good part, or at least the more important part, and that the material aspect, the body, is the evil or less good part, or at least the less significant aspect of the human person. Instead of seeing human beings as animated bodies or embodied spirits, dualists see us as imprisoned souls. For the anthropological dualist, the human soul is reduced to its present diminished or sin-filled state largely because of its imprisonment in material flesh. It strives to return to its original pure state of spirituality.

Other forms of dualism may be connected in various ways to this body–soul dualism. "Original dualists" hold that the split in human persons between soul and body is explained by the fact that there are two equally powerful creator gods, one good who creates spirit, and the other evil who creates matter. Thus, for the Manichaeans, salvation is the return of the good soul from the evil body to the good god of light.

Similarly, sexist dualists, who hold for the inherent superiority of man to woman, often identify man with soul, spirit, and intellect, and woman with body. Woman is inferior to man as body is inferior to spirit. Sexism pervades human social and economic systems, including systems of health care. The large discrepancy in income between doctors, who until recently have been mostly men, and nurses, who have been mostly women; the unnecessary surgery sometimes performed on women; and the tendency in some approaches to medical ethics for men to tell women what they may and may not morally do with their bodies are examples of practices where sexism is apparent.

Then there is the kind of dualism that so separates humankind from the rest of creation as to reject any notion of interdependency and interaction. This is the dualism that is often charged against the biblical idea that humankind has a "dominion" over nature. It arises when dominion becomes exploitive domination. Like all dualisms, it implies that the mind and the technology it creates should take precedence over material creation, the "body" of our universe. This destructive form of anthropocentrism is also often coupled with sexism. Men are said to be the ones capable of changing nature with their minds and technology; women are seen to be more like the body of nature. Feminist ethics correctly criticizes this form of patriarchy.

Finally, there is a dualism in our theological understanding of divine and human causality where these are seen as two separate and even opposing principles. Theologies that oppose grace to human freedom are examples of this. This dualism is treated later in this chapter.

The opposite of dualism is holism. This emphasizes the integrity of the human person and opposes any attempt at those kinds of dichotomies that would diminish the dignity of human persons by splitting us up into superior and inferior parts. It is true that the term "holism" is sometimes used to avoid the complex analyses necessary for an adequate theology and ethics of health care. "Holism" can become a modern and rather pedantic word for everything good, noble, true, and beautiful. It rejects criticism and questioning because it is "whole." When used this way, the term "holistic" is applied to ethics or to medicine in a way that covers up sloppiness and hinders good ethics and good health care. Nonetheless, as an antidote to the truly destructive forms of dualism that so often arise in theology and in health care, the contemporary emphasis on human integrity is essential.

We have already seen that the Hebrew Scriptures present a generally holistic view of the human person. There is little anthropological dualism and no original dualism in the main Hebrew tradition, although sexism is apparent in the patriarchal system of the Hebrews, and some later Old Testament books show the influence of body–soul dualism. It is the whole person who is created in the image of God, not just the soul or spirit. The Hebrews did not think in terms of distinctions or separations within the human person. There are no words in biblical Hebrew that can correspond correctly to later notions of "body" and "soul." Indeed, most of the Old Testament does not include with any real clarity the idea of an afterlife. There is no notion of an individual "immortal soul." Human life is here and now embodied as God wants it to be. The *nephesh*, or human person, is animated by God's *ruah*, the Spirit or divine force of God that returns to God when the *nephesh* dies.

Pauline anthropology is generally similar. Paul thought primarily in Hebrew terms. His basic understanding of the person is holistic. His famous discourse on the struggle between the spirit and the flesh in his letter to the Romans does not refer to the soul and body of the human person but, in keeping with the Hebrew practice of using terms to apply to the whole person under differing perspectives, refers to the whole human person because that person is or is not empowered by Christ's Spirit and grace. It is not the soul that wars against the body but the cosmic order of God's grace that wars against the cosmic order of evil and death.

Greek philosophy, with its emphasis on distinction and analysis, brought along with its great contribution to Western thought a tendency to reduce the bodily aspects of men and women to second-class status. Platonic, neo-Platonic, and Stoic schools were especially influential in this. Whereas in Hebrew thought almost any "part" of the human person could represent the whole, in Greek thought the human being was indeed split up for analysis. And in many schools of Greek thought, the body was considered ontologically or essentially inferior to the spirit. For Plato, for example, the real world was not this world, with its material reality, but the world of ideas of which this world was merely an imperfect image. Body and matter were inferior to mind and idea (Plato 1991, bk VII, 514a–521b).

It is interesting to note that this dualism led to two opposite extremes concerning an ethic of the body. For both hedonists and Stoics, the body was unimportant, insignificant when compared to the spirit. The hedonists concluded from this dualism that people ought to pursue pleasure with abandon, since whatever they did with their bodies counted not in the least, whereas the Stoics argued for an ascetic life, since the body ought to be suppressed and disciplined in the service of the soul.

This dualistic emphasis entered Christian theology early in its development. To reject all Greek influence as if Christian theology would have been better without it is too simplistic. It is in any case quite impossible to determine what Christian theology would have been like without Hellenism, since its influence has been central and not peripheral. But it is possible, and indeed necessary, to point out and to counteract the inadequate theologies that have resulted from this influence.

The dignity of the human person is a dignity based on God's plan that humans be created in the divine image with a destiny to live with God. But what is it of the human person that images God, and what is it of the human person that has such a destiny? Unfortunately, many Christians have been apt to answer that it is our souls or our minds or spirits that image God, and that only they have an ultimate destiny. Bodies are of no ultimate importance.

Early in the development of the theology of the human person, church authors (the fathers of the church) began to develop the idea that the human person was created in God's image. They asked what it was about the human person that imaged God. They even asked what aspect of God the human being resembled. Varying answers to these questions showed varying implications concerning the integrity of the human person (O'Grady 1975, 16–18). For Irenaeus of Lyon, the entire human person was created in the image of Jesus of Nazareth, who was the image of God the Father. There is here no sense of dualism. For Origen (who castrated himself to remove sexual temptations) and for Clement of Alexandria, on the other hand, our spirits were created in the image not of the incarnate Jesus but of the preexisting Word of God, the Platonic Logos, the Son as he was in the perfect world of ideas, the spiritual world. And for Augustine, who emphasized the depravity of human nature resulting from original sin, it was our minds that imaged the eternal Trinity. Thus, in much of Christian theology, the soul took precedence and the body became diminished.

Though no orthodox Catholic theologian has ever held that the body was created evil by God—Augustine himself was adamant in rejecting the Manichaean heresy that thought so—there has been a general tendency in Catholic theology to downplay the body's goodness and importance. Scholastic theology included tendencies toward a separation of body and soul, and of natural and supernatural orders. Thus, the Catholic religion was seen as "saving souls." In comparison, other tasks were secondary.

Contemporary theologians are in the process of counteracting this trend. Drawing on contemporary philosophy with its "turn to the subject," today's theologians are more apt to stress the integrated mystery that is the human person. Because the body is a human, enspirited body, and because the soul is a human, enfleshed soul, the human person in his or her totality is worthy of respect. We are free and noble not because of our souls but because of our created humanity. Even the idea of our eschatological destiny has shifted with the realization that it is not so much our "immortal souls" that are saved in a spiritual afterlife as it is our total human selves in a future that is here and now as well as in a more definitive state where God and we will fulfill our created destiny. The Christian dogma of the resurrection of the body takes on greater meaning in this context. Heaven becomes less an unhuman place where souls float around and more the realization of human hope as revealed to us by God.

Implications for health care are apparent. Health care practitioners are not performing secondary functions as they heal bodies instead of souls. The integrity of the human person means that it is indeed impossible merely to heal a body, as if that body belonged to a person who existed somehow apart from it. Sensitive and ethical health care professionals learn this from their experience with those whom they serve. Theology agrees. As God has created us, and as God has predestined us, we are whole beings who deserve to be treated and healed as such. The alien dignity of the human being is the dignity of an integrated person.

Divine and Human Causality

One sort of theological dualism needs further exploration. Throughout the history of the development of Christian theology, one of the most difficult theological issues has been the relationship between divine and human or "natural" causality. We have already discussed aspects of this. Sometimes the issue has been framed in the context of the relationship of grace and nature or of grace and human freedom; here the central issue becomes whether grace and nature are two separate or even opposing forces or whether they are two interconnected dynamics in God's original creating will, a question we have already briefly explored. Or the issue can be seen in the context of original sin,

with its effects on human nature and on the world; here the issues become the relationship of sin to natural causality and created finitude, the degree to which sin has altered
or destroyed God's original plan, and the problem of how much of what we experience
as growth and as decay is due to sin rather than to the inherent limits of creation. We
have also briefly developed these areas. We need now to turn more directly to the issue
of causality itself.

The problem is easy enough to describe, though the theological and human mystery it presents is unfathomable in its richness and depth. What is the relationship
between divine and human causality? What does God do and what does "nature,"
including human nature, do? How actually does God work in human affairs? Does God
directly create disease? Is disease a divine punishment for sin? Is the healing of disease
cooperation with God's creative plan, or is it rather a contradiction of that plan, a
usurpation of God's sovereignty, a removing of what God has sent? If God causes and
wills cancer, then are we contradicting the divine will when we try to cure it? Does God
heal disease or do we? Has God established a "nature" that God wills to be closed to
human transformation? Or is human causality, transforming the world and even
humanity itself, acting in cooperation with God's will?

It is easy to see how a dualistic answer to the problem of divine and natural causality gets us into trouble. The very way we ask the question causes problems, if we see
divine and natural causality as separated from each other. Some of the questions in the
previous paragraph may appear bizarre to us, but they are questions demanded by a
dualistic approach to this issue of causality. If God's acting is seen as intrusive, as an
opposition to the created causalities of the world and of human beings, then this kind
of problem emerges.

We can easily enough reject two extremes that fall outside any acceptable Christian
theological spectrum: the extremes of a reductionist naturalism and of a reductionist
supernaturalism. The former extreme is an atheistic denial of all divine causing; it
allows only for natural causality and denies altogether the existence and relevance of
God's creative activity and providence. It has seldom been a temptation for Christianity.
The latter extreme has at times found its way into Christian theology and piety. It is a
supernaturalistic rejection of all natural processes of causality. It tends to lead to a
rejection of science and medicine, to insist on "faith" as the only acceptable process for
healing, and to see God's immediate choice in each and every event. Natural disasters
are seen as God's punishments for the sins of those hurt in them, and disease is seen
as an immediate punishment for the sins of the person who is sick.[1]

Yet if it is easy to reject the extremes of the spectrum, it is harder to develop an
adequate theology of the relationship of divine and natural causality. It is hard to
remember that these causal dynamics are in fact not separate, and so we are tempted
to identify certain events as "God's will" while we stress the human or natural causality
in other events. Nonetheless, a correct theology will continue to emphasize the inseparability of these aspects of creative causality, refusing to allow either to eliminate the
other.

The Old Testament includes various approaches to the relationship of divine and
natural causality. At times the Bible tends to see God's direct hand in events that we
would be less likely to describe as directly caused by God. Thus, the prophets often see
natural disasters and sickness as God's punishment. Wars that afflict the Israelites are

seen as God's wrath against their infidelity, and the prophets often reject any attempt the people make to form alliances to protect themselves against their attackers. Jahweh himself will destroy their enemies; they are not to trust in natural alliances. Thus, the prophet Hanani criticizes King Asa for his alliance with Aram; Isaiah and Jeremiah both reject alliances with Egypt. God himself has caused the war; God alone can save the people from its devastation (2 Chr 16:7–9). Medical help may also be rejected. For example, King Asa is criticized for turning to doctors and not to Jahweh in his final illness (2 Chr 16:12). And Deuteronomic theology rejects Israel's attempts to develop a kingdom with secular rulers, insisting that God alone rules in Israel.

But there is also a different theme in the Old Testament, a theme in which human or natural causality cooperates with the divine will. The Jahwist tradition, in its theology, accepts Israel's attempts at establishing a kingdom. This approach emphasizes God's trust in the people of Israel; the king rules with God's confidence and is God's representative who transforms the land in accordance with God's will. Here the people continue the task entrusted to them in the beginning. Within the limits of creatureliness, women and men carry on God's work. It is in this line that the book of Sirach (Ecclesiasticus) praises the physician and his skill: "The skill of the physician shall lift up his head; and in the sight of great men he shall be admired. The Lord created medicines out of the earth; and a prudent man will have no disgust at them" (Ecclus 38:1–3).

The same two approaches to the relationship of divine and human or natural causality continued into Christian theology. Sometimes the emphasis was placed on a more immediate divine causality, at other times on natural causality. Those who stressed the latter might be accused of secularizing Christianity, of neglecting the immediate importance of God's presence, while those who stressed the former might be charged with denying the goodness of God's creation or with hindering scientific and social progress. It is probably impossible to avoid an overemphasis on one or the other aspect as long as we see these two modes of causality as separate. When we do, we are likely to reject divine causality altogether if we are not believers, or to reject human causality if we are. Thus, for example, the early Christians Tatian and Tertullian argued against the use of medical care, as did the tenth-century ascetic Nilus, who insisted on trusting in God and not in doctors (Entralgo 1969, 79). Bernard of Clairvaux, in his twelfth-century letter to the monastery of Anastasius, rejects at least some use of medical treatment for monks, since "those who live the life of nature cannot be acceptable to God. . . . The proper medicine is humility and [prayer to be purged of guilt] . . . because vain is the help of man" (Bernard of Clairvaux 1953, 458–59, letter 388). One further example is the nineteenth-century condemnation of inoculation against poxes, which were explained as God's punishment (Schillebeeckx 1982, 117–18).

But the central tradition of Catholic theology has not been opposed to medical care. Indeed, even in some of the examples just cited, it is hard to be sure whether the opposition was based on bad theology or on a correct avoidance of ineffectual and even harmful medical treatment. Catholic theology has generally supported health care as a properly Christian task, and even as a special Christian vocation. Catholic theology has developed the necessary basis for allowing the possibility of health care as pursued by human art without seeing it as contradicting God's own purpose. In the process of doing this, various theological stages have been important.

We have already mentioned the work of Hippocrates, the Greek physician and philosopher of the fifth century BC who contributed to the advance of medicine by pointing out the patterns in nature, patterns that would enable the student of anatomy to understand disease and its cure through a process of analysis, diagnosis, and prescription. Modern medicine is based on this process. But Hippocrates did not really secularize medicine, as so many have believed (Entralgo 1969, 60-62; Pompey 1968, 17-20). Rather, the advance he made in the understanding of nature was as much theological as scientific. Instead of seeing in disease and its cure the more or less whimsical decisions of supernatural beings (the Greek gods and goddesses), he saw in these things the workings of nature. He did not, however, reject the supernatural aspects of causality, since for him nature was a sacred, not a secular, reality.

Philosophers and theologians recovered the tradition of Greek medicine in the High Middle Ages. Here Thomas Aquinas was of particular importance. Basing his theology on the philosophy of Aristotle, Thomas stressed nature in a way somewhat similar to that proposed by Hippocrates. Nature is not opposed to grace. Rather, grace builds on nature. Similarly, divine and natural causality need not be seen in opposition to one another but are instead compatible. It is easy for us to underestimate the importance of Thomas's claim that "the perfection of divine providence requires intermediary causes for its fulfillment" (Thomas Aquinas 1945, II, 144, *Summa contra gentiles*, bk 3, ch 77). Thomas distinguished primary and secondary causality (ibid., ch 72). Though God is the ultimate or primary cause, God works through created secondary causes that we can study and learn to manipulate. These are patterns embedded by God in creation, patterns that God expects us to learn about and to work with. Processes such as disease and healing are not the immediate result of God's free choice but are rather mediated by the patterns of causality placed by God in the created world (Entralgo 1969, 87). "Just as the divine providence does not altogether banish evil from the world, so neither does it exclude contingency, nor impose necessity on things" (Thomas Aquinas 1945, II, 133, *Summa contra gentiles*, bk 3, ch 72).

Similarly, Aquinas's notion of "conditioned necessity" helped in the process of integrating divine and natural causality. Certain realities, events, and processes were to be seen as only conditionally necessary and not as absolutely necessary. Although caused by God as primary or ultimate cause, these events need not be seen as absolutely willed by God but only as conditionally willed. We may rightly alter them by learning to use the patterns God has embedded in creation (Entralgo 1969, 87-94; Thomas Aquinas 1945, I, 198-200, *Summa Theologica* I, q. 19, a.3).

Thomas was interested in medicine. He writes about the causality that moves the human heart, and, more important, he spends a great deal of effort to determine the kind of human endeavor medicine is. For Thomas, medicine is not a science like physics as much as it is an art. Yet it is an art that must use the knowledge of physics and of other sciences, "for the practices used in the art must be based on the properties of natural things" (Thomas Aquinas 1986, q. 5, art. 1, ad 5, p. 22). That is, medicine is an art in the sense of a skilled art, a *techne* in the Aristotelian sense. It draws on knowledge of the patterns of natural causality that God has embedded in creation to do God's work in transforming creation according to God's plan (Larkin 1960).

Thomas's development for Christian theology of the complex relationship between divine and natural causality was thus an important step forward toward providing an adequate theological basis for health care and for health care ethics. Divine and natural causality could be seen as cooperating. Medicine could be accepted as an art in its own right, without any sense of conflict with God's active providence. Contemporary Catholic theologians have furthered this process by insisting even more on the inseparability of divine and human causality. Despite the advances he made in stressing their compatibility, Thomas still tended to think in terms of two more or less separate levels or orders, one human and the other divine, one natural and the other supernatural, one of nature and the other of grace. Today Catholic theology has moved toward a rejection of this separation. The mystery of the meaning of human life is such that it is impossible to separate what is human and what is divine.

This inseparability does not mean that we can act as if either causality had been eliminated by the other. This is often a danger in "holism"—we keep only the part we like and we call it the whole. The history of the Christian tradition may have wrongly separated the two kinds of causality, and it may sometimes have seen them in opposition to one another, but it is important not to lose sight of the insights gained when these "two" causalities are seen in creative tension with one another. Though it is true that they can never be separated, never even known apart from one another, it nevertheless remains helpful for us to allow these two aspects of creative causality to teach us their "separate" lessons. From human or natural causality we learn our nobility, our freedom, our creative energies, our capacities to transform the universe. Thus, if we stress only divine causality as if it were a rigid and confining thing that we dare not challenge by any effort at creative change, we fail to fulfill God's destiny for us as human persons. But from divine or supernatural causality we learn of our limits, of our sinfulness, of the fact that we are not, after all, God. We are warned against the kind of stress on human causality that leads us to hubris, that prompts us to do anything and everything our knowledge makes possible.

The human person, in each individual's dignity and destiny, is a whole, not a duality. When we care for the body, we care for the spirit; when we minister to the spirit, we minister to the body. And our task is both human and divine. Our excitement at learning and practicing the art of health care is an excitement that participates in the creative energies of God.

Note

1. The blasphemous suggestion by some American Christian preachers that AIDS is a punishment for homosexuality, well deserved by gays, is a particularly odious form of this approach.

CHAPTER 4

THE IMPLICATIONS FOR HEALTH CARE

WHEREAS THE PRECEDING CHAPTERS have developed a basis in theological anthropology for health care, this chapter and the next explore the implications of this anthropological basis more specifically for ethics. Here we ask in somewhat more practical terms how what we have learned in theological anthropology is and ought to be applied to health care ethics.

Sanctity and Quality of Life

The anthropological themes discussed thus far support the unique dignity, destiny, and integrity of human life. In a word, human life is sacred; it is holy because it participates in God's own holiness. Human life is characterized by its sanctity.

But when ethicists talk about the sanctity of human life, they may use this term to imply something a bit different from what we have thus far discovered theologically. For some moralists, the term "sanctity of life" designates one pole of an axiological spectrum used in ethical analysis. At the other end of the spectrum is "quality of life." Ethicists use these concepts to ask whether human life is to be judged and evaluated on the basis of its quality, or whether its intrinsic sanctity means that quality or lack of it is irrelevant to ethical decisions about health care.

While it is often difficult to make these decisions in individual cases, an adequate ethical application of theology can help us eliminate the two extremes of the spectrum. One end is an absolute sanctity-of-life position, which requires that all possible actions be taken to save a human life. No cost is too great if there is even a remote chance of prolonging or saving a person's life. Men and women may never be allowed to die if they might live on, despite the lack of quality that their lives would have or the brevity of time that might remain to them. Even if they are unable "to pursue life's goals and purposes, understood as the values that transcend physical life," their lives must be prolonged (Shannon and Walter 1988, 636). Those who hold for this absolute sanctity of human life are often called "vitalists," since for them a person's physical life is itself of ultimate value. Thus, no other value, however important, can ever justify the taking, or the giving up, of a human life.

Very few moralists adopt this extreme position. But some approach so closely this end of the spectrum as to refuse cessation of treatment in cases where further medical invasion seems useless and even harmful. Human life must be sustained at virtually all costs. Catholic moral theology has not accepted this approach, though some Orthodox Jewish scholars tend to do so (Dorff 2000a, 313), and surveys have indicated that physicians sometimes find this emphasis compatible with what they perceive as their medical role, though this is far from universal among doctors and has clearly changed in the last few decades.

The other extreme end of the spectrum is a totally lax quality-of-life position. Here the argument is that human life loses all value when certain qualities are lacking. This position permits cessation of treatment, or active killing, for trivial and even hedonistic reasons. The qualities considered may be those connected with efficiency and material productivity. Only the strongest and the fittest have sufficient quality of life to merit health care. Attempts have been made to list a number of indicators of human personhood, some of which are overly quantitative while others are not sufficiently well defined. They lend themselves easily to abuse. Joseph Fletcher has made attempts in this direction, but it is not always clear whether his indicators—an IQ of at least 20, self-awareness, self-control, a sense of time, a sense of the future and the past, the capacity for relationship, concern for others, control of nature, curiosity, idiosyncrasy, and upper-brain function—are intended to mean that if any are lacking there is no person at all, or that such a being is a person but need not be cared for, or that a person should strive for the optimal development of these human dimensions (Fletcher 1975).

Again, very few moralists argue for the most extreme position. But there are some who come close enough as to allow for cessation of treatment or active killing even in cases where there is a likelihood that a meaningful and dignified human life can be sustained by reasonable medical effort. The reductionist argument that the morality of abortion depends on the woman's choice, the argument that infants with virtually any handicap should be allowed to die if the parents so choose, the approach to suffering that denies it human value, and the position that the morality of suicide is purely a personal matter are typical of this view, where nearly any reduction in the quality of our lives is seen as a morally valid reason for ending them.

Although it is easy to reject these more extreme approaches, it is far harder to try to determine ahead of time what exactly the theological principle of the dignity of human life requires in this context. Both the sanctity of life and the quality of life are important. Each emphasis brings necessary warning and witness. Each corrects the excesses of the other.

The Roman Catholic tradition has recognized both the sanctity of life—life is indeed sacred—and the ethical import of at least some degree of quality of life—at some point, a lack of quality means that life can be let go. This humane application of the theology of human life to health care ethics is clearly found in the distinction between ordinary and extraordinary means of preserving life. The distinction goes back several centuries, though it is most often attributed to Pope Pius XII, who repeated it and stressed it during his pontificate in the 1940s and 1950s (Pius XII 1957, 1958). According to this tradition, it is never obligatory to make use of medical measures that are morally "extraordinary" in order to preserve life. This principle will be examined in detail in chapter 13. For now, it is enough to note that it is based on *both* sanctity *and* quality of life. In the words of the *Catechism of the Catholic Church*, "If morality requires respect for the life of the body, it does not make it an absolute value" (1994, 2289, p. 551).

It is true there is a danger that the distinction between ordinary and extraordinary means of preserving life may tend toward too lax a quality-of-life position. This is especially problematic when social and economic factors are included in the decision-making process. It is far too easy a temptation for health care providers and institutions, and for politicians and voters, to decide to eliminate health care opportunities for the poor and the powerless as a means of "solving" the problem of scarce resources. On the other hand, resources are not infinite, and the Catholic tradition has been wise in its insistence that a variety of factors must be considered in the attempt to determine what is ordinary and what is extraordinary. Quality of life must be considered (Ashley 1988).

This Catholic approach, which has insisted on sanctity of life and quality of life, is based on the theology of the meaning of human life in its dignity, its destiny, and its integrity. Human life is sacred, yet its sacredness resides not in the mere prolongation of physical or even of psychic or spiritual activity. The very freedom of the human person—our created destiny to move beyond ourselves, our unique status in God's creative providence, and the existential unity of ourselves as body–soul—calls for more than mere continuance in life. But this same theology of the human person condemns the attitude that human life consists in a quantitative accumulation of easily defined and measured characteristics, the absence of which would be reason to deny life's meaning and goodness. We return to this more explicitly in the next chapter, but it is becoming clear that the theological concepts and symbols of the Christian understanding of human life do not give simple unidirectional answers to specific issues of health care ethics. What they do is require us to avoid simplistic answers because they unfold to us more adequately, but never completely, the mystery of human life as God creates it.

In a similar way, theology provides no easy answers to the question of exactly when human personal life begins or ends. We have stressed the integrity of the human person as a unity of body–soul. Even when earlier approaches to theology tended at times to separate these into two distinct aspects, there was no complete agreement on when precisely the being we have come to call a human person began or ceased to be in this life. The Catholic Church has never officially decided when the soul "enters" or "leaves" the body. In its Declaration on Procured Abortion, the Vatican Congregation for the Doctrine of the Faith says this explicitly: "This declaration expressly leaves aside the question of the moment when the spiritual soul is infused. There is not a unanimous tradition on this point and authors are in disagreement" (CDF [1974] 1999, n19). Nor can contemporary theology answer the question of when full human life with full basic human rights begins or ends. Both the more dualistic and the more holistic approaches to the human person have recognized that the human being, in this life at least, needs both body and soul to be alive. Each must be apt for the other. Each must be sufficient for the other. Some of Catholic tradition speaks from a Thomistic-Aristotelian base and argues that there must be enough matter for there to be a form. Contemporary theology prefers to avoid phrases that imply separation but agrees that the human person is neither soul nor body but a unity where the body is enspirited and the spirit enfleshed. For neither approach is it easy to determine when human personal life begins or ends. This theological tradition ought to make us more hesitant than we sometimes are in coming to easy judgments about abortion or euthanasia. But this does not make the-ology useless. Quite the contrary. Adequate theological principles allow us to reject easy solutions to difficult mysteries. They argue against a too simplistic identification of the completeness of human life with the moment of conception, an identification that ignores the complexity and the uniqueness of the human person along with other human values. They argue equally against the attempt to deny the value of early human life altogether, to make it automatically secondary to other considerations, or to make it depend extrinsically on social or parental choice.

Human Life as Individual and Social

Another set of concepts that, like sanctity and quality of life, are sometimes seen by ethicists as being in opposition to one another are those of individuality and collectivity or social corporateness. An adequate theological basis for health care and health care ethics must recognize and support the human significance of both society and individual.

We have already briefly noted the shift in emphasis in contemporary moral theology from an excessive and sometimes restrictive focus on individual sin to an emphasis on social and structural sin. Unlike Protestant ethics, Catholic ethics developed in the context of individual confession. This practice began in the sixth and seventh centuries among the Celtic monks in Ireland, who then spread it in their missionary journeys to continental Europe. Until then, reception of the sacrament of reconciliation had been public and usually limited to one time per person. The penitent would confess to the bishop and then enter a period of public penance followed by public reconciliation before the Christian community. For various reasons the practice had fallen into disuse. Often Christians would put it off until just before death, since then the penance could not be imposed and there was less chance of their falling back into sin when the sacra-ment would not again be permitted (Mahoney 1987, 4–5).

The Irish development had its advantages and symbolized well that the forgiveness of God in Jesus and the Church was always available to the contrite. But its effects on the developing discipline of moral theology were not all benign. Priests now needed to be told, or so it was believed, how to judge individual penitents and individual sins. The penitential books were lists of sins with their penances, and from them developed later the summas for confessors and the manuals of moral theology. Emphasis turned more to individual actions of individual persons (Mahoney 1987, 5–17).

This occurred even more in medical ethics than in other areas. The wider array of topics discussed in pastoral medicine was largely neglected, and the individual daily professional practices of medical personnel were more and more stressed. Catholic med-ical ethics was interested in what individual patients and individual doctors and nurses did medically.

This restricted emphasis has been challenged in the decades since Vatican II, a challenge that correctly rejects the individualist bias in the definition of the earlier tradition. And the challenge is itself part of a wider recognition in contemporary ethics (and, indeed, in other disciplines such as sociology, psychology, philosophy, and polit-ical science) of the inadequacy of trying to understand the human person, and the meaning of human life, from a purely individualist perspective. This has been the temptation in Western medicine and in Western philosophy since the Enlightenment. Many of the Enlightenment thinkers saw "man" essentially as an individual whose rights and aspirations were open to abuse by others and by society. The human person was seen more or less as a separate atom, a little world apart from others. True, most individualists recognized the need for some kind of social interaction, but there was the sense that such interaction, and the structures needed for it, were secondary to the individual and were morally subordinate to the individual's needs, priorities, and goals. Sociologists argue that this trend has been most pervasive in the United States, where the development of the individual's personhood is seen to require the removal or the overcoming of social influences. Church, family, and state are thus privatized, leaving the individual free to choose among them, to accept or reject their influence as he or she thinks right. Commitment is treated with suspicion, and the larger society is neglected for the sake of the individual, resulting in personal loneliness and in structural injustice (Bellah et al. 1986).

Nothing of what we have discovered from the Christian understanding of the human person leads in this direction. God created not so much an individual man, Adam the individual, as *ha-adam*, humankind, in the divine image and likeness. God chooses us as a people, a society, a chosen race, a royal priesthood. Grace is not a thing acquired by individuals, but God's own communication to his human creation through which we become symbols of God to one another, sacraments of God's presence in humankind itself. Just as the "supernatural existential"—the order of grace in creation—has a social dimension, so does the order of sin. We are born into a dynamic of sin that transcends the individual, just as we are born into a dynamic of grace that transcends the individual. Christianity, like Judaism, proposes a people of God, not just a loose and private collection of individuals.

This means that we have responsibilities to one another that are based on essential human solidarity and not just on individual agreement. Society is not ontologically (metaphysically, essentially, in its real nature) a free agreement among individuals who might just as well have decided to stay separate. In a real way, this kind of individualism is another kind of dualism, a dualism that separates what cannot be separated, that divides individuals from one another and from the larger whole that includes them all. The recent reemphasis in Catholic moral theology on questions of social justice is but one example of how contemporary theology is aware in a renewed way of this social dynamic at the heart of the human mystery.

But there are dangers present in this emphasis if the importance of the individual person is neglected. Reductionist individualism, both ontological and ethical, is rightly rejected. But this rejection is sometimes done too easily, without the proper nuance, as if it could rightly be replaced by its opposite, by a kind of reductionist collectivism or corporatism. While it is true that the individual cannot live in isolation and may not rightly neglect the common good, it is also true that the corporate whole of society—the collective, the state—may not rightly trample on individuals. Again we have an example of how a dualism can cut both ways. The separation of individuals from society, so that individuals are led to neglect social commitment and the common good, can bring with it the equally devastating separation of society from the individual so that the collective neglects the persons that constitute it.

It was this insight that led to the admittedly one-sided individualism of the Enlightenment. Enlightenment philosophers saw the destruction done by the social structures of the time, including the church. "Coherence," "solidarity," and "community" can be oppressive, and both church and state have brought tyranny in their name. Individualist philosophy reacted against that by emphasizing the potential of the individual and by trying to create structures where the individual could not only survive but could thrive. Sociologists are right when they decry the alienation and the rootlessness that follows from an individualistic society. Ultimately, no human person can thrive alone. But it is dangerous to react so totally against individualism as to fall into collectivism. Neither the individual nor the collective is ultimately prior.

Thus, individualism and corporatism should serve in some sense as correctives to one another, not as synonyms for evil and good, as is often implied in contemporary social ethics. In health care ethics, this is especially important. Too much emphasis on the individual can lead to decisions that neglect the common good; a misplaced emphasis on the corporate whole can lead to unethical decisions. Two areas in medical ethics can serve as examples: organ transplants and the "right to health care." More is said of each in later chapters; here I merely make a few points about the individual and corporate whole.

For some time, Catholic medical ethics argued against the morality of organ transplants. The argument was based on a restricted interpretation of the principle of totality, according to which a human body might be "mutilated" by the removal of an organ only if such a procedure were for the good of the individual's own body. Because this condition would not be met if the purpose of the mutilation were for another's body, most Catholic moralists wrote, for a time, against the procedure. This teaching was changed when Bert Cunningham, a student of moral theology at The Catholic University of America, suggested that the mystical body of Christ might serve as the basis for a wider interpretation of "totality" (Cunningham 1944). The totality would be corporate and not individual. Organ transplantations would be licit.

But Cunningham tended in some of his conclusions to neglect the individual donor. He would have permitted the transplant of an eye from a living donor, even from a one-eyed convict sentenced to life in prison, and thus "not needed by anyone" (Cunningham 1944, 106). It is clear that Cunningham's move toward corporatism entails a lack of respect for the individual person. It is true, of course, that a "valid" corporatism would reject this kind of imbalance. But we need to guard against it precisely by using individualism and corporatism as correctives to each other's excesses. Contemporary medical ethics does this when it insists on the donor's rights as well as on the responsibilities each of us has to give, sometimes of our own bodies, to the health of others (Kelly 1988).

Another area where questions of the relationship of individual and corporate whole are apparent in health care ethics is the area of the right to health care. Included here are questions of access to care; cost containment; managed care; medical insurance; socialized medicine; economic and budgetary priorities; private, public, and for-profit hospitals; the incomes of health care practitioners; and a host of other questions that seem to defy ethical analysis. To what extent is health care a right? Again, theological principles do not bring us easy answers. The claim that an overemphasis on either the individual or the collective makes for bad health care is true enough, but it does not solve these often excruciatingly complex issues.

Christian theology must indeed argue that health care is a human right. Because health in all its manifestations is such an essential part of the dignity and indeed the destiny of human life, we have an obligation, to the extent that this is reasonably possible, of providing each other necessary health care. Health care is not just another commodity that can ethically be left to market forces. Both larger governmental bodies, through their powers of taxation, and smaller voluntary units, have roles to play in this process. Health care practitioners themselves are obliged to contribute to the effort.

But the right to health care is not an absolute right; there is no right to an infinite amount of health care. We often hear that no price can be put on the value of even a single human life. This is true, but it means that human life is not measurable in terms of dollars; it does not mean that human life is measurable in terms of an infinity or an indefinite number of dollars. It does not mean that society is obligated to provide unlimited funds for health care.

Priorities in these areas are notoriously difficult to establish. Is it morally right to transplant a heart while people starve in Africa? The problem is often phrased this way, or in the context of arguing about military and domestic budgets (how can we train a soldier or build a tank while people die from lack of medical care?). Though questions like these may help with their shock value, they are not ultimately helpful in leading to answers. We might also ask if it is morally right to spend money on symphony orchestras, or televisions, or on the education of chaplains, instead of on starving peoples. Economies are more complicated than that, and health care does not exhaust the morally right expenditure of society's wealth.

But health care is a human right, and even if the more specific questions of resource allocation defy simple ethical analysis, Christian health care ethics must insist that wealthy societies meet their obligations to provide medical care to those who need it. The ability to pay cannot be the basic criterion for health care. Economies generally and health care institutions specifically exist to serve the common good and must not make efficiency or profit the ultimate priority.

CHAPTER 5

THEOLOGICAL PRINCIPLES IN HEALTH CARE ETHICS

THE METHODOLOGY OF Roman Catholic medical ethics has undergone an important and controversial transformation in the decades since the Second Vatican Council. We attend in considerable detail to the whole area of methodology in part II, but it is helpful to speak of it just enough here to introduce one final specifically theological question: the question of the proper role for theological principles in health care ethics. This is ultimately a theological question more than it is a methodological one, at least as we speak of method in part II.

Prior to the 1960s Catholic medical ethics had developed a finely specified method that enabled it to offer clear solutions to the kinds of medical ethical issues that constituted its array of topics. These were largely limited to individual medical interventions by doctors and nurses. To deal with them, Catholic medical moralists applied a kind of ethical cause-and-effect analysis, whereby each procedure was subjected to a diagnostic scrutiny through the application of the principle of double effect, which is discussed at length in chapter 12. The act itself was analyzed and broken down into its various causal relationships, and this analysis of the act-in-itself became the principal tool that Catholic moralists used to reach their judgments as to the rightness or wrongness of the act. Answers given were seen to be universal, applicable to all cases involving the same physical act. Although psychological, social, and spiritual aspects might have been included in the discussion, the final judgment usually depended on the analysis of the physical biological properties of the act itself—the act of birth control, of direct or indirect sterilization or abortion, of mutilation, and so on (Kelly 1979, 251, 259–74). Many, though not all, of today's Catholic moralists criticize this "physicalism" as too restrictive.

In addition, especially during the 1940s and 1950s, Catholic medical ethics tended in practice to contradict its theoretical insistence on the natural law (the law of God as known to all persons through natural reason and not dependent on any directly supernatural revelation or supernatural authority) by emphasizing the role of the church magisterium in medical ethics decisions. Morality, according to consistent Catholic tradition, does not depend on ecclesiastical proclamation. If a procedure is wrong, the church merely recognizes that fact and teaches it; the church does not establish the procedure's wrongness. During the decades prior to Vatican II, however, the official pronouncements of the hierarchy became more and more important, and the supernaturally guaranteed authority of the magisterium came to supplement, and at times to replace, the tradition of natural law. Thus, a kind of "ecclesiastical positivism" whereby church officials in fact "posited" or established medical morality joined "physicalism" as the central methodological frameworks in Catholic medical ethics. In technical philosophical language, to which we return in part II, a positivist metaethical theory joined a physicalist deontological normative theory. The resulting combination allowed moralists to arrive at precisely specified conclusions based on cause-and-effect analysis and backed up by a teaching body whose authority could not be questioned (Kelly 1979, 311–20).

Other principles were also mentioned by Catholic moralists, principles that were more theologically evocative and that came from the kinds of basic themes in Christian anthropology we discuss in the preceding chapters, but these were in fact subordinated to the two more pervasive approaches of physicalism and ecclesiastical positivism. Chief among these theological principles were the principle of divine sovereignty over life and the principle of redemptive suffering.

It is clear enough that these two principles, or sets of principles, are of great importance in health care ethics. They present to us in a different perspective a theme that we have already discovered in Christian anthropology. They are two aspects of one theological axis that grapples with the issue of our relationship as creatures with our creator. Are we "simply" creatures, intended by God to accept things as they are, creatures whose sufferings take on meaning when joined to those of Jesus? Or are we cocreators or at least coagents with God, with the task of eliminating suffering whenever we can? What are the relative ethical weights of cocreativity and creatureliness in ethical application? What is the relationship of divine and human causality, of grace and nature?

As long as physicalism and ecclesiastical positivism were dominant in Catholic medical ethics, theological principles of divine sovereignty and of redemptive suffering were not really very important. Catholic moralists did appeal to these principles as secondary arguments to support moral judgments already reached through physicalist and positivist methods. They also used them for pastoral and moral motivation. Thus, if a procedure was forbidden (a direct sterilization, for example), that procedure would be said to violate God's dominion over life, and patients would be urged to accept the resulting suffering as redemptive. But if a procedure was permitted (an indirect sterilization, for example), then the physician was said to act in God's creating image when relieving the patient's suffering.[1] The theological principles of sovereignty and of the meaning of suffering, and thus the whole theological issue of the creator–creature relationship, were not of any practical ethical importance since they were consistently subordinated to the master frameworks of physicalism and ecclesiastical positivism (Kelly 1979, 443–44).

These methodological frameworks are no longer dominant in much of Catholic health care ethics. Many moralists have moved toward a more holistic methodology where the precise physicalist application of the principle of double effect and the positivist application of official magisterial statements are no longer decisive. Although controversy about this revision in method continues, it is clear that there has been a shift, at least among many Catholic scholars, toward a more teleological or proportionalist method where a priori judgments about acts themselves are of less importance than considerations of the consequences that flow from them, and toward a more personalist method where psychological, social, and spiritual factors are of more significance than the physical or biological aspects of the action itself.

This methodological revision is a theological advance for health care ethics. No longer are theological principles rigidly subordinated to physicalist and positivist method. They are now freed to exercise their proper role. But how should we apply them? What role should they play? It is true that they were too long misused as theological proof-texts. But a more direct, less subordinate application in health care ethics will be equally objectionable unless their proper theological character is safeguarded.

The principles of divine sovereignty and redemptive suffering are principles of Christian anthropology. They deal with the relationship of creature to creator and with the human person's role as creature and as coagent with God. Thus, their proper place in theological health care ethics is not as ethical rules that can answer specific health care questions but as helps in interpreting the meaning of the human person. They are hermeneutic themes, not ethical rules. They serve not so much in the context of specific moral issues—is this procedure right or wrong?—as in the context of the "biosignificance question": what is the meaning of human life (Kelly 1979, 437, 446)?

This context preserves the proper character of these theological principles by helping us to avoid an either/or dichotomy that would not sufficiently consider the dimension of paradox, symbol, and mystery inherent in these principles. We are both creatures and coagents with God. Suffering is an essentially mysterious reality in human life, and no one-dimensional answer to the question of suffering, evil, and sin in God's creation has ever been adequate. Thus, neither the subordination of these themes to rigid ethical systems, as was done for so long, nor their immediate application as moral rules to individual ethical problems, as is sometimes the current temptation, is acceptable.

As hermeneutic themes, theological principles are applied to health care ethics in a manner both more and less direct than was the case within physicalism and positivism. Inasmuch as they are no longer subordinate to these frameworks, they can be of more direct influence. They are no longer distorted by these intervening and dominating systems. On the other hand, their use is a less direct one in that their context is more properly that of Christian anthropology than that of precise moral distinctions between medical procedures. It is in this wider context that the mystery-filled aspect of theological themes becomes more compelling. Here, in the context of human life as a whole, it is more immediately apparent that women and men are both creatures and coagents, called both to accept suffering and to fight against it. Neither pole of the creature/cocreator axis can stand in isolation from the other to demand or forbid a specific medical procedure. When the proper stress is given to the creative tension inherent in theological principles as hermeneutic themes, wider latitude is granted to the range of health care procedures that are recognized as licit in at least some cases. Theological principles as hermeneutic themes are not rightly used as reasons for judging human acts to be intrinsically evil. It becomes less easy to arrive at universally applicable or absolute material norms, while limits to the range of morally acceptable behavior are retained and theologically supported (Kelly 1979, 443–44).

Medical ethicists sometimes seem unaware of the creative dialectic inherent in these theological themes. Often one pole of the axis is stressed and the other neglected. This can result in the same kind of restrictive legalism found in Catholic health care ethics prior to its recent development. Thus, some contemporary ethicists emphasize only the evil found in the human person. They tend to see human endeavor, especially if related to creative technology, as contrary to God's will and to divine sovereignty over nature and human life. Technology to them is dehumanizing and escapist; it is humankind's invalid and ultimately useless attempt to avoid the suffering that ennobles us and through which we share in the redemptive suffering of Jesus. They thus forbid certain human interventions that might be judged licit if proper weight were also given to humanity's coagency with God (Kelly 1979, 444–46).

Other ethicists, together with some scientists, tend to see technological development only as signs of human creativity and sovereignty. They believe in automatic progress. They tend to think that all suffering can be eliminated by the right quick fix, by the right expert with the right technique. Especially now, with recent developments in genetic technology, humankind itself becomes for them a kind of experimental object, open to limitless manipulation. They forget that the dignity of the human person is inherent in us from God our creator. They thus permit or even command activities that destroy human life and jeopardize the future of humankind. People become commodities.

The theological principles of God's dominion over life and of redemptive suffering, when seen as hermeneutic themes within the context of the "biosignificance question," serve to confront us with the mysteries that underlie the dilemmas of medical ethics. Theological principles cannot solve health care ethics questions as mathematical rules solve for the value of an unknown algebraic expression. Instead, they contribute to theological health care ethics precisely by denying to us the always tempting escape of ethical shortcuts. By refusing to permit facile judgments, theological principles as mystery-filled hermeneutic themes recall the mystery of humankind and help us to avoid destructively rigid policies (Kelly 1979, 446–47).

This is true not merely for the principles of divine sovereignty over human life and of redemptive suffering but also for the entire theological basis of health care and health care ethics. Theology at its best confronts the Christian with a creative tension that rejects shortcuts and easy answers. We have seen this same creative tension in the dialectic between sanctity and quality of life, in the balance of individual and corporate whole, in the relationship of nature and grace, in the very processes of growth and decay inherent in created finitude, and even in the struggle between created goodness and inherited sin. Christian anthropology cannot of itself yield simple rules for health care ethics. That is not what theology is.

Studies in linguistics and hermeneutics have emphasized this "tension theory" or "interaction theory" as a more adequate method for interpreting religious metaphor than literalist or fundamentalist approaches (Tracy 1975, 124–31). Today's systematic theologians are recognizing that the human mystery demands this kind of approach. Nothing less is adequate to express who it is that we are.

The conclusion reached here, that theology should not function to give specific answers as to the rightness or wrongness of medical procedures and practices, is somewhat different from the answer usually given regarding the role of theology in bioethics (Chapman 1999, 255–56). Here the question is usually asked in terms of the role of theology in public, secular bioethical discourse. It is usually assumed that that role is different for believers than it is for nonbelievers. For example, Lisa Sowle Cahill distinguishes between "faith language" and "faith commitments" (Cahill 1990, 11). When faith language is used as the only reason for a judgment in bioethics, she says, it will convince only members of that faith. But faith commitments can motivate a consensus even among persons from different traditions.

This is doubtless correct as far as it goes. It seems simply common sense, for example, that only Christians will be convinced by an argument from the passion and death of Jesus that we ought to accept suffering as he did. But there is an unproven assumption here. It is assumed that theology works one way for believers and another way for nonbelievers. Although there is obviously a sense in which this is true (any particular theological symbol or faith statement is presumably more powerful within a given faith community than outside it), there is also an important way in which it is false. If what we have seen so far is correct, it is false in its assumption that faith statements or specifically theological themes and principles will of themselves give believers the correct answers to particular medical ethical questions—that, to use Cahill's words, "faith language . . . as the sole warrant for moral conclusions will convince . . . members of that tradition" (Cahill 1990, 11). Theology does not work that way.

An Example: Physician-Assisted Suicide

It may be helpful here to suggest how this might play out in practice. We ought to be able to show how theology might apply to real-world health care questions. The issue of physician-assisted suicide (PAS) will serve as an example. Complete details about the ethical and legal facts and implications of PAS follow in chapter 19. The purpose here is to hint at some ways in which theology might play a role in the ethical analysis of PAS.

Anna Quindlen, liberal back-page commentator for *Newsweek* for a number of years, wrote in early 2002 a piece on PAS and euthanasia (Quindlen 2002). In it she argues for the legalization of PAS. Arguments against this position are developed later, especially in chapter 19. Her position is not the one we will advocate later in this book. But the reason for treating her column here is not so much her argumentation; it is that something seems to be missing.

Quindlen's piece is not merely cut-and-dry. She begins with the story of Chester and Joan Nimitz and their suicide pact, and this story evokes—as it should—a sympathetic response. But her analysis of PAS is incomplete. She states that the greatest advance in health care has been the consumer movement: "Americans have increasingly demanded more information and more control." She cites a poll showing that two-thirds of Americans support legalizing euthanasia. She cites "the American ethos of self-determination and the right to be left alone." The points she makes are valid, but some important facts are left out. She forgets to tell us that patients and surrogates can withdraw life-sustaining treatment when it is of little or no human benefit to the dying person (she paints a picture of persons tied to tubes they do not want as their death is prolonged). And she forgets to say that pain can always be eliminated in the dying patient (she shows how much pain and humiliation attends the dying process).

But what is of interest here is to note that she might have written differently had she attended to some theological images. Very briefly, we can note the following.

First, there is not the slightest hint here that suffering might be noble, even redemptive. Now this is a dangerous idea—all theology, all religion, all faith is dangerous. It is all too easy to see God as some sort of sadist inflicting diseases we should bear up under to prove our faith and merit heaven. But the theologian, the believer, might want to slow Quindlen down just a bit and ask whether there might ever be meaning to suffering.

Second, there is no sense here of God's sovereignty. Again, these theological principles draw us both ways: we are called to do some things to preserve our lives (ordinary means) but not all things (not extraordinary means). We are sometimes permitted to take life, but not always. Is this one of these times? How does God's role as creator and sustainer and giver of life fit in here? Perhaps theology might have given Quindlen a bit of hesitation.

Third, there is no sense here of a *people*. Now this is strange for a liberal, who is supposed to worry about society as a whole, especially about the poor. Perhaps if she had thought a bit about God's choosing a *people*, Quindlen might have remembered that legalizing PAS might pose real risks to the poor and to the disenfranchised among us. She might have worried some about how we have obligations, even at some cost to ourselves, to protect the vulnerable. She might have shown concern about the temptation to eliminate some health care costs by eliminating some of the dying. She might have worried about a social ethos developing that would support an obligation to die before one's time.

Fourth, there is no sense here of sin. There is no sense that we are indeed in some real ways alienated from God and from each other. Had Quindlen thought of this, she might have worried about how old dying people are often concerned about being a burden to their children and about how at least some of the children support this by refusing care for their parents. The right to die with a doctor's help might all too easily become a kind of duty to die, a duty to die perhaps even before sickness took its final grasp (Hardwig 1997). She might have worried a bit about how the sins that divide us might be "solved" by suicide, by getting out of the way. And she might have shown concern, as liberals usually do, about minority populations. These, especially African Americans, already fear and distrust the health care system. Sometimes when doctors tell minority families that there is nothing more medicine can do and suggest that it is time to withdraw treatment and allow the patient to die, minority families refuse, fearing that this is just one more way to deny them proper care and respect. Making it legal for doctors to assist in the suicides of their patients might just add another concern to those already experienced by minority populations. And the same concern is very often found among persons with handicaps and their advocacy groups.

Doubtless there are other ways as well in which theological symbols might have helped this public discourse about PAS. It is important to note, however, that none of this offers us definitive moral warrants against PAS. Theology cuts both ways. These same four themes call us the other way as well. Although suffering can be redemptive, it can also be destructive, and God wants us to relieve it when we can and should. Although God has ultimate sovereignty over our lives, God gives us a great deal of control; we are not only creatures but also stewards, coagents with God. Although we are social beings, we are also created in God's image as individuals and have some degree of autonomy; we are not just nameless, faceless parts of the whole. And finally, although we are affected by sin, we are also—indeed, more importantly—graced and saved.

It is true that the same insights about who we are as persons that we gain from theological images and symbols can, at least in theory, be gained from other sources. Atheists can know that some suffering encourages growth, that we are social beings, that there is evil and division in the world. But there is no reason in health care ethics (not even in public, secular discourse) not to include the richness, depth, and thickness of the religious tradition in speaking about these anthropological claims. When all is said and done, however, if we are to be true to the fullness of Catholic theological anthropology, we will not try to use these claims as complete proofs for or against any particular proposal. That is not the way they work, within the tradition or without.

This conclusion might seem to be weak one. This is all we can do theologically. The real work is always rational and secular. But it can also be seen as a strong conclusion. Look at what we can do! We can help forestall simplistic ethics. We can add caution where it is needed, saying that human persons are not that simple. There is a complexity in the human person that our fix-it society too often overlooks. There is multidimensional beauty that we ignore at our peril. And, yes, there is sin and we ignore *it* at our peril, too. That is what Catholic theology does best in theological ethics. And it is an essential contribution.

From a Catholic Christian perspective, health care and health care ethics must be based on the best possible theological anthropology. If we are to make the proper moral judgments, we need an adequate understanding of the meaning of human life on which to base them. The kind of theological basis we have explored in these pages will not itself answer our ethical questions in health care. Health care ethics is not complete when its theological basis is established. Yet when used as helps for interpreting the meaning of human life, theological principles as hermeneutic themes are suited to the task of health care ethics. They best provide the proper theological basis and serve to symbolize the meaning of human life in its dignity, its destiny, its integrity, and its creative mystery.

Note

1. Direct and indirect sterilization and other similar distinctions are treated at length in chapter 12.

Method

THE LEVELS AND QUESTIONS OF ETHICS

PART II HAS TWO MAJOR SECTIONS. The first is an introduction and analysis of the key terms and approaches used in secular philosophical ethics in general and bioethics in particular. It is divided into four chapters. Chapter 6 presents an introduction to the basic areas and questions of ethics. Chapter 7 examines the human person as moral agent. Chapter 8 discusses how to judge right and wrong. Chapter 9 deals with metaethics.

The second section of part II analyzes the methods used in Roman Catholic medical ethics. Chapter 10 is a historical and analytical overview of the methodological debate in Catholic moral theology. Chapter 11 deals with the methodologically important issue of contraception. Chapter 12 is a detailed consideration of the important principle of double effect, and it applies that principle to a number of medical ethics issues. These chapters, although located in the section on method, are also about application and they present the official teaching of the Catholic Church on many bioethical issues.

The Levels and Questions of Ethics

We begin by exploring the basic questions that ethics examines. Obviously ethics does not ask what bus I take to get to school (though that might be considered part of an ethical question if I wanted to go to school to steal its computers). Nor does ethics ask how a proton differs from an electron (though what scientists do with their electronic discoveries *is* of ethical importance, as is the very investigation of electrons, since that study involves time and energy, money, and so on, that might be used for other purposes; in that sense, there is no such thing as a "value-free" science). Ethics does not ask about whether God exists, though that question, too, has ethical implications.

The Two Levels of Ethics

What then *does* ethics deal with? What kinds of questions does one look at when doing ethics? The next three chapters discuss these basic questions as they are presented by secular or "philosophical" ethics, using one of the most widely proposed structures for this purpose taken from Richard B. Brandt (1961). We will see that there are two general levels of ethics that philosophers speak of: normative ethics and metaethics. But these two levels of ethical issues are treated not only by secular or philosophical ethics but also by theological ethics or moral theology. So we will consider both secular philosophical and religious theological approaches to medical ethics. It is impossible to make a clear distinction between the two. Although "normative ethical theory" and "meta-ethics" are technical terms used in philosophical ethics, religious ethics, including Roman Catholic moral theology, treats the same two sets of issues. Theologians often do not use the same terms and make precisely the same distinctions in the same ways, but the same questions are investigated. Somehow and somewhere every ethicist has to touch on these two levels of thought.

The first and more basic level is normative ethics or normative ethical theory. The word "normative" in the context of ethics refers simply to "oughtness." It has to do with "oughts" and "ought nots." Normative ethical theory deals with the core questions we usually think of when we think of ethics: Are people morally accountable? Is this action right or wrong? What ought we to treasure?

The second level of ethics, which received most of the attention of twentieth-century philosophers, is "metaethics." This word, which comes from the Greek, means simply "beyond ethics." It deals with the problem of verification of meaning in ethics. Metaethics is the epistemology of ethics; it asks if it makes any sense to do ethics. It asks if ethics and ethical judgments have any meaning, and if so, how that meaning is verified. We return to metaethics in chapter 9. Here we briefly discuss the questions of normative ethics.

The Three Questions of Normative Ethical Theory

Normative ethics asks three questions. Question 1 examines whether, in principle, humans are praiseworthy or blameworthy. Are we moral agents? Are we ever morally accountable for what we do? Are we always morally accountable (and thus praiseworthy or blameworthy), or are there times when, for one reason or another, we lack that accountability and are therefore not praiseworthy or blameworthy? Are there factors that limit our capacity as moral agents?

Question 2 considers when an action or a pattern of behavior or a social structure is right or wrong. This is the question we usually think of when we think of applied ethics, and since health care ethics is applied ethics, this question will be given special consideration. How does one determine what must be done and what must be avoided? Why are these acts right or wrong? Why is this pattern of activity right or wrong? Why is this kind of social structure (for example, the present American system of health insurance) morally right or wrong?

Question 3 asks about ultimate value. A value is a loved truth, a truth that is cherished or desired. What is the ultimate good? What "ought" we to love and seek above all other goods? What we treasure affects how we live.[1] Some of the most evocative works in health care and health care ethics have looked at the healing professions with this question in mind (Pellegrino 1979; Pellegrino and Thomasma 1996; May 1983; Drane 1988). It may be helpful to present two cases to illustrate how these questions work.[2]

Case 1: The Grant Competition

Let us suppose that you, the reader, and one other person are applying for a scholarship grant for doctoral work in bioethics. This other person is a friend of yours. There is only one grant available. The scholarship is restricted in such a way that the two of you are the only persons eligible and you both know this. You have both received the application materials, and you have read them and know that all materials must be posted no later than this Friday. Your friend comes into your room, and she happens to tell you that she is applying and is now filling out the forms and will get them in by next Monday. You know that if she does this, she will be too late, and you will win the scholarship grant.

We have noted three questions in normative ethics. It is true, of course, that the questions overlap each other, but we will take them again in the order used above.

Question 1 asks whether you would be blameworthy if you did not tell her that she should get the forms done in a hurry. This depends a great deal, of course, on whether you are obliged to tell her, which is question 2. But there is a real sense in which the two questions can be distinguished. Perhaps you are preoccupied (or drunk) when she drops in on you. You do not really understand what she said. Now perhaps we could say that you are not free to perform a truly good act or a truly evil act, since your freedom is impaired. Thus, the question as to whether you are blameworthy must be based on this factor, along with the objective situation. In the next chapter, we find a number of factors that reduce human freedom in just this way.

Question 2 asks if the action, in this individual circumstance and in this situation, is right or wrong. Is it wrong not to tell her the truth? Assuming no drunkenness or other impairment of free will, is it wrong? What if we were to change the situation a bit and say that your opponent was your enemy rather than your friend? Would this make any difference to the obligation on your part? What if she had previously done you some serious injury? Does this make it any different? Or what if you know that you are really intending to goof off all through school and use the money you saved on a car, whereas she is a serious student and will become a great scholar? Does that make a difference in the current situation of whether you tell her? Or reverse the case. She is the goof-off and you are the hard worker. Does that make any difference to the rightness and wrongness, to the obligation connected with telling her or not telling her? An ethicist may not be able to give concrete answers to all of these questions. Some ethical situations have no easy answers (this case is interesting because it can perhaps be argued that reading directions and replying on time is part of the competition and you have no responsibility to do your friend's work for her). But ethics gives us at least a way of looking at the case.

Question 3, the question of ultimate values, is less immediately apparent in the case. What, in a more ultimate sense, beyond the immediate action involved in this case, is of value here? What intrinsic values are at stake? Do intrinsic values exist? An intrinsic value is some reality, event, or quality that is properly desired for its own sake, apart from any further consequences. What is of intrinsic value in this case? Would it be pleasure—my pleasure in going to school and working hard, or in owning the car and goofing off? Her pleasure in getting the scholarship? How about the virtue of honesty? Would that be of ultimate value (virtue is its own reward)? Or is it happiness that is of ultimate value? If so, how is happiness best achieved here? By my telling her, or by my not telling her? If happiness is of ultimate value, what kind of happiness? Physical, financial, moral, spiritual? Happiness in this life, or in the next, or both?

Case 2: The Patty Hearst Bank Robbery Case

Another, widely known case is helpful in making the distinctions of the three questions a bit clearer: the Patty Hearst bank robbery case. It happened back in the 1970s, and it is a good example of how to see the difference between the first two questions of normative ethical theory. Patty Hearst was the heiress of William Randolph Hearst, a wealthy newspaper publisher in California. She was kidnapped by members of a radical group known as the Symbionese Liberation Army (SLA). The police and the FBI were unable to find her until one day when the SLA, Patty Hearst among them, robbed a bank. There was Hearst with a gun in the bank. They were all ultimately caught, and Hearst was put on trial along with the rest of them.

Question 1 asks whether Hearst was blameworthy for her role in the robbery. More specifically, was she forced somehow or brainwashed into doing it? Or had she indeed converted to the radical cause and freely joined the SLA? These are "question 1 questions." They ask about blameworthiness, about moral accountability and guilt, about freedom.

Question 2 is about the rightness and wrongness of robbing banks. More specifically, is bank robbery by rebels who want to change society right or wrong? Does it depend on the goodness of the society and the intention of the rebels? Does it depend on the consequences in this particular case or in cases like this in general, or is it rather the case that bank robbery is always wrong regardless of circumstances and consequences? (In that case, robbing Hitler's bank to slow down his war effort would also be wrong.)

Question 3, as always, is harder to get a sharp focus on. It asks what is the ultimate reason or value or goal of a person's life that might help us know what the good life is. What ought the SLA to have valued in this way? Justice, power, happiness? What light does this shed on bank robbery? Perhaps life is simply absurd, of no reason or value or importance whatsoever. Perhaps there is no meaning to any human actions. Then there would be no basis for claiming that bank robbery—or anything else—is right or wrong.

These, then, are the basic questions ethics asks. In the next two chapters, we examine the first two questions in some detail: the question of moral accountability and the question of right and wrong.

Notes

1. Various answers are given to the question of ultimate value, and no list can be complete. Some of the candidates proposed by philosophers and theologians include: pleasure (hedonism); happiness—for Aristotle, happiness is acting rightly, a theory known as "eudaimonism" (Aristotle 1962, bk X); God—for Thomas Aquinas, our true end is happiness, and we achieve this end in the beatific vision of God after death (Thomas Aquinas 1948, ST I-II q. 1, art. 7); rational conformity to nature—the Stoics held this; and life itself (vitalism). Other candidates might include love or friendship, knowledge or wisdom, beauty, peace, health, good order, power, and so on.

Finally, there are pluralist systems, which hold that many goods are of intrinsic value, and nihilism, which claims that there is no ultimate good because life is absurd.

2. The first of these cases is especially helpful in drawing out students' opinions and thinking processes. Various student answers can be labeled—relativism, deontology, utilitarianism, and so on—anticipating later chapters.

CHAPTER 7

FREEDOM AND THE MORAL AGENT

I N THIS CHAPTER AND THE NEXT, we examine the first two questions of normative ethical theory in greater detail, beginning with question 1: blameworthiness
and praiseworthiness of persons. The central question here is human freedom. Is a
person ever free to choose between alternatives, some of which are right and some of
which are wrong? And, if we answer yes to the first question (and some philosophers
do not), then are there factors that might eliminate or reduce freedom in certain situations? Is the act done then really free? In Thomistic terms used by the Catholic tradition, is it a "human act" or is it simply an "act of a man," an act that a person does but
in which there is no personal engagement of reason or will (Thomas Aquinas 1948, *ST*
I-II q. 115, art. 4)? The solutions proposed to the question of whether human persons
are blameworthy or praiseworthy for their actions are generally divided into two types:
determinist theories and free will theories (sometimes called libertarian theories).

Determinist Theories

In general terms, the proponents of determinism hold that the individual is not free to
choose between one set and another set of acts but instead is determined to act in this
way rather than in that way. All human behavior is caused entirely by factors over which
we have no control. Each act and behavior pattern of any individual is thus theoretically
predictable. There is no room for free will. A scientific determinist position would
argue, for example, that a correctly developed scientific method could, and perhaps
someday will, be able to predict and control all acts of all people. For our purposes
here, we need not go into detail about varying "strengths" of determinisms. We need
only describe "strong" or reductionist determinist theories, those that utterly reject the
possibility of free choice and with this, it seems, reject altogether the possibility of
ethics. Determinism of this type eliminates any possibility of free consent, personal
autonomy, and similar values on which, as we will see in part III, so much of bioethics
rests. Determinism can be divided into two general categories: "natural" determinism
and "nonnatural" determinism. The terms are somewhat awkward, but the differences
between them are important.

Natural Determinism

Most determinists subscribe to one of the natural determinisms, which are often said to fall into three types. Under a theory of psychological determinism, one has no freedom of choice because one is determined by one's own personal psychological history, family life, prenatal life, childhood, and so on. Sociological determinism claims that we are never free but are always determined to act unfreely according to what our society has manipulated us into doing. Genetic determinism claims that each person is forced to act according to the specific DNA genetic code received from his or her biological parents.[1] These types can be combined, claiming that some combination of external factors over which we have no control are entirely causative of all human behavior. The behaviorist psychologist B. F. Skinner was a determinist who claimed that all human actions are caused by environmental stimuli that elicit in us conditioned reflexes reinforced by society. He was not shy about his resulting claims that humans were really only complicated animals, with no claim to freedom or dignity (Skinner 1971, 175–206).

Ethics requires some possibility of human choice. But this does not mean that humans have unrestricted freedom. As we saw in part I, we are finite beings. We live in space and in time; we live in a world where sin affects us. Our freedom is not that of God. Our environment, our genetic inheritance, our society, and our families all affect how we behave. Skinner and other reductionist determinists are wrong when they altogether reject the possibility of choice. They are not wrong when they point to all the factors that influence us and sometimes control us. In part III, when we speak of "free and informed consent," we will have reason to note again the situatedness of human freedom

Nonnatural Determinism

There are a number of determinist theories that claim some otherworldly or nonnatural factor or factors as the cause of our behavior. Some persons seem to believe that their actions are caused by the position of the stars and the planets, which might be called astrological determinism. Others believe in some form of influence from spirits of the dead. Still others seem to believe that our actions are caused by what we did in previous incarnations or by choices we made in our true, "metaphysical" state between incarnations, where we decide which experiences to have the next time around. But the nonnatural determinism that interests Christian theologians and religious ethicists most is divine determinism, the idea that our actions are caused by God.

Some people believe that their God or gods control each and every individual act of the human person, so that we are not free with respect to our actions. Others, and this applies to some approaches to the Christian faith to a significant degree, hold that human beings are not really free with respect to our final destiny, heaven or hell. This lack of freedom with respect to our final destiny, as we saw in chapter 2, is called predestination: we are destined ahead of time to go to heaven or to hell, and there is nothing we can do about it.

There are many complex issues that we need not discuss here, but a few remarks will be helpful in suggesting some theological directions. First, within Christianity there is the belief, at least in general, that God is the creator of all that is, not only in the sense that God made it, but also in the sense that God preserves it and keeps it in existence. If God stopped thinking about us, we would simply cease to exist, like an essay that disappears from a computer's RAM if the electricity goes off. This is true not only of objects but of activities, including human actions. God's activity is necessary not only for our continued existence but for each of our actions as well. Some people worry that this means we can have no freedom to choose. Perhaps it is God who acts, not we ourselves. The best Christian answer to this, while complex in its details, can be simply stated. God keeps us and our actions going according to our human nature as God has created that nature and is creating it. That is, God creates us and sustains us as free persons, since this is God's creative desire. This theology fits with what we saw in chapter 3 about divine and human causality. It is also in keeping with the Catholic Thomistic tradition.

Second, when Christians add the concepts of original sin and grace, a further problem emerges. Christian theology generally agrees that without grace it is impossible to do any truly good action. For some theologians, even actions that appear to be good on the outside are in a real sense evil and sinful if the person doing them has no grace. This approach tends to limit grace to believing Christians. Original sin is said to overwhelm us so much that we are not able to act rightly unless we receive the grace of baptism. Otherwise we cannot do anything "salvific," "saving"—anything truly righteous.

This is not exactly the same as natural determinism, in that natural determinism applies to each act, which is said to be caused by genes, society, environment, or psychological factors. Christian predestinationists generally accept the idea of some free choice in human actions. But predestinationism is still a determinism in that our behavior on the whole is determined to fail if we have no grace or, in some versions, to succeed if we do.

A somewhat similar approach comes from those who, like Lutheran theologian Helmut Thielicke, underline the depravity of humankind coming from original sin to the extent that it is sometimes, though by no means always, necessary to sin. And for these sins there is real guilt (Thielicke 1966, 594–98). Situations arise in which one must choose among different options, each one of which is wrong; whatever the choice—and a choice must be made—the person still sins (Thielicke 1966, 485–88). In a sense, this is a kind of determinism to do wrong.

There are various approaches to this problem, and a detailed discussion is impossible here. But we can briefly recall from chapter 2 three theologians who have been important in this context. First, Augustine, in the fifth century, put a great emphasis on original sin and on its effects, especially on how it diminishes and perhaps even destroys human freedom. From Augustine's perspective, persons are so corrupted by original sin that, without the grace that only Christians receive, humans are doomed to sin constantly. Even if non-Catholics choose actions that seem right, they are really evil actions, and all non-Catholics are inevitably damned (Augustine 1887a, 3, 14).

Second, Thomas Aquinas, in the thirteenth century, gave a greater emphasis to human freedom. Original sin does not totally destroy our freedom. We are still free in our created nature, at least to some extent (Thomas Aquinas 1948, *ST* I-II q. 83, art. 1). Since Catholicism has followed Aquinas more than Protestantism has (which has historically tended more to base its theology on Augustine), there is in general a greater emphasis on the capacities of human freedom in the Catholic tradition than in Protestantism.

Third, Karl Rahner, a twentieth-century German Catholic theologian, argued that grace is not limited to Christians. The proof that grace is present to all persons is in the very capacity we have to act freely and to transcend who we are. Only God's grace could make this possible. This approach allows us to stop making facile distinctions between those who "have grace" and those who do not. And, as we saw in greater depth in chapter 2, it helps us eliminate the kinds of dualism that lead to the problem of predestinational determinism in the first place (Rahner 1969, sec. 3).

In the final analysis, the exact relationship between God's grace and power on the one hand and our freedom on the other is a mystery. But it is better understood as a mystery of cooperation than of opposition. The great Christian traditions have in one way or another insisted that humans are accountable and responsible for their actions. The human person, empowered with grace, is surely called to choose to act rightly.

Free Will Theories

Libertarian or free will theories hold that the human person is capable of free choice. Human behavior may be influenced by other factors, and may sometimes be determined by them, but reductionist or strong determinism is rejected. Free choice is possible.

For some free will theorists, the will is a faculty of the human person, a power, like the faculties of speech or of reason. Because we have free wills, we are able to choose one act and reject another. Thomas Aquinas, Aristotle, and the tradition of Catholic moral theology hold to this notion of freedom. For others, freedom is the very definition of who the human being is. This is closer to the thought of many existentialist philosophers. The human person *is* freedom, almost by definition. Rather than defining the human being as a thinking or rational animal, existentialists such as Martin Heidegger define the human person as "thrownness." The individual is thrown into the world and is not the world but rather is a being together with others in the world (Heidegger), or a *pour-soi* (for oneself) where all other things are *en-soi* (in itself) (Jean-Paul Sartre). The human person is not like other things, which are not free. The human person is freedom itself. Only humans are able to look beyond. We alone are not determined to be; we *exist*, are out of, are away from, are a negation of the simple deterministic laws that govern all other kinds of reality.

Free-will theorists often distinguish, as Thomas Aquinas and Aristotle do, between the kinds of laws that govern nonhuman beings, such as stones, and even to a large extent animals (we will not debate that here), and the kinds of laws that govern people. Aristotle, in the *Nicomachean Ethics*, insists that whereas stones move only from without, if some outside force lifts them up, a human person can act from within, by choice (Aristotle 1962, book II). One moves oneself. Thomas repeats this idea in the *Summa theologica* (Thomas Aquinas 1948, *ST* I-II q. 83, art. 1).

Modifiers of the Voluntary

Free-will theorists generally admit that there are factors that modify or limit human freedom, thereby reducing blameworthiness. The term "modifiers of the voluntary" comes from the Catholic tradition. Catholic theologians have always been more interested in this question than have secular philosophers because of the need to deal with penitents in the sacrament of penance. Philosophers have tended to emphasize question 2 (right and wrong), question 3 (ultimate value), and metaethics. But Catholic theologians and philosophers have had to deal with guilt and innocence and with questions of when and how a person might or might not sin. Different authors give different lists, adding or combining, but the following four "modifiers of the voluntary" are usually included (Davis 1946, 1:16–33).

1. Force or fear

Here the direct physical threat or action of another really does "cause" me to act. Patty Hearst claimed that she had been forced to participate in the bank robbery. It would be ethically right for us to "help" a thief steal a car if the alternative was that he would do us a serious injury. The thievery itself does not become right, but the "helper" is surely not responsible for it, or at least not as much responsible for it as he or she would be had he or she initiated the theft. Physicians do wrong when they refuse to care for persons with AIDS; their blameworthiness may be diminished, however, if they are not able to control their fear of contagion.

2. Ignorance

For many centuries the Catholic moral tradition has insisted that one must always follow one's conscience. This is true even if that conscience is indeed erroneous—if, for example, a person, after real reflection and examination of his or her conscience, decides that a particular action is right when it is indeed objectively wrong. If we are unaware that a chosen is wrong and are convinced in our conscience that this is the right thing to do, then morally, though not necessarily legally, we are not blameworthy for performing the action. We must follow our own conscience. James Hanigan calls conscience "the ultimate subjective norm of morality" (Hanigan 1986, 120). It is not the ultimate objective norm; it can and often does make mistakes. But it is the ultimate subjective norm. We might say that conscience "rules" question 1. We are not blameworthy when we follow our conscience. This does not mean, of course, that we are allowed by the Catholic tradition to rationalize what we know to be wrong simply by pretending that we think it is right. We are supposed to form our conscience carefully, listening to what others tell us, sifting this out, being truly serious about it. For Catholics, one of the sources to listen to is the official teaching of the magisterium, that is, the pope and the bishops. But assuming all this is done carefully, we are obliged to follow our conscience. If we have developed virtue through good living, it is likely that our conscience will guide us well, and growing in virtue is a prerequisite for a well-developed conscience.

If we choose wrongly, and our ignorance is later corrected, we are obliged to change our behavior. For example, a person might think that sexist exploitation of female workers is right. This ignorance, if it were real, would excuse the agent from being morally blameworthy. But once he found out it was wrong, then if he continued to do it, he would be accountable. (There is a great deal of literature showing that nurses are mistreated by doctors and hospital administrators, and it seems obvious that much of this is due to the historical fact that most physicians and administrators have been men and most nurses women.)

Catholic moral theology makes two helpful distinctions concerning ignorance. First is the distinction between ignorance of the fact and ignorance of the law (the law here does not refer to civil law but to moral law, to what is in fact right and wrong). We may be unaware of the situation. This is ignorance of the fact. We may truly think, for example, that a patient has not made an advance directive. We have tried to find it, and no one thinks there is one. After we have agreed to do what the patient's closest family members request, we discover an advance directive that tells us to do the opposite and appoints a different proxy. We are not blameworthy for what we did. We acted in good conscience. We were ignorant of an important fact in the case. On the other hand, if we never really tried to find out about the advance directive and just did what we felt like doing, then our ignorance would not be real; it would be fictitious or pretended ignorance, and we would be blameworthy for what we did.

Ignorance of the law is ignorance about the rightness or wrongness of the action we do. We honestly believe that it is right to lie to a patient who asks us whether he has cancer. Even when we read books and articles in medical ethics that insist it is almost always wrong, we think it is right. Even though we know we open ourselves to legal action, we remain convinced that in this case it is right. So we lie to him. Even if indeed it is wrong to do so (and it seems clear that in almost all cases it is wrong), if we do so and are ignorant of the law (ignorant of what is morally right and wrong) we are not blameworthy (do not sin).

The second distinction Catholic moral theology makes about ignorance is between vincible and invincible ignorance. If we can "conquer" our ignorance, if it is vincible, we are obliged to do that. If we do not, our ignorance may not protect us from being morally culpable. But invincible ignorance, whether of the fact or of the law, can well mean that our actions, even if they are objectively wrong, are not blameworthy. In religious language, we do not sin. It may be helpful to say that invincible ignorance is when we don't know we don't know, or when we know we don't know but we can't find out. Vincible ignorance, on the other hand, is when we know we don't know and we can find out. In this case we are obliged to correct our ignorance before we act. All this is really only common sense. Persons cannot be held morally responsible for what they honestly do not know. Nonetheless, it seems often to come as a shock that Catholic moral theology places such a high stress on conscience. Nor is this a recent revision in the Catholic tradition, though it has sometimes been underemphasized and even forgotten. A person who does wrong truly believing it to be right is not subjectively blameworthy, even though what is done remains wrong.

3. Overwhelming passion, desire, or concupiscence

If a person is indeed overwhelmed by desire to the extent that she or he cannot resist a certain behavior, then that act is not morally blameworthy. For example, a true kleptomaniac may well not be blameworthy for each act of stealing. Of course, such a person is morally obliged to seek help to try to overcome this desire. But acts that are in this sense forced are not free and thus are not morally blameworthy.

4. Habit

The final modifier of the voluntary often listed in Catholic texts is habit. When we have behaved in a certain way for a long time, we tend to do it rather automatically. To that extent, our attention to what we do is limited, and it becomes very difficult to stop the habit. This might be applied, for example, to smoking (along with desire for nicotine, which, if truly addictive, could well be an overwhelming desire). We are morally obliged to try to break the habit, but if it becomes terribly hard, or if we find that our attempts to do this cause too many bad side effects, then we may not be blameworthy for smoking. (Actually this last factor, bad effects from stopping, fits in more with question 2 on right and wrong. We can see that in real-life cases these questions overlap.)

Catholic ethics insists that there cannot be a case where a person is required or determined to sin. Unlike Thielicke, Catholic ethics insists that the power of sin in the world does not overwhelm human freedom. Sin must always be a free choice, a "human act," an act that engages at least to some degree our freedom and our reason. There can be no forced sins.

We have now completed our typology of proposed solutions to the first question of normative ethics, the question of whether the individual is free, and thus whether one can be blamed or praised for one's actions. We saw two kinds of theories: free will or libertarian theories, with their modifiers of the voluntary, and determinist theories, which hold that the individual is never really free to choose because all actions are determined by environment, genes, stars, God, or a combination of factors we cannot control.

One final point is important here. Catholic moral theology has insisted that no person may accuse another of sin. This is because no one can really be certain about the internal disposition of the person we might be pleased to judge. Serious or mortal sin has traditionally been said to require a "full consent of the will." In today's theological language, this is often expressed by saying that the serious sinner must make a fundamental option or choice, must truly engage himself or herself in evil. No other person can judge that this has been done. Although we often hear it said that such-and-such an action is "a sin" or even "a mortal sin," the Catholic tradition really should not phrase it this way. We should rather say that an action is "wrong" or "seriously wrong." Only if one has engaged oneself in the action by consenting to what one knows to be wrong can we speak of a sin. And since this can never be known with certainty by others, no one can accuse another of sin.

But we can judge the rightness and wrongness of actions, behavior patterns, and social structures. In the next chapter, we look at some of the approaches proposed for doing this.

Note

1. Genetic influence on human behavior is now receiving a great deal of attention. For a particularly insightful description and analysis of recent research in this area, and on its implications for human freedom and equality, see Parens 2004.

CHAPTER 8

RIGHT AND WRONG

W E TURN NOW TO THE proposed solutions to the second question asked in normative ethical theory, the question of rightness and wrongness of acts or patterns of behavior or social systems and structures. Apart from whether a physician may be afraid of treating patients with AIDS, is it right to refuse to do so? Apart from whether a dying patient fears the loss of control that comes with a terminal illness, is euthanasia right or wrong? Is it sometimes right and sometimes wrong? Should it be legalized? How do we tell?

Philosophers often distinguish two main approaches to answering this question: deontology and consequentialism. Not all medical ethicists use these approaches, and today there is a good deal of debate about whether they are helpful. But this distinction remains an excellent starting point for discussion.

Deontological or formalist theories (or deontologism, formalism, or simply deontology) refer in general to an approach that looks to rules and duties. "Deontology" comes from the Greek word for "obligation." There are certain things we simply are obliged to do or not to do. This approach is sometimes called a "formalist" approach because of the sense that some acts are considered wrong in themselves, wrong by their very form or quality, hence formally wrong. Rather than looking outward to material contexts and consequences, deontology looks within, to the formal makeup of the action in question.

Consequentialist theories, or consequentialism (sometimes called teleological ethics, and sometimes but not always equated with utilitarianism), refer in general to an approach that looks to consequences or effects of an action, behavior pattern, or social system to find out whether it is right or wrong. The word "consequentialism" is easy enough. "Teleology" comes from the Greek word "telos," which means aim or goal, and refers to the goals of actions. There is often a significant difference between consequentialism and teleology. Some forms of teleological ethics can be more deontological than consequentialist. For example, when sexual acts are said to have as their goal or "telos" the procreation of children, a resulting judgment may be made that all sexual activity must be open to procreation, so that all other sexual acts are intrinsically or formally wrong regardless of other circumstances or consequences. Contraception thus becomes an "intrinsically evil act." So, although there is some congruence between the idea of goal or end (people act for goals or purposes) and the idea of consequences (this is what results and is what people presumably act for), and although teleology and consequentialism are sometimes seen as the same approach, careful thinkers make a distinction between them (Shannon and Walter 1988, 636). We will consider utilitarianism later. In general, then, this consequentialist approach looks to the effects of actions.

Introductory Remarks on Deontology and Consequentialism

It would be far easier to learn the meaning of the terms "deontology" and "consequentialism" if they were used consistently by scholars. Unfortunately, that is not always the case. Different scholars over the years have changed them, added subdivisions to them, and debated about them so that when they occur in scholarly and popular articles, it is often hard to know exactly what authors mean by them. But they remain essential terms, and despite those who claim that other approaches to ethics should replace them, the basic differences between them are important to medical ethics. When we examine method in Catholic medical ethics in chapter 10, we will see that a significant difference between the two currently controverted positions in Catholic moral theological method is indeed the difference between deontology and some form of consequentialism. Also, since for the purpose of applying these terms to Catholic method we are going to define these two terms in a particular way, and since that way is not universally accepted, it is important to start out with an introduction as to why they are difficult to define and why different medical ethicists define them differently.

But it is possible to start more simply and give a general description and comparison of the two approaches to the question of how to determine right and wrong. Deontology and consequentialism are easy enough to understand in general, since certain characteristics are universally attributed to these two approaches:

Consequentialism insists on results. Deontology either ignores results or does not insist as strongly on them. Consequentialism looks to the future for consequences, for effects, for results. Deontology looks to the past for rules, for precedents.

Consequentialism tends to be a posteriori: it works from the bottom up. Deontology tends to be a priori: it works from the top down. That is, deontology tends to be deductive; once we have the principle or the rule, we can apply it directly and get the answer as to whether an action is right or wrong. Consequentialism tends to be inductive; it starts with the actions and all there is to know about them, and the judgment of right or wrong follows from that.

Deontology tends to be more absolute than consequentialism. It tends to hold that rules apply more widely and more strictly than consequentialism does; it allows for fewer exceptions.

Reasons That Definitions Are Controverted

So far so good. But when we try to give a more precise definition or description of these two terms, disagreements emerge. There are at least two different reasons for this controversy. The first is that some persons wish to consider themselves deontologists and others want to consider themselves consequentialists. The deontologists do not like the term "consequentialist," or they honestly are not consequentialists. They normally tend as a result of this to define consequentialism in rather narrow terms, making it less likely to attract support, and they tend to define deontology in broader, "nicer" terms, making it seem more attractive. The opposite is true for those who like the word "consequentialist," or even the word "utilitarian," which we discuss later, and who want to be considered consequentialists. These persons do not like the term "deontology," or they honestly are not deontologists. They tend as a result of this to define deontology in rather narrow terms, making it less likely to attract support from others, and they tend to define consequentialism or utilitarianism in broader, "nicer" terms, making it seem more attractive.

All this suggests an interesting point. Definitions are seldom totally "value-free," and this kind of definition is almost inevitably value-laden. All of us tend to define an opposing approach in restrictive terms to make it less attractive and define "our" approach in inclusive terms to make it more acceptable. There is no way to get around that entirely, and the authors of this book will doubtless do it here to some degree ourselves. Since in the methodological approach defended in this book there is a greater degree of consequentialism than what is found in most earlier Catholic moral theologians, and since there seems to be no conclusive reason to avoid the term "consequentialism" (though there is significant reason for hesitation about the word "utilitarianism," which we will come to), deontology may well be defined here in a restricted way and consequentialism in a more open way. This does not mean that the definitions given here are false ones, or useless ones, or are not found in the literature. They are perfectly acceptable definitions and occur often in the literature. But they are not the only ones found there, and it is necessary to be aware of that.

The second reason these definitions are controverted is that there are two different ways of viewing the relationship between deontology and consequentialism. One can view deontology and consequentialism as two compatible and complementary approaches, both of which are needed some of the time, or one can view them as incompatible alternative approaches, so that if we accept one, we will not and cannot accept the other. Unlike most writers in practical bioethics, we will use them in this second sense; that is, they will be considered alternative and incompatible. This is the way they were originally conceived, and there is good reason to use them this way.

Much of the philosophical literature in bioethics, however, uses deontology and consequentialism as complementary approaches. And this provides an opportunity for introducing some very important concepts often used in bioethics that will demonstrate how some ethicists view deontology and consequentialism as complementary alternatives. These concepts are often called the "four basic principles" of biomedical ethics.

Four Basic Principles of Bioethics

Many bioethicists talk about four important concepts in approaching the moral rights and wrongs of medical practice: beneficence, nonmaleficence, autonomy, and justice. These four basic principles form the structure of the commonly used textbook by Tom Beauchamp and James Childress titled *Principles of Biomedical Ethics* (2001). They are important concepts and, if properly used, can serve as checkpoints when we examine specific cases. There is now considerable debate about whether these principles, or the approach that has come to be called principlism, is the proper one to take in bioethics.

Alternative approaches are often suggested: narrative ethics, casuistry, feminist ethics, liberation approaches, hermeneutic ethics, and others (DuBose, Hamel, and O'Connell 1994). These other approaches are all helpful, even essential, in uncovering morally relevant aspects of real-world situations. But principles are also essential, and these four have stood the test of some decades of time, providing checkpoints for clinicians and ethicists. The four principles can be described simply:

- "Beneficence" means the obligation to do good for the patient and others.
- "Nonmaleficence" means the obligation not to harm the patient or others.
- "Autonomy" means the right of the patient to decide what is to be done.
- "Justice" means treating people fairly.

There is much more to it than this, of course, but this is the basic idea. Now people who use deontology and consequentialism in a complementary way (they are both-and; one needs both) argue that beneficence and nonmaleficence come from consequentialism—the results, the consequences for the patient (and for others), determine what is right and wrong. And they argue that autonomy and justice come from deontology—something other than results determines right and wrong. It is the patient's a priori right to choose, or it is the obligation of fairness and equality. But those who view deontology and consequentialism as incompatible alternatives, as they will be used for our purposes here, think that all four of these concepts (beneficence, nonmaleficence, autonomy, and justice) can fit into whichever approach they consider to be the right one. For example, respecting patient autonomy seems essential to bringing about good consequences for the patient; prolonging physical life is not the only thing to be seen as a consequence. Patients are badly treated—the consequences are bad for patients—when their autonomy is overridden, since patients are more than bodies. Similarly, justice has to do with what the consequences are for society as a whole and for the various people within it. So all four of these basic concepts (beneficence, nonmaleficence, autonomy, and justice) can be accepted and upheld within at least some versions of consequentialism. Of course, how consequentialism is defined and what is meant by it will be important; some versions of consequentialism, and especially of utilitarianism, subordinate autonomy and justice to a weighing of immediate and limited consequences. These versions of consequentialism are not acceptable. What we mean by consequentialism and the special kind of consequentialism that can be defended will become clearer in this and subsequent chapters.

The way these terms are used here, as incompatible alternatives, is the way these terms were often used historically. For example, when C. D. Broad first defined deontology and teleology, he saw them as contrasts. For him, deontology holds that an act "would always be right [or wrong, presumably] . . . no matter what its consequences might be" (Broad 1959, 206). This is the definition of deontology we will use. But it is not the most common approach in contemporary bioethics. The other way to use the concepts, seeing deontology and consequentialism as compatible complements, is more common and perfectly acceptable. It is the way Beauchamp and Childress use these concepts, and this has had a great influence on their use in American bioethics (Beauchamp and Childress 2001, 340–55, 376–77).

The basic reason for viewing these approaches as incompatible alternatives and for accepting a form of consequentialism and rejecting deontology is that within Roman Catholic moral theology, and especially in Catholic medical ethics, these two approaches, although often given different names, do operate as incompatible alternatives. There are Catholic moral theologians who subscribe to a deontological approach in the sense of the definition given here. And we disagree with that approach. We support something else. Many Catholic theologians today also support something else. Most of them do not call that something else "consequentialism." They call it "proportionalism" or "mixed consequentialism." But there seems no reason not to call it "consequentialism," if that term is properly defined. We will spend some time on these questions of Catholic medical ethics later, in chapters 10 through 12.

There is another reason for avoiding the practice of seeing autonomy and justice as somehow opposed to beneficence and nonmaleficence—the former as deontological and the latter as consequentialist. This is because, in contemporary philosophy as in official Catholic ethics, deontology almost always trumps consequentialism. In American secular bioethics, this often means that autonomy trumps everything else. This is not, I am convinced, what Beauchamp and Childress have in mind. But since deontology depends on strict rules, and since autonomy in the Kantian sense is said to be deontological, the autonomy of the individual often seems to win out over other considerations. This can lead to claimed refutations of substantive theories of justice (Engelhardt 1986, 66–102), to underemphasis or no emphasis on the good of nonpersons and of entities such as embryos and fetuses that may or may not be persons (Robertson, Kahn, and Wagner 2002, 35–37), to automatic acceptance of advance directives that seem to be hurtful to the present patient, to court decisions that neglect the real needs of marginally competent patients by allowing them to refuse essential treatment (Schneider 2004), and so on. We will return to these issues in detail later. But when autonomy is weighed and balanced with other goods in a consequentialist or proportionalist approach, judgments reached are more likely to be valid. Recall what we have already seen in part I: the human person is both individual and social. To anticipate what we will discuss in the section on Catholic method, autonomy becomes one of the aspects of "the human person adequately considered" (Janssens [1947] 1988, 13), not the only one or even necessarily the most important one.

This approach to these concepts is not idiosyncratic. The way these terms are defined here is more or less the same as the approach used by Bruno Schüller, a German Catholic theologian who, basing his approach on his own substantial research, uses these terms the same way. Schüller's context is that of defending proportionalism against prior approaches to normative ethics and arguing that even the word "utilitarianism" can be understood in a way that merits defense (Schüller 1986, 169–97). On the other hand, the definitions and interpretations we will give of the theories differ from those of American Catholic moral theologian Charles Curran. Aspects of Curran's approach to moral theology and medical ethics are very similar to our own. Indeed, we learned much from him. Yet Curran wants to refute utilitarianism and to deny that he is a utilitarian or even a consequentialist. Thus, he interprets consequentialism more restrictively than we do (Curran 1999, 69–73).[1]

This introduction to the problem of defining and using deontology and consequentialism has been rather theoretical, but it shows how and why these two terms are not easy to define. Reading bioethics literature requires that we discern what each author means by them. And we need to be aware as well that many authors use these terms without carefully attending to what they mean, which causes additional confusion. Now we are ready to turn to more precise definitions of these two terms.

Deontology

Deontology or deontologism, as this concept is used here, proposes that an act is right or wrong according to whether it meets or does not meet some intrinsic requirement by itself, apart from any kinds of consequences. Deontologists propose that some actions are always wrong in themselves regardless of consequences. Such actions are wrong because of some intrinsic quality in the act itself, some formally wrong-making quality, such that it is never right to do any act that belongs in this category.

Generally, deontologists point to three actions (or kinds of actions) that they claim are always wrong. The first of these is killing innocent people. Regardless of consequences, it is always morally wrong to directly kill an innocent person (we will come back to the term "directly" when we discuss the principle of double effect in chapter 12). There are never any exceptions. A general caught by the Nazis with information that will lead to the deaths of thousands, who knows he will be forced by drugs and torture to reveal the information, may not kill himself. Euthanasia is always forbidden, even if the patient is in great pain with no possibility of relief (we discuss this issue in detail later and argue that with proper medical care, this ought never to be the case). These and other acts of direct killing are deontologically proscribed. Regardless of the consequences, they are always morally wrong.

The second act that deontologists often absolutely forbid is lying. Regardless of the circumstances, it is always wrong to lie. The captured general may refuse to say anything beyond giving his name, rank, and serial number, but he may not give false information about battle plans.

The third set of actions often included in the "absolutely wrong" category are acts of genital sexuality. Different deontologists differ as to which acts fall in this category. Some may include only adultery as absolutely forbidden. Others include all nonmarital sex. The official teaching of the Roman Catholic Church includes in this category any act that arouses sexual pleasure outside of marriage, and forbids as well any marital action where the couple interfere with the possibility that the act may be fertile (the proscription against birth control). All these actions are said to be intrinsically evil, absolutely forbidden by the nature of the acts themselves, which are seen as violations of the meaning of human sexuality.

Immanuel Kant

Immanuel Kant is the philosopher most commonly thought of as a strict formalist or deontologist in this sense. Difficult to understand, and far better in theory than in practice, Kant does present one of the best examples of what formalist ethics means.

In his 1785 *Foundations of the Metaphysics of Morals*, Kant gives his deontological or formalist theory of morality. An act is right or wrong, he says, not because of its consequences in any sense of that word but according to whether it is or is not in conformity with duty, or the good will. The good will, according to Kant, is not good because of what it accomplishes. It is good only because of its willing. That is, it is good of itself. It is formally good, not good because of any material effects it brings about.

For Kant, "the first proposition of morality is that to have moral worth [to be morally right and not morally wrong] an action must be done from duty" (Kant 1981, 12). Duty, in turn, is "the necessity of an action executed from respect for law" (ibid., 13). But, he asks, what kind of law? And he answers: law-as-such. That is, universal law. When I act, I should act in such a way that I would want what I do to be a universal law, binding in all similar circumstances.

Kant speaks of what he calls the "categorical imperative" (ibid., 24–30), by which he means an absolutely unconditional requirement. There are three "forms" to this categorical imperative, but for our purposes here only the first form is needed: "Act only according to that maxim [rule, norm] by which you can at the same time will that it [the maxim] should become a universal law" (ibid., 30). It is important to note here that Kant holds (assuming this interpretation of him is correct) that actions are right or wrong apart from their consequences; they are right or wrong only because they do or do not have this quality of good will or duty attached to them.

One essay that Kant wrote late in life demonstrates his deontological ethic. In his "On the Supposed Right to Lie because of Philanthropic Concerns," Kant presents what has become a classic case about lying (Kant 1993). Here the case is enhanced a little for effect, but the basic idea is Kant's. A man is home and his friend is visiting him. Thugs come to the door and ask the man if the friend is there. The man knows that the thugs want to murder his friend, and he knows that he will not be able to defend against them because they are too many. What "ought" he to say? If he keeps silent, the thugs will know why and will kill the friend. He can hardly say, "I don't know"! Kant insists that he must say, "Yes, my friend is here." Lying is always wrong. If we lie, we must admit that a maxim allowing lying should become a universal law. Few contemporary philosophers would agree with Kant's conclusion in this case. Yet Catholic moral theology, perhaps following Augustine (who himself made the same judgment about the case Kant uses), has traditionally forbidden all lies in just this way (Hoose 2001, 67). When we come to the medical ethical applications of the principle of double effect, we will see how some Catholic moralists have tried to get around this absolute prohibition.

Consequentialism

Consequentialism proposes that the rightness or wrongness of acts (and of behavior patterns and social structures) depends on the reasonably foreseeable consequences of the act, pattern, or system. Acts are right or wrong only according to their effects. An act is a right act if its effects are positive, good ones; it is a wrong act if its effects are negative, bad, harmful ones. Those who reject consequentialism sometimes argue that no one can foresee actual consequences, but it seems perfectly valid for consequentialists to answer that one can recognize foreseeable effects and that morally sensitive persons do properly worry about the likely consequences of their actions. In any case, even strict deontologists do not claim that all actions not included in their list of always-wrong acts are always right. Deontologists, too, have to worry about consequences. As we will see when we analyze the principle of double effect, even that deontological principle includes a consequentialist requirement.

There are two kinds of consequentialism. The first, egoistic consequentialism, claims that an act is right or wrong according to its good or bad effects on the agent alone. If an act is beneficial for the agent, it is a right act. If it is harmful to the agent, it is a wrong act. Although some scholars still propose a moderate form of this view, most reject it altogether and no bioethicist that we know of accepts it as a valid approach to health care ethics.

As an aside, it is interesting to note one confusing factor that shows how an egoistic consequentialist might end up with a very strict ethic. An egoistic consequentialist might possibly argue this way: An act is wrong if it keeps me from happiness. But this act (premarital sex, for example) will bring me the pains of hell. Therefore, the act is wrong. This is still an egoistic consequentialism. The act is wrong (in this case) simply because it brings the agent pain or excludes the happiness of heaven and the presence of God. But this conclusion is not what we might expect from an egoistic consequentialist. We might expect the answer: "Sure, it's fun for me, and no one else need be considered." But in this case the answer to question 3 (what is of ultimate value?) is such that it demands the conclusion that the act is wrong because of its consequence, hell, which is against the agent's own best interests. Thus, the judgments reached by the various theories need not always be what are expected. Also, of course, persons with different theories may well reach similar conclusions.

The second kind of consequentialism is universal consequentialism. Universal consequentialism insists on considering the consequences for some sort of whole, not just the consequences for the agent. So it is more likely to be a valid approach to bioethics than egoism. Universal consequentialism is often called utilitarianism. That is, some—but not all—scholars identify the two and use the two terms synonymously. Bruno Schüller defends this usage and supports this approach to ethics (Schüller 1986, 173-78). But other philosophers and many theologians consider utilitarianism to be a restrictive subdivision of universal consequentialism. They see utilitarianism as limiting the consequences it considers to immediate or measurable consequences. Utilitarianism in this sense is identified with a simplistic interpretation of "the ends justify the means." As long as one has a good end in view, it does not matter what one does to get there. If that is what the word means, or if the relevant consequences are limited to easily visible or measurable ones, then utilitarianism is clearly insufficient as an approach to bioethics. But other philosophers use the same word to apply to an approach that takes into consideration not only immediate and easily quantifiable consequences but also intrinsic and less easily measurable effects. This is sometimes called ideal utilitarianism, and it seems that this is less easily dismissed. It is a kind of "intrinsic consequentialism" and similar to what some Catholic theologians now call "proportionalism." This approach, we think, is a valid method in bioethics.

Another helpful perspective on this question is to go back to the general definition of universal consequentialism. It insists on looking at the consequences not just for the agent but for the "whole." The problem of how to define that "whole" remains, and here we have a number of different suggestions:

- Classical utilitarianism (the original theory as proposed by philosophers Jeremy Bentham and John Stuart Mill) proposes that rightness and wrongness depend on the effects of the act (or behavior pattern or system) for the "greatest good of the greatest number" (of people). This is dangerous if not interpreted properly. It may give too little importance to the rights of minorities. It may suggest that it is simply a question of numbers. Is the heinous crime of slavery justified, for example, if the "greatest number" (the white majority in a slave-holding nation) can be said to benefit from the practice? For Bentham and Mill, utilitarianism was in fact a progressive method. They insisted that practices were wrong if they benefited only the royalty or the nobles or the very wealthy. Bentham and Mill saw utilitarianism as a way to make sure that everyone counted. For them, each person counts as one, but only as one. This was a real advance over the notion that practices are right if the autocrat decrees them to be such since they are for his or her personal benefit. And the theory is less problematic when intensity and duration of the greatest good are included along with the greatest number of people, as classical utilitarianism claims to do. But there is still the danger that the utilitarian calculus (weighing and measuring effects for the largest number in some presumably quantifiable way) is too facile to serve as a basis for ethics.
- Other consequentialists suggest that the "whole" is all people seen both as individuals and as a society. This, I think, is better. This is what Catholic moral theologian Louis Janssens said was the norm of morality: "the human person adequately considered in regard to self and in relation with others' (Janssens [1947] 1988, 13).
- Or one might want to insist that it is not just human beings who need to be included but animals as well.
- Finally, for some, all reality needs to be included, since all of creation, including inanimate objects, ought to be considered. Rocks and rivers have rights, too.

The best of these approaches is "the human person adequately considered." Animals and inanimate objects are not equal to people—the theological foundation for this is discussed in chapter 2—but this does not imply that persons can run roughshod over the rest of God's creation. To consider the human person adequately includes a proper regard for animal life and for the ecosphere. But it is not true that all that ultimately counts is the ecosphere such that it becomes almost irrelevant whether it is people or cockroaches that ultimately survive.

Another problem with classical utilitarianism needs a short discussion here, even though it properly belongs in question 3 (what is of ultimate value?). Both Bentham and Mill, the originators of classical utilitarianism, answered question 3 by proposing that pleasure is of ultimate value. That is, in philosophical terms they were hedonists. The greatest good we must seek, they said, is the presence of pleasure and the absence of pain. Thus, many persons who reject hedonism as an answer to question 3 reject utilitarianism as an answer to question 2 for that reason. Yet others, such as ideal utilitarians and some other schools of consequentialists and teleologists, reject hedonism as the ultimate value but remain in some sense consequentialists. The two need not go together. Still, utilitarianism (universal consequentialism) suffers from its connection with hedonism.

Act and Rule Utilitarianism

Early on in the debate about whether utilitarianism (we are using this now as synonymous with universal consequentialism) is a workable theory, the question was raised about the role of rules. If deontologists, in the sense in which we have defined them here, make some rules absolute, what role do utilitarians give to rules? Do they reject them altogether? If so, it would seem that utilitarianism is either too permissive (anything goes) or, paradoxically, impossible (one must measure all the foreseeable effects each time there is an ethical decision to make). So utilitarians have come up with a distinction that tries to answer this question. They distinguished between act and rule versions of utilitarianism.

Unfortunately, however, just as is the case with the terms "deontology" and "consequentialism," so too with this distinction there are different versions both of act utilitarianism and of rule utilitarianism. This can be frustrating. One can argue with considerable plausibility that technical terms such as these ought to retain precise meanings. But even though they do not, the terms are often used in bioethics, for example, by Beauchamp and Childress (2001, 343–48), and the distinction can provide some clarity about the variety of approaches that exist in contemporary health care ethics. These terms help us see various positions on a spectrum of approaches and, when properly understood, help us to situate and thus to sharpen our own approach. For example, we have suggested a preference for a moderate form of intrinsic consequentialism to the kind of deontology defined here. But there is a need to worry about whether this bias is one that can be defended and used consistently. If we allow ourselves the flexibility of moderate consequentialism but require a strict adherence to rules from everyone else, then there is something wrong with how we "do ethics" as well as with our moral character. By helping us examine our approach to ethics and our individual biases in this way, these kinds of distinctions help us know what we think and why we think it.

There are two different meanings given both to act utilitarianism (AU) and to rule utilitarianism (RU). This means there are really four different positions. To make it easier to keep them straight, adjectives are added here to modify them, but these adjectives are never used in the literature. We have to decide for ourselves which meaning an author is employing. Hint: authors usually think that they are "moderate" and that those they disagree with are not. Although this does not always work, it usually does. The four positions are as follows:

- "Strict" rule utilitarianism holds that some rules are absolute. They bind always. This sounds just like deontology, and in practice it often is. But it differs in one important way. For deontologists, as we have defined deontology, the reason some rules always bind and some acts are absolutely wrong is that there is some intrinsic wrong-making quality in the act itself. But rule utilitarians, even "strict" ones, are still consequentialists. Their reason for saying that some rules always bind is their claim that violating these rules would, in the long run, always produce more bad effects than good ones for society as a whole. There is another difference that follows from this one. Whereas deontologists claim that their judgments can never change—what is intrinsically evil has always been such and always will be such—strict rule utilitarians can admit that if society should change radically enough (or if some other society is sufficiently different), some rules that always bind now (or here) might not bind in that future (or in that other) society.

- "Moderate" rule utilitarianism holds that rules are indeed important—often very important. There are, however, some exceptional cases where a rule should be violated since in those cases the consequences of following the rule are very bad.
- "Moderate" act utilitarianism holds that rules are indeed important. There are, however, some cases where a rule should be violated since in those cases the consequences of following the rule are worse than the consequences of violating it. Yes, this definition is the same as the one for moderate rule utilitarianism, except here we have less hesitation to make exceptions to rules.
- "Radical" act utilitarianism is at the other end of the spectrum from deontology. Radical act utilitarianism holds that rules are worthless or almost worthless. Each situation is so totally new that we should jettison the rules and look at each case in a new light. This approach fails first because it is not true to human experience—there *are* similarities among cases—and second because it makes the theory nearly impossible to use in practice.

Summary of Approaches

We end up, then, with six approaches. On one end of the spectrum is deontology. Next come the four types of utilitarianism or universal consequentialism in the order in which we have just seen them: strict RU, moderate RU, moderate AU, and radical AU. At the other extreme end of the spectrum, so extreme that almost no one defends it, is egoistic consequentialism, which considers only what is good for the agent and ignores everyone else.

Legalism and Situationalism

Before ending this chapter on right and wrong, it is helpful to introduce two more sets of important terms. The first is the contrast between "legalism" and "situationalism." These two terms are often used as less technical ways to answer one of the questions answered by the spectrum of approaches we have just seen: How widely do rules apply? For example, to how many different kinds of killing does the rule "Thou shalt not kill" apply? All would doubtless agree that it is wrong to murder a defenseless robbery victim. But can we also say that capital punishment is wrong? Would we also say that euthanasia is always wrong, or that for a physician to assist in a patient's suicide is always wrong? How widely does the rule apply?

Again we have a spectrum. "Legalism" is a name given (critically) to the approach that insists that the rule applies whenever the action is the same. This is more or less the same as deontology in the way in which we have defined it, and possibly the same as strict rule utilitarianism. Killing is always wrong. No situations alter this judgment. Some persons (pacifists) hold to this absolute rule, but most do not. Most argue that in at least some situations of self-defense, killing is unfortunate but right. We have already seen that many deontologists hold that all direct killing of innocent persons is wrong. For them, there are never any consequences or situations that would allow such killing to be judged right. Yet, in a sense, even that deontological rule is not as universal as it might be. "Innocence" introduces a situational element. In the situation where the person I kill is an unjust aggressor, I may kill. In any case, the term "legalism" is often used, usually as a criticism, to apply to an approach that insists there are no exceptions to the law.

Radical situationalism is at the other end of the spectrum. Here there are never any rules at all; it depends on the situation. This is identical to radical act utilitarianism. The extreme situationalist says that there are never any rules that apply to a wide number of cases. Each case, each situation, is *entirely* different, and therefore each case must be seen on its own merits. Joseph Fletcher is often seen as holding this view, and in some of his writings he clearly does, though there are also places where he seems not to go quite so far (Fletcher 1966). It is hard, after all, to teach or write much about ethics if all one can say is that it totally depends on the situation.

Thus, the extremes are legalism and radical situationalism. Legalists hold that rules always apply when a given type of act is committed. Radical situationalists say there are no rules at all. Most medical ethicists hold positions somewhere in between. Other terms might be proposed for a more moderate approach. Perhaps "moderate situationalism" would work. "Moderate legalism" does not work, since the word "legalism" is really a word of rejection; it denies any moderation to the approach it rejects.

Formal and Material Norms

There is one final set of terms to define in the context of how widely rules apply. Sometimes there is confusion about this because of the failure to distinguish between formal norms (or rules) and material norms (or rules). The term "rule" and the term "norm" can usually be interchanged without any real danger. Some philosophers distinguish them according to their form, the way they are expressed. The norm might be "Euthanasia is wrong," and the rule would be "Do not perform euthanasia." But while "rule" and "norm" are interchangeable, formal norms or rules and material norms or rules are not the same.

It is perhaps easier to give an example than to start with definitions. One example of a formal norm is "Murder is wrong." If we take a look at the meaning of the word "murder," we easily see that "murder" *means* "wrong killing." So the norm does not give us very much in the way of explanation of what is right and what is wrong, because everyone agrees that murder is always wrong. If someone kills an attacker in self-defense, the word "murder" is not applied to the action. Similarly, people who hold that capital punishment is right do not think it is murder to execute criminals, though they do think it is killing. Only those who oppose capital punishment claim it is murder. So "Murder is wrong" is a formal norm. Formal norms apply everywhere and always.

On the other hand, the norm "Killing is wrong" is a material norm. The word "killing" does not necessarily mean wrong killing. Not all people hold that killing is always wrong, though everyone holds that it is sometimes wrong and most of us hold that there is a good reason to presume it is wrong until it can be justified. But "killing" is a material term, and "Killing is wrong" is a material norm. Material norms do make claims about what is right and what is wrong. They explain something to us.

There are more technical definitions of formal and material norms that may be helpful. A formal norm is a norm in which the moral quality attributed by the predicate is already present in the subject. "Murder is wrong" merely states that wrong killing (the subject) is wrong. The predicate "is" attributes "wrongness" to a subject that already includes wrongness in it.

A material norm is a norm in which the moral quality attributed by the predicate is *not* already present in the subject. "Killing is wrong" is a material norm. It is not a priori clear that it is automatically true all the time. Strict pacifists claim that it is true all the time, that all killing is murder. We have seen already that strict pacifism is usually an example of deontology. The material norm is thought to bind always and without exception because the act "killing" is said to be intrinsically wrong. "All killing is murder" is thus an absolute material norm. Not everyone agrees. But the norm "Murder is wrong" is a formal norm and is automatically true. Everyone knows that murder is wrong.

Other examples of formal terms such as "murder" are "injustice," "unchastity," "sloth," "greed," and so on. "Greed is good" is an oxymoron, an internal contradiction. "Desire for more wealth is good" is something we can discuss: maybe yes, maybe no; it depends. But if it is really greed, it is wrong. Formal norms are thus tautologies ("same-words"). The predicate adds nothing to the subject. But this does not mean that formal norms are useless. They serve as reminders, as exhortations to do the right thing. "Unchastity is wrong! Don't do it!"

It is important to note that the distinction between deontology and consequentialism, and the one between legalism and situationalism, has to do with material norms not with formal norms. All formal norms bind all the time because they are tautologies. There is no reason to debate this. What deontology and strict rule utilitarianism hold is that some material norms bind all the time too. Other consequentialists and situationalists (radical and moderate) say they do not.

The distinction between formal and material norms is helpful to keep in mind. Claims that some actions are always wrong are sometimes ambiguous. Authors may try to reject situationalism or consequentialism, for example, by including formal norms as examples, implying, for instance, that because "unchastity" or "murder" is always wrong, there are at least some absolutely exceptionless norms. The real debate is about whether there are any absolutely exceptionless material norms, and that is a very different question.

Note

1. Timothy O'Connell, on the other hand, did use an approach in the first edition of his book *Principles for a Catholic Morality* that was the same, more or less, as the one proposed here. In the first edition (1978), he accepted the term "consequentialism" or "macroconsequentialism" as applying to his theory (O'Connell 1978, 146–49, 165–73). But in his second edition (1990), he changed his method and rejected even "macroconsequentialism" (O'Connell 1990, 202–5, 278nn5–6). He came to hold that certain actions are always wrong regardless of consequences (ibid., 193–96). Thus, he was at least in this respect a deontologist.

CHAPTER 9

METAETHICS

Introduction

THE TECHNICAL TERM "metaethics" means "beyond ethics" and refers to the area of ethics that deals with the possibility of meaning in and knowledge of ethics. It is the epistemology of ethics. Epistemology is the science of knowledge, the branch of philosophy that asks about human knowledge. How do we know? How much is illusion? How much depends on our individual and social biases and even prejudices? What are the sources of our knowledge? How much comes from us and how much from "reality"?

The term "metaethics" is quite recent and comes from the analytic school of modern philosophy. That school, or at least the more reductionist or radical versions of that school, hold that the entire task of philosophy is to analyze statements. Thus, metaethics analyzes ethical statements. This would not be of concern to our study except that the questions that metaethics asks have been important for a long time, even before anyone heard of analytic philosophy. Metaethics asks questions about whether knowledge of ethics is even possible, and if so, how.

The word "metaethics" is also at times used in relation to analytic questions other than the specifically epistemological ones I deal with in this chapter. Beauchamp and Childress, for example, say that metaethics "involves analysis of the language, concepts, and methods of reasoning in ethics. . . . It addresses the meaning of ethical terms. . . . It also treats moral epistemology" (Beauchamp and Childress 2001, 2). However, I think it is better to reserve the term for what I take to be its central task: the analysis of the possibility of ethical knowledge. Does ethics have any meaning, and if so, how is that meaning verified? If we limit metaethics to this core area, we can later more easily distinguish between normative and metaethical tasks. I have found this distinction to be extremely helpful in reading and critiquing ethical claims and arguments. At the end of this chapter, for example, I show how situationalism, with which I have already dealt, and (meta)ethical relativism, which I describe here, are very different, though they are often confused.

Health care presumes a certain epistemological realism. Epistemological realism is the approach to the theory of human knowledge that holds that there is some kind of valid relationship between our knowledge and reality or "the real world out there." What we think we know about reality is indeed to some extent what reality is. It is clear that health care professionals presume that there are patterns in human nature, in the way the body will react to disease and to its treatment. All of us claim that we know these patterns, and that they actually exist, despite the fact that often they are not entirely the same in different cases and are very complex. We claim that we know ahead of time, at least with a decent degree of certitude, how bodies will act and react. We do not have to start anew with each new patient. We know enough, I hope, to be humble about all of this. Sometimes we make mistakes. Some diseases have no cures. Our ignorance is great. But our knowledge is great, too. We claim there are things we know about the body and about its treatment. If we could not make this claim, we would have to abandon the attempt to study and practice scientific medicine. Thus, in philosophical terms, we make certain "epistemological presuppositions" without which we could not practice medicine.

The same problems arise in ethics, but ethics is different from the more immediately empirical and experimental areas of human knowledge. Few people would want to argue that it is just a baseless opinion that appendectomies help in the treatment of appendicitis. Many do argue, however, that ethics and moral judgments are matters of baseless opinion. No one can say what is right and what is wrong. So metaethics asks whether there is any meaning to ethics and ethical statements or judgments. Does ethics have any meaning, and if it does, how do I verify that meaning?

Metaethics asks, for example, about the meaning of the ethical judgment "X is wrong." Does this statement mean anything at all? If it does, what does it mean? And how can I verify that it means something? In the last chapter, we spent some time asking how widely rules apply. Is a rule absolute? Does it apply in all cases, in many cases, or just to this one case? Does it have any exceptions? Now in metaethics we will be asking a different question: Granted the exact same act and circumstances X, what does it mean when I say "X is wrong"?

Consider the following example: "The killing of Jews by the Nazis in the Holocaust was wrong." Very few persons would disagree with that judgment. Some of us might want to say "All killing is wrong," others to say "Most killing is wrong" or "Killing is wrong except when it is in self-defense," and so on. But these are more general than the judgments about the Holocaust, and, as we have already seen, there are differences between deontology and consequentialism, and between legalism and situationalism, that account for differences in these more general judgments.

In metaethics, the generality or specificity of the judgment is not the issue. Whether we make a specific judgment about an indefensible incident of medical experimentation or a more general judgment about killing, metaethics wants to ask about the meaning of that judgment. Does ethics have any meaning, and if so, how do we verify that meaning?

Metaethical Theories

What does it mean when I say "X is wrong"? The answers given to this question can be divided into three general types. This typology comes from a 1973 article by bioethicist Robert M. Veatch titled "Does Ethics Have an Empirical Basis?" (Veatch 1973a). I have found this typology to be easily understood and more or less comprehensive in noting the principal varieties of answers to the question of verification of ethics.

First Type: Noncognitivism or Emotivism

For radical noncognitivists, when someone says "X is wrong" (for example, "This medical experiment was wrong"), or when someone makes a more general ethical judgment (such as "Euthanasia is wrong"), it means nothing verifiable at all. It means nothing that I can understand, nothing meaningful. It is thus "noncognitive"; it has "no meaning." The most I can say for it is that it means "Boo for the murder of Jews in Nazi Germany." It does not mean "Murdering Jews was wrong." It does not mean even that "I think it was wrong." It is a meaningless statement, merely an emotional outburst. Hence noncognitivism is often called "emotivism" or "ethical emotivism." Ethical judgments are only emotional reactions people have. They are similar to rooting for a particular sports team or reacting to a foul odor.[1]

Second Type: Metaethical (or Ethical) Relativism

In the context of ethics, the word "relativism" should always be given a metaethical meaning. Metaethical relativism asserts that when I say "X is wrong" it means only "I think it is wrong" or "My society thinks it is wrong." There are thus two kinds of ethical relativism: individual metaethical relativism and social metaethical relativism.

Individual metaethical relativism claims that when someone makes an ethical judgment—when someone says the Holocaust was wrong, for example—that means only that he or she thinks it was wrong. That much can be verified. But if someone else claims it was right, there is no basis for rejecting that claim. The ethical relativist claims that we cannot verify rightness or wrongness from any source at all. There is no way to go any further. It is all relative. Different people think differently. There is no more to ethics or morality than to find out what people think.

The more common kind of ethical relativism is social ethical relativism or, more technically, social metaethical relativism. This theory holds that when I say "X is wrong" (again, for example, "The Holocaust was wrong"), all this means is that my social group has come to believe that the Holocaust was wrong. Other groups may agree or disagree. That is all that can be verified. No universal verification is possible. Jews think it is wrong to be killed; Nazis think it is right to kill them. Neither judgment can be said in itself in any way to be right or wrong, since nothing more can be verified.

This, of course, applies as well to more general judgments. Conservative Christians say euthanasia and abortion are wrong. Liberal thinkers say they are right. All we can do with this is to say that conservative Christians say one thing and liberal thinkers another. There is no possibility of verifying whether euthanasia or abortion is right or wrong. It is all relative.

It is very important here to distinguish between relativism and situationalism. For example, one might claim that euthanasia is wrong and still claim that killing convicted murderers is right. Or one might argue that the bombing of London by the Luftwaffe was wrong (because the war conducted by Hitler's Germany was an unjust war) and still claim that the bombing of German submarine pens in France was right (because this was a just defensive war on the part of the Allies). In these cases, we might say that moral judgments have to be "related to the situation." This is (some form of) situationalism as we have defined that term. But relativism is different. Relativism claims that all ethical judgments and norms are only opinions. It is important, then, not to use the word "relativism" to mean situational differences. Situationalism has to do with the question of universality of applicability of rules or norms. Here, in meta-ethics, we are looking at the possibility of verifiability of ethical judgments, rules, or norms. The two concepts are often confused, but they are not the same.

There is one more way to clarify what relativism is. Ethicists talk about descriptive ethics and prescriptive ethics.[2] Descriptive ethics is simply the process of describing what various people think about certain ethical issues. We will be doing that in this book. All ethicists do that when they write about what different groups think about physician-assisted suicide, for example. Authors describe what various groups think. Prescriptive ethics, on the other hand, is the actual making of an ethical judgment. When one concludes that physician-assisted suicide is right, or wrong, or sometimes right and sometimes wrong depending on the situation, one makes a judgment. One prescribes rightness and wrongness. We will also be doing this in this book.

The true ethical relativist can never prescribe. Since ethical relativists claim that moral judgments cannot be verified, that they are simply a matter of opinion, all they can do is descriptive ethics. They can never really prescribe because prescribing (saying that physician-assisted suicide is sometimes right, for example) implies that the one making the judgment thinks there is some basis for it. Otherwise why make it? So ethical relativists, if they are to remain true to their theory of relativism, can never actually make an ethical judgment. It is in fact silly of them to do so. If they say "Ethnic cleansing is wrong," what they are really saying is "My opinion of ethnic cleansing is that it is wrong, but this opinion of mine has no basis at all. The opinion that it is right is just as good an opinion, so really I have no judgment to make in the first place because there is no basis for any judgment." It seems reasonable to claim that if either (radical) noncognitivism or (radical) ethical relativism is the correct answer to the metaethical question, we should all give up on ethics.

The arguments for and against the possibility of verification of ethical judgments and norms and systems are very complex, and we have only scratched the surface. Epistemology is terribly difficult. Modern thinkers, and especially postmodern thinkers, have learned to distrust certain bases for the claim that our knowledge is true. In the Enlightenment, the West learned to distrust certain religious bases; in the Romantic movement, we learned to distrust certain scientific bases. In postmodernism, some distrust all bases. There is, of course, some good reason for distrust. Tyrants, whether religious or scientific, have used knowledge systems as the bases for their tyranny. Everyone "knows" that kings are chosen by God to rule, so we must obey. Everybody "knows" that the future of economics is determined to be stateless Communism, so we must obey. Still, few of us are willing to reject all (or most) claims to true knowledge.

Certain contemporary ethicists have made an argument that seems plausible. They claim that the bases for rejecting the verifiability of ethical judgments work equally well as bases for rejecting the verifiability of all judgments. This seems correct, though it is probably impossible to prove it. If we cannot claim to make valid ethical judgments, then we cannot claim to make valid empirical or scientific judgments either. The same epistemic capacities needed for empirical judgments suffice for the making of ethical judgments. For example, why do we think we have a better basis for saying "I know that the volcano does not contain an angry god; the natives who think that are ignorant of the truth," than we have for saying "I know that female genital mutilation is wrong; the cultures that do that are ignorant of the truth"? We can no more prove, in purely empirical ways, the first claim than we can the second. Yet we tend to think we "know" the first on scientific grounds, and to think the second is less well supported.

The differences between ethical and empirical or scientific judgments are real but perhaps are not as important as we think. Ethical judgments are sometimes very hard to make. But scientific judgments are also hard to make. We forget that we used to "know" that the earth was flat; we had clear empirical proof for it: if it were round, we would fall off if we traveled too far over the curve. Ethical judgments often vary depending on the situation, but scientific judgments (and, surely, medical judgments) also vary depending on the situation. Different people hold to differing ethical judgments, but different people hold to differing scientific judgments, too. This is not to claim that we can arrive at the same *kind* of certitude in moral matters as in empirical or scientific ones. To use the classical distinction, there is a difference between speculative reason (pure reason for Kant) and practical reason. They arrive at different kinds of certitude. It seems plausible, however, that the supposed weaknesses in our capacity to know ethical truth, the ones used by noncognitivists, turn out to be weaknesses as well in our capacity to know any truth. Health care workers assume we can arrive at some kinds of empirical or scientific truth. We can really know some things, not perfectly, not comprehensively, but enough to be able to make judgments about them and act on those judgments. The same is true in ethics. If this claim is valid, then health care professionals, whose art of healing depends in significant measure on the knowledge of anatomic patterns scientifically understood, ought to be open to the possibility of ethical knowledge as well. Neither scientific nor ethical knowledge is immutable; neither is certainly free from error. And both in ethics and in scientific medicine, there are better-founded truths and less-well-founded opinions. It is sometimes very hard to determine which is which, but neither in medicine nor in ethics is there an a priori reason for rejecting the possibility of valid judgment and of its verification. This leads to the third and last type of metaethical theory.

Third Type: Metaethical Absolutist Positions

For metaethical absolutists, ethical judgments do have meaning, and that meaning can be verified. Metaethical absolutists hold that the judgment "X is wrong" actually means what it says. It means X is wrong. It does not necessarily mean Y is wrong, even if X and Y are somewhat similar, or even if they involve the same physical act, as long as they are also different in a morally relevant way. That is, despite the word "absolutism," metaethical absolutism is not the same as "absolute rules"; it is not the same as legalism. Metaethical absolutists may be legalists or they may be situationalists. They may be deontologists or consequentialists or something else entirely in their answer to question 2 of normative ethical theory (the question of right and wrong). But they do hold that the judgment "X is wrong" means X is wrong, and that it is possible, at least in principle, to verify that judgment.

Now there can still be disagreement about X being wrong. Perhaps some of us will claim that X is right, or that X is sometimes right. Metaethical absolutists claim only that judgments like these do have meaning and can be verified, not that everyone will reach the same conclusion or verify his or her judgments correctly. Theoretically, of course, metaethical absolutists think that everyone really ought to arrive at the same correct judgment, but they recognize that that is not going to happen in many cases, and they may also realize that their own judgments are often tentative and may in fact change as they learn more. Thus, metaethical absolutism does not require the (obviously nonexistent) state of affairs where everyone agrees. Indeed, the very fact that differing ethical judgments are taken seriously and can be debated presupposes that the debaters hold that their varying judgments can be verified. Each debater thinks that the other has reached the wrong conclusion; she or he does not claim that all ethical judgments are meaningless and unverifiable but only that the other's judgment is invalid.

Obviously, neither noncognitivists nor relativists need to answer the question of how ethical judgments are verified, since they claim they cannot be. But metaethical absolutists do have to answer this question, and, according to Veatch's typology, there are four different sources claimed for this verification.

Four Types of Metaethical Absolutism

Supernatural Metaethical Absolutism

Supernatural metaethical absolutism holds that ethical judgments do have meaning and can be verified. They are verified on the basis of some (supposedly supernatural and specifically definable) source of divine revelation. X is wrong because God says that it is wrong. And God says this in some specific source of direct revelation. This last is important because, as we will soon see, there is another kind of metaethical absolutism that also relates verification ultimately to the law of God but does not claim any specific source of revelation as its basis. Proponents of supernatural metaethical absolutism see the basis for ethics in a source that we would call directly religious, and these sources are usually ones claimed by one or another religion to be available only through faith.

Perhaps the most obvious candidates for this would be the sacred writings of different religions. The Christian Bible, including both Jewish and Christian Testaments, is a source often claimed by Christians. Jewish Scriptures are claimed as a source of norms or judgments by some Jews, as is the Qur'an by some Muslims. Not all Christians see the Bible this way, however, nor do all Jews or Muslims view their scriptures as the main or privileged source of specific ethical norms or judgments. Many believers claim that the source for verification is really God's creation: human nature and all of created reality. Those Christians who do claim that the Bible is the source for verification of all (or most, or perhaps just some) ethical norms and judgments are often said to hold a theory called "biblical positivism."

The second most obvious candidate for a source of direct divine revelation is the church itself—most often the leaders of the church. Certain church leaders have claimed to have received direct revelations from God about ethical matters. In Roman Catholicism, the theory that we know God's law primarily through the teachings of the magisterium (the teaching authority of the pope and the bishops) can be called "ecclesiastical positivism" (Kelly 1979, 311–20).

Other candidates could be suggested as well, such as divinely inspired dreams and visions or direct apparitions of Jesus, Mary, saints, or prophets. In principle, Catholic moral theology does not subscribe to supernatural metaethical absolutism. The tradition has more generally held that moral knowledge is available to all through the use of natural reason (natural law). We will return to this subject after touching on two more metaethical absolutist theories.

Intuitional Metaethical Absolutism (Intuitionism)

Intuitionists also claim that ethical judgments have meaning and can be verified. For them, the source of verification is a universal and valid common moral sense or moral intuition. X is wrong because everyone (or at least almost everyone) can tell by some sort of moral sense that X is wrong. Everyone intuits that the Holocaust was wrong.

This theory has a good deal of validity. People do have a moral sense. We tend to disagree about difficult issues, but at least most people seem to agree on at least some of the basics. And it does not seem intolerant or "judgmental" in the negative sense of that word to claim that those who do not agree on these very basic ethical issues are sociopathic or amoral. They do not have, or have not developed, that valid common moral sense that people usually have. We are not likely to debate the morality of serial murder. We simply know that the serial killer lacks common moral sense. Still, there is a problem with intuitionism. It is too easy to move from there to an easy kind of metaethical relativism. Perhaps your moral intuition is different from mine. I think serial killing is right. And I claim that my moral intuition is as good as yours is. In addition, if there is no other basis for verification than intuition, it will be hard to converse and debate about ethical issues.

Rational Metaethical Absolutism

The theory of rational metaethical absolutism claims that we verify moral judgments on the basis of some rational system. X is wrong because that is the only rationally correct thing to hold. Perhaps a Kantian ethic could be said to adhere to this theory.

Empirical Metaethical Absolutism (Natural Law Theory)

Veatch calls the last of his four types "empirical metaethical absolutism." This theory, like the other versions of metaethical absolutism, claims that ethical judgments have meaning and can be verified. Here the source of verification is reality. That is, we verify by studying reality, especially the human person and human society, and on this basis we can work toward valid moral norms and judgments.

This theory does not claim that we can decide what to do simply by looking at what is actually done. It may be true that most people lie from time to time, but that does not make it right. Nor does this theory claim that it is always easy to answer ethical questions or that such answers are inevitably right. Nor does it claim that judgments are necessarily valid across cultures or across time. The relationship of "ought" to "is" is more complex than that.

It is not possible to prove that this is the best approach. Many, probably most, contemporary philosophers do not agree that we can learn enough about people to be able to discover what is right and wrong. However, this is the metaethical theory held over the centuries by Catholic moral theology, and the authors of this book are convinced that it continues to be the best basis for verification of ethical judgments. Indeed, we worry that any other basis, or lack of basis, can too easily lead to tyranny.

When Catholic moral theology asks about the basis for verification of ethical norms and judgments, it uses the term "natural law." In the next chapter, when we discuss Catholic medical ethics, we will see how that same word has been used for a specific kind of normative ethic that many Catholic moralists reject. Natural law in this other sense is a restrictive kind of deontology. But natural law theory on the metaethical level is, we think, the best approach to the problem of meaning and verification.

A good definition of natural law from a theological perspective is this: Natural law theory is a metaethical theory according to which people discover right and wrong by using their reason and experience to investigate, individually and collectively, the emergent patterns of creation as God is creating them. Traditionally, Catholic moral theology has tended to overemphasize deductive reason and underemphasize human experience, and it has seen created nature as stagnant and unchanging. This definition of natural law tries to change that. But it is still true to the basic Catholic insight about how we learn God's law for us. We learn what God wants us to do and be primarily by learning who we are and who we can become. This natural law approach is true to the kind of theological basis for health care ethics reviewed in part I.

We learn ethics by learning about reality, especially by learning about ourselves. It is here, in this context, that the Bible and the magisterium are especially important for Catholics in the area of ethics. They help us to learn about ourselves and our relationship with others and with God. Catholics must not overlook these sources. But the bases we use for our ethical judgments are not in principle hidden to non-Catholics or to non-Christians, as would be the case were they limited to specifically Catholic or Christian sources of revelation. All human persons can discover right and wrong. As Lisa Sowle Cahill puts it: "This is what the 'Catholic' (Aristotelian-Thomistic) ethical tradition is essentially about: a confidence that reasonable reflection on human experience can lead us not only to recognize and condemn injustice, but to persuade others that they can recognize and condemn it more or less on the same terms we do" (Cahill 1970, 69). This basic insight of Catholic moral theology is essential to good ethics.

Foundationalism

Philosophers and theologians often use the term "foundationalism" in this context. The basic question is whether ethics has a discoverable foundation. Probably most philosophers who use this term argue against it. That is, as we have already seen, they think that we cannot know enough about human beings to be able to found or base an ethic. They are, in some form or other, noncognitivists (usually not the radical kind). The metaethical theory that we propose here—"empirical metaethical absolutism" or "natural law theory"—is foundationalist.

It is interesting to note, however, that foundationalism can mean at least two very different things. One form, which for the purpose of making these distinctions easier to grasp we will call "deductive foundationalism," is said to hold that all ethical norms and judgments can be deduced from one primary principle. Three candidates are sometimes proposed for this honor: the principle of utility, Kant's categorical imperative, and the so-called primary principle of the natural law (good is to be done and evil avoided). But natural law theory should not be seen as a deductive foundationalism. The kind of "intrinsic consequentialism" (or proportionalism) proposed in chapter 8 is not primarily a deductive process; nor do most utilitarians hold that their ethics are simply deduced from the principle of utility. And no natural law thinker (at least in the sense of natural law as a metaethical theory) claims that rules and norms are deduced from the primary principle of the natural law. Rules and norms may be developed instantiations of that principle, or more precise examples, but they cannot be deduced from that more general principle. Thus we reject deductive foundationalism.

The second form of foundationalism that many philosophers claim to reject is a wider "metaethical foundationalism." Because we cannot know enough to base our ethical knowledge on any foundation in reality, they claim, we must be antifoundationalists. If foundationalism means metaethical foundationalism, then natural law as a metaethical theory is indeed foundationalist. Contrary to the thinking of many contemporary thinkers, Catholic health care ethics claims that there is a foundation in created reality for ethical judgments and principles.

An Illustrative Case

We have now introduced the basic questions with which ethics deals and the main approaches suggested for answering them. The following case is one to which we might apply some of these terms and concepts for further clarity.

In Alaska and the Canadian Arctic, indigenous peoples, so the story goes, used to go off into the cold to die when they were old. The younger people helped their elderly relatives onto the ice floes. A Christian missionary, according to this story—whether true or not is irrelevant for our purpose—went to an Inuit village to evangelize the people with the Gospel and was horrified when he saw the elderly committing what he saw to be suicide. These people, he thought, had no sense of caring for the old, and since they assisted at suicide they were really murderers. So he convinced them at length that this was murder, that it was against God's law. He left the village and went on his way. When he returned years later, he discovered that the tribe had been almost wiped out. He was able to find out what had happened. The clan had followed his advice, keeping the elderly with them. This slowed down the migration process and required more food than was available. The children began to die. Ultimately the whole tribe, or most of it, died.

In somewhat parallel fashion, an American man named Joe wanted to inherit his mother's money. When she grew old, he put her on a raft and sent her off into Lake Michigan in midwinter.

Now we need to imagine asking an ethicist about these cases. His name is Dr. Jones. All we know about Dr. Jones is that he makes two statements. Dr. Jones says: "What the Inuit did was right. What Joe did was wrong." Then Dr. Jones goes away and says no more. Our task is to write down in one column all the terms we think can be applied to Dr. Jones, and in another all the terms we think cannot be applied to Dr. Jones. What kind of ethicist is Dr. Jones? What normative theory does he hold? What is his metaethical stance?

A number of answers can be given, but it is most important to emphasize that Dr. Jones is not a relativist. He is some kind of situationalist, at least as we have defined this term. He is not a deontologist in the sense of strict deontology; at least he is not a deontologist relative to this case—he does not think that helping people kill themselves is necessarily wrong. But he does make ethical judgments. And that makes him some sort of metaethical absolutist. We do not know whether he bases his judgments on the word of God (e.g., God told him in a dream that the Inuit were right and Joe was wrong), though this is unlikely, or whether he is an intuitionist—quite possible—or whether he has based his conclusions on his understanding of reality (this may be the most likely). But he is not and cannot be a relativist. Had a relativist been told the same two stories, she would have to have answered only that the Inuit thought they were right, and that the police who arrested Joe and the jury who convicted him and the media who wrote about him thought that Joe was wrong. Perhaps even Joe himself later repented of his crime. What the (radical) ethical relativist cannot say is that what Joe did was wrong. Relativists, if they are to be consistent to their theory, can only do descriptive ethics; they cannot prescribe (judge) what is right and what is wrong.

Having finished our discussion of the methodology of bioethics in the terms used by secular philosophers, we now turn to Catholic moral theology and medical ethics. Here the theory is more immediately practical; as part of this next section, we discuss a number of medical ethical issues and show how traditional Catholic medical ethics answered (and still answers) them.

Notes

1. We have been considering here only the most radical or "reductionist" kind of noncognitivism or emotivism. There are more moderate forms as well. One of these, often called "coherentism," argues that ethical judgments of right and wrong are posited by moral agents or rational persons thinking reasonably. They think reasonably by achieving "coherence." To the degree that the process of achieving coherence does indeed assume that the reasonable thinkers are able to know what human individual reality and human social reality are, the process of achieving coherence can be seen as consistent with natural law theory. But those who espouse coherentism often reject any correspondence theory of truth; they reject even moderate forms of realism. They are skeptical of our capacity to understand reality. This metaethical form of coherentism is not, it would seem, based on reality, but rather is based only on the thinking (and possibly the feeling) processes of the moral agent. Thus, we could call this metaethical theory "rational positivism." Ethical judgments are posited by rational persons. Beauchamp and Childress, who also reject this approach, call it "bare coherence" (Beauchamp and Childress 2001, 400) and propose instead a "common morality" theory (401–8). "Certain normative views are wrong not merely because they are incoherent. . . . They are wrong because there is no way, when starting from 'considered moral judgments' in the common morality, that one could . . . wind up with anything like" this kind of clearly wrong belief (Beauchamp and Childress 2009, 385). For a development of these issues in the context of bioethics, see Veatch 2003, Turner 2003, DeGrazia 2003, Brand-Ballard 2003, Beauchamp 2003, and Gordon 2011. In their discussions of coherence and common morality, none of these theorists claim to base their ethic on human teleology or on patterns discoverable in reality; none even mention natural law metaethics.

2. What is meant here by "descriptive" differs from what some philosophers mean by "descriptivism" (see Brand-Ballard 2003, 232–33).

CHAPTER 10

METHOD IN CATHOLIC MEDICAL ETHICS

THIS CHAPTER AND THE TWO THAT FOLLOW examine method in Catholic medical ethics. Unlike chapters 6 through 9, however, chapters 10 through 12 include a great deal of application as well. The present chapter traces a brief history of the key methodological shifts in Catholic medical ethics. Chapter 11 considers contraception, perhaps the best example of what has been happening in the recent and ongoing discussion about how Catholics ought to do health care ethics. Chapter 12 introduces the important principle of double effect and applies that principle to a number of different medical ethics topics, thus presenting the received tradition (the "official teaching") of Catholic medical ethics on those issues.

Methodological Shifts

A number of methodological shifts have occurred in Catholic moral theology since the mid-twentieth century. Those that are of importance for medical ethics are described here.

Natural Law

The previous chapter, on metaethics, presented four kinds of metaethical absolutism: supernatural, intuitional, rational, and empirical. Roman Catholic moral theologians have traditionally been natural law moralists. We defined natural law as the theory that responds to the metaethical question by claiming that, yes, moral judgments can be verified. Human persons discover right and wrong through reason and life experience by examining, collectively and individually, the emergent patterns of creation as God creates them. This is a theological version of empirical metaethical absolutism. That is, ethical judgments do have meaning, and we can verify them, and we do this by looking at what is, by looking at the actual ethical reality.

Unfortunately, however, "natural law" had, and has, another meaning as well. (The word "unfortunately" implies a judgment that this other meaning is invalid; some scholars defend this other meaning.) This second meaning is on the normative level, not the metaethical level, and is more or less the same as "deontology" as we have defined that term. In this normative sense, natural law implies that there are acts according to nature and acts against nature. Natural law has a specific notion of what kind of nature human beings have. Certain acts are considered natural and others unnatural. Those judged to be unnatural are wrong because of some intrinsic quality in the acts themselves. They are "against nature" (*contra naturam*) and hence against the natural law. They are "intrinsically evil acts."

The history of how these judgments (that this or that act is intrinsically evil) came about is complex, and we need not examine this in any great depth. In the next chapter, we look at one issue, contraception, in detail because of its historical importance in the history of Catholic medical ethics and, indeed, in the early phases of secular American bioethics. But for the sake of the present discussion we can say that there was a tendency in traditional, pre-Vatican II (pre-1960s) Roman Catholic moral theology, especially in sexual and medical ethics, to emphasize the physical nature of each act and of each human power and faculty. For example, the purpose of the sex faculty was seen to be procreation. That was its primary, natural purpose. Anything done to oppose that natural purpose was seen as unnatural. Thus, contraception is called an "intrinsically evil act."

These two meanings of natural law, one metaethical, the other normative, each have their own historical development. The metaethical meaning comes from Aristotle, and from him to Thomas Aquinas, who defined natural law as "the participation of the eternal law of God in the rational creature" (Thomas Aquinas 1948, *ST* I-II q. 91, art. 2, and q. 94, art. 1). That is, for Thomas, we humans were to use our right reason to discover God's plan for us in God's creation of us. The other "natural/unnatural" normative meaning has its roots in Ulpian, a third-century Roman jurist. Ulpian, a pagan, defined the natural law as that law that is common to human beings and other animals (Curran 1970b, 8–13; 1970c, 105–10). He contrasted this with civil or human law, laws made by humans. For Ulpian, therefore, natural law was something instinctive, something static, something built into the physical nature of all animals, including people. There was nothing specifically rational about it. This approach to natural law is also present in Thomas Aquinas (Curran 1968, 116; 1970a, 76–79), primarily in the sections where he deals with specific moral questions, especially sexual issues.

These two strains of natural law are often called "natural law according to reason" (the Aristotelian metaethical strain) and "natural law according to nature" (the Ulpianist normative deontological strain). Natural law according to nature supposes a fixed, static human nature whose purposes are set into the physical reality of who we are. There is little room for the more human dimensions of our personhood.

Physicalism and Personalism

This second normative approach to natural law has been called "physicalism" (Curran 1968, 1970c). Physicalism is the approach that emphasizes the physical properties of actions and does not worry as much about the other aspects of human interactions, such as the psychological, spiritual, and social aspects (Kelly 1979, 244–47, 421–29). Each act is analyzed by itself according to its physical properties. If an act fits into one kind of category, it is right; if it fits into another, it is wrong. Physicalism is close to legalism as we have defined it. It is also close to strict deontology. The acts themselves, in their physical structure, are what count—at least primarily—in determining whether a behavior is right or wrong. Consequences, situations, and intentions are at most secondary.

In the 1960s, the time of Vatican II, Catholic moralists started questioning this approach. As a reaction against physicalism, they proposed an approach many called "personalism." Instead of focusing on the physical or biological properties of the act in question, they began emphasizing the personal and human dimensions of the act in its circumstances, including its consequences (Kelly 1979, 416–20). Thus, personalism is an emphasis on persons instead of on the physical acts themselves. Louis Janssens proposed that the norm is "the human person adequately considered in regard to self and in relation with others" (Janssens [1947] 1988, 13).

Proportionalism and Consequentialism

The name often given to this approach as a normative method is "proportionalism" (Hoose 1987). This term probably goes back to a 1967 article by Peter Knauer, who suggested the importance of proportionality, arguing that any evil caused by our actions must be counterbalanced by a proportionate reason (Knauer [1967] 1979). This shift from physicalism to personalism, or from traditional (deontological) method to proportionalism, is a shift from legalism to at least a moderate form of situationalism—though it is certainly not a radical situationalism because rules are still of great importance.

It is, moreover, a shift from strict deontology to a theory closer to consequentialism, and at least partly consequentialist. Proportionalist Catholic moralists usually insist that proportionalism is not the same as consequentialism or utilitarianism (Curran 1977; 1999, 69–71; Janssens 1972–73). But it is not clear that this is the case (Kelly 1979, 417–21, esp. 418n24). Whether it is the same as consequentialism depends on how one defines consequentialism and on how one views the influence of the intention of the agent on the rightness or wrongness of the action. Consequentialism considers only consequences. Clearly intention plays an essential role in Catholic moral theology. For Janssens, for example, it appears to be the major factor (Janssens 1972–73, 117; Selling 2002, 7). For Curran, it is one of the key reasons for rejecting consequentialism (Curran 1999, 70–71). It is certain that the intention of the agent is an essential operative factor, that it counts toward the determination of the moral quality of the action. How it counts, however, is not easily determined.

Here we suggest briefly how intentionality can be seen to play its essential role and still allow us to call proportionalism a special type of consequentialism (a type that a student suggested should be called "intrinsic consequentialism"). As we saw in chapter 8, Catholic moral theology cannot be utilitarian in the usual connotations of that term. It cannot look only to aggregates; it cannot ignore the demands of justice. But in the limited context of arriving at judgments of right and wrong, it seems that proportionalists do form their judgments consequentially.

The one exception is, perhaps, the intention of the agent. It is clear that if the role of intentionality in determining right and wrong is not used consequentially, then proportionalism cannot be said to be a type of consequentialism as we have defined it: "Consequentialism proposes that the rightness or wrongness of acts (and of behavior patterns and social structures) depends on the reasonably foreseeable consequences of the act, pattern, or system. Acts are right or wrong only according to their effects."[1]

But how is intentionality really used? Consider two kinds of cases. In the first, an agent does something that is generally considered morally wrong, but the agent's intention—what the agent seeks—is good, something right to intend. A man gives money to the Ku Klux Klan. He does so not because he wants to support racism and violence against blacks and other minorities but because he honestly believes that the KKK is an environmental organization trying to save an endangered species of African antelope called the Ku Klux. This makes him invincibly ignorant. But his action remains objectively wrong. The fact that he is ill-informed does not change the fact that it is wrong to give money to the Klan. What he has done remains wrong (question 2), but the voluntariness of his action has been modified by his ignorance (question 1). His culpability is reduced. He does not sin. In this case, intention applies not to the determination of right and wrong but to the determination of personal blameworthiness. In this case, there is therefore no reason to claim that the use of intention means that proportionalism cannot be consequentialist. This is because proportionalism/intrinsic consequentialism, as a method, works only in the context of question 2 of normative ethics, the question of how to determine right and wrong. It is not appropriate in the context of questions 1 and 3. It does not apply to virtues, character, sin, conscience, or conversion; it is not a way to discover values. This means that consequentialism and deontology are not really "models," as Charles Curran calls them (Curran 1999, 60–73), since that term implies more than what these methods are: ways to determine right and wrong.

The reverse case is much harder to judge. Now a woman performs an action that is usually and properly considered morally right, but she does so with an evil intention. She becomes an usher in her parish church and her intention is to steal from the Sunday offerings. She goes to medical school to become a physician with the intention of refusing treatment to homosexuals. Here the traditional answer to the role of intention is that intention changes the moral quality of the action from right to wrong. And this is indeed a perfectly valid way to look at it. And if we look at it this way, we must conclude that proportionalism is not and ought not to be a species of consequentialism.

But there is a technically better way of looking at this type of case. What we have in cases of this type are two actions, one accomplished (she does become an usher; she does go to medical school) and the other either accomplished (she does steal; she does refuse treatment to gays) or intended but not accomplished (she never gets the chance to be alone with the money; she fails medical school). These two actions are connected, but it seems plausible to claim that they are not connected as two aspects of the same act. They are separable for purposes of determining their rightness or wrongness. It is right to be an usher and wrong to steal; right to become a physician and wrong to refuse to treat gays. And it is wrong to choose to try to steal or to choose to try to reject gays, even if the agent never gets to do this. These choices, these actions of will, have consequences, and they can be properly judged as wrong on the basis of those consequences. That is what is meant by "intrinsic consequentialism." These choices, these actions that may never be accomplished, may never have effects. Immediately, the effects are on the agent. She supports her greed; she strengthens her bigotry. But it is easily foreseeable that these actions will affect others as well and will have bad consequences on others. Unless the usher converts, she is now more likely to steal when she gets the chance. If she becomes a paramedic, she is now more likely to refuse to treat homosexuals than she was before she made the homophobic choice. It is not only accomplished acts that have consequences, though these are easier to see. Interior choices change the chooser, strengthening virtues and deepening vices. As John le Carré puts it in *The Secret Pilgrim:* "Please don't ever imagine that you'll be unscathed by the methods you use. The end may be used to justify the means—if it wasn't supposed to, I dare say you wouldn't be here. But there's a price to pay, and the price does tend to be oneself."

This way of looking at intention is consistent with the Catholic tradition of virtue and character ethics. And it allows us to say that, within the admittedly narrow context of question 2 of normative ethical theory—in the context of determining whether an action is right or wrong—proportionalism is indeed an "intrinsic" consequentialism.

A student of Dr. Kelly's wrote a course paper in which he, like his professor, criticizes various forms of deontology and finds utilitarianism inadequate if it is seen as relying merely on external, supposedly quantifiable consequences. There has to be something intrinsic that guides us in the way we evaluate the consequences. He puts it this way: "Teleological methods are unable to provide justification for consequences apart from an appeal to some principled end" (Henderson 2003, 35). That seems to be right. And the principled end is best described in Janssens's terms as "the human person adequately considered" (Janssens [1947] 1988, 13). Hence, *intrinsic* consequentialism.

Stages in Catholic Medical Ethics

For purposes of showing the change in method in Catholic medical ethics, which is our present task, we can divide the history of Catholic moral theology into three periods. It will be immediately apparent that these periods are inexact and unbalanced—the first is far longer than either of the others, but for our purposes this division will be helpful.

The first period, the "traditional" period, runs from about 1100 up to the beginning of the 1960s, the start of the Second Vatican Council. The second, the "transitional" stage, goes from approximately 1960 to 1970, a period of ten years or so. The third, the "contemporary" period, starts in the early 1970s and continues into the present.

The development of Catholic moral theology has, of course, a very long history, which we cannot investigate in detail here. But as a systematized discipline, it began in conjunction with the development of canon law and scholastic theology and philosophy in the twelfth century, or thereabouts. Its roots go back before that, and the early fathers of the church, as well as the scriptures, have much exhortation to give regarding the activity that befits a Christian. Nonetheless, the systematic development of the discipline began in the twelfth century when Alain de Lille first made the distinction between dogmatic and moral theology. Some think that this was a major mistake, and since the Second Vatican Council, moral theologians have been united in calling for a reconnection of moral with speculative or dogmatic theology, especially with spirituality. In any case, the twelfth century saw the beginning of what we will call the "traditional" approach to moral theology. Note, of course, that the word "traditional" is fraught with danger. Today's "revisionist-proportionalist" school is also part of the "tradition" in that it, too, is handed on or transmitted for future peoples. And the tradition of Catholic moral theology has been far from monolithic; major changes and clear contradictions have all emerged within the "tradition." But the word is useful here to designate Catholic moral theology as it has been received from earlier centuries. It is helpful in describing these three stages or periods to go back once again to the basic distinction between normative ethics and metaethics, drawing on what we have just seen about the natural law and its two meanings.

Metaethics

On the metaethical level, all three periods are, at least in theory, the same. All claim to follow a natural law metaethics. The traditional approach to moral theology was to discover in "nature," that is, to discover in creation through the use of reason, certain principles or rules or norms for moral living. From these rules or norms, applications were made to specific actions. In the transitional period and in the contemporary period, precisely the same thing is happening. Catholic moralists still claim that we discover, with our reason, who the human person is as God creates us to be. From this reflection, certain norms or principles or rules are discovered, and these are applied to specific actions. Metaethically, at least in theory, nothing important has been changed.

It is important to start by reiterating that we are where we were, even though it seems we have said nothing. The shift that took place in Catholic moral theology and medical ethics around the time of Vatican II is not in any sense a rejection of the idea that we, as God's creatures, are supposed to find out what God wills for us. This shift, important as it is, is not an acceptance of relativism or of "Godless humanism." Catholic medical ethicists are united in our insistence that God's will is to be taken seriously and that there are indeed objective moral norms. Catholic medical ethics proceeds by taking seriously the idea that the God who redeems us is the same God who created (and creates) us and who reveals the Divine Self and the divine law in who we are. Catholic medical ethics thus remains faithful to a natural law metaethics. Admittedly, natural law metaethics has not always been as clear in practice as it has been in theory. Later in this chapter, we note that in practice Catholic medical ethics has sometimes given precedence to the decisions of the magisterium, thus tending toward an ecclesiastical positivism that stands in some tension with a natural law metaethics. Thus, on the metaethical level, at least in theory, all three stages of Catholic medical ethics have adhered to a natural law metaethics, to a form of empirical metaethical absolutism.

Normative Ethics

It is on the normative level that the changes have taken place since the 1960s and the Second Vatican Council. During the 1960s, which we have labeled the transitional stage, the shift occurred from physicalism to personalism. Whereas the traditional period tended to analyze medical (and sexual) issues in a physicalist way, a number of moral theologians in the 1960s began to question and to reject this approach. In the transitional and in the contemporary stages, personalism has come to replace physicalism, or at least to contend with it, as the general normative method of Catholic medical ethics.

To restate this in terms of what we have seen of the two meanings of the natural law, we can say that while on the metaethical level "natural law according to reason" was kept and, indeed, reclaimed by transitional and contemporary medical ethicists, on the normative level "natural law according to nature" was questioned and ultimately rejected. That is, the criteria used to determine what is human nature, and thus what is according to the natural law, shifted from an emphasis on the physical and biological aspects of actions to an emphasis on the human person adequately considered.

Traditional Stage

When the traditional moralist—there are still those who support this approach, of course, but for ease of reading we will use the past tense here—looked at human nature with his reason, enlightened by the revelation of God found in scripture and in the teaching of the church, but not limited to those modalities of revelation, he emphasized the biological or physical nature of the act in question. He (virtually all were men, and virtually all were priests) asked basically what was the purpose of the act (*finis operis*) in the strictest and most restrictive sense of the term. Of course there were issues in which the traditional moralist granted far greater latitude. But in most of the areas that we have come to think of as pertaining to medical (and sexual) ethics, the traditional moralist asked what was the purpose of the act biologically and/or physically.

The question of contraception, which we examine in greater detail in the next chapter, was the specific issue around which the methodological debate coalesced, and we use it as an example here. For the traditional moralist, the purpose of human sexuality was seen as identical to the purpose of the physical transfer of semen from man to woman, that is, procreation. Thus, any sexual actions that were not directly intended to be procreative were considered immoral. Originally, especially in the thought of Augustine, it was immoral to have sex for pleasure or for love, even if one did not actually oppose procreation by a positive act. Thus, intercourse during pregnancy, after menopause, and so on, were included as gravely wrong acts. Later, and especially with Pius XII's permission for the use of the rhythm method of family planning, it was deemed permissible to have sex for "secondary ends" such as the expression of love or the "allaying of concupiscence," as long as nothing "artificial" was done to hinder the biological purpose of the action. Thus, artificial contraception was considered gravely wrong, an objectively grave matter, and a mortal sin for those who did it knowingly and willingly.

Transitional Stage

When the transitional moralist (from the time of Vatican II through the end of the 1960s) looked at human nature with reason, also enlightened by scripture and church tradition, he began to emphasize the personal or human dimensions of acts in their circumstances. He asked basically what was the human meaning and what were the human, social, spiritual, physical, and psychological consequences of the act or behavior pattern in question. Yet he generally came to the same conclusions as the traditional moralist.

One of the best examples of this can be found in the work of Louis Janssens, professor of moral theology at the University of Louvain in Belgium and one of the most important moral theologians around the time of the Second Vatican Council. His analysis of contraception was arguably the beginning of the birth control controversy (Noonan 1967, 549–54, 559–61; Janssens 1963; Swift 1966). When Janssens looked at this issue, he came generally to the same conclusions (at first) as his predecessors, the traditional moralists. With the important exception of the anovulant pill, which he considered allowable because it duplicated the natural process of the woman's body, Janssens considered artificial birth control to be gravely wrong. This is what he taught his students in the early 1960s (Janssens 1963–64, 65–69).

Janssens's reasons, however, were quite different from those of the traditional moralists. For him, it was no longer a question of respecting the biological end of the act (*finis operis*, as traditionally understood).[2] Rather, the key consideration was that the use of other means, such as condoms, diaphragms, spermicidal agents, and so on, hindered the personal meaning of human sexuality. For Janssens, the purpose of sexuality in humans was not primarily physical procreation. Rather, the purpose of sexual intercourse was to be a symbol of unreserved, unrestricted self-giving in marriage. It was because Janssens thought that the use of contraceptive devices disrupted the personal dimensions of the marriage act that he judged contraception to be forbidden (Janssens 1963). In the early and mid-1960s, other moralists said the same thing (Curran 1964; Swift 1966, 42–45). The reasoning process had changed, but the conclusion (except with respect to the pill, which was new) was the same.

Contemporary Stage

When the contemporary moralist (from the 1970s on) looks at human nature with reason, enlightened by the scriptures and the wisdom of tradition, he or she supports the personalist approach, emphasizing the personal or human dimensions of the act in its circumstances. Continuing the shift that began in the 1960s, the contemporary moralist asks what are the human, social, spiritual, physical, and psychological consequences of the act or behavior pattern in question. Unlike transitional moralists, however, contemporary (revisionist, personalist, or proportionalist) moralists tend to allow their reasoning process to follow through into their conclusions. Or, to be more exact, revisionist moral theologians are apt to find that when they examine the personal dimensions of human nature and of human behavior, the conclusions they come to are not the same as those arrived at by the traditional or transitional moralists.

Thus, when contemporary proportionalist moralists examine the question of contraception, they will be likely to conclude that it is not valid to make an absolute moral rule against such a practice because often the human and personal growth—the holiness if you will—of the people involved demands or at least permits the use of contraceptives. Janssens himself has extended his original judgment on the pill to include other methods of contraception. Indeed, he started doing this as early as 1966 (Janssens 1966). He no longer sees these methods as contrary to the human meaning of sexuality. It seems that his original judgment that condoms and other barrier methods violated the human personal symbolism of human sexuality was itself too physicalist. Married couples often testify that these barrier methods are more human for them, better than abstinence, rhythm, or the pill, enabling them to express their love for one another in an important and sacramental way. And many of the moralists who rejected Janssens's approval of the pill argued that this would open the way to approval of other contraceptive methods as well (Swift 1966, 42–45). The basic point here is that once the method shifted from physicalism to personalism, many traditional conclusions, which had been derived from physicalist premises, came to be questioned and even rejected by the revisionists from their personalist approach of deciding about right and wrong based on the human person adequately considered (Janssens's phrase). What we have seen about the three stages in the development of Catholic medical ethics is summarized in table 10.1.

Why the Delay in Changing Conclusions?

We have one more methodological question to ask. We have seen that transitional moralists reached the same conclusions as traditional moralists, even though they used different methods and reasoning processes. Then we noted that contemporary moralists reach different conclusions, even though they use the same reasoning processes as the transitional moralists. Why? It seems there are four reasons for this. The first is the most complex; the others are simple.

Respect for and Submission to Church Authority

Transitional moralists tended more to ecclesiastical positivism than contemporary moralists do. In other words, they gave a greater emphasis to the force of Church tradition as that tradition is handed down by the magisterium. In this approach certain moral conclusions are considered to be true essentially because the Catholic Church, representing God, declares them to be true. The decade of the 1960s followed the papacy of Pius XII, who was very much interested in medical ethics and who spoke and wrote often on medical issues. We have noted, and will note again in the next chapter, that it was he who changed what had been the traditional ("official") teaching on the rhythm method (periodic abstinence), explicitly permitting what once had been clearly forbidden. So it was natural that the Catholic moralists of that time would be hesitant to

Table 10.1: Stages in the Development of Catholic Medical Ethics

	Traditional Stage 1100–1960	Transitional Stage 1960–1970	Contemporary Stage 1970–present
Metaethical Approach	Natural Law (& Eccles. Pos.)	Natural Law (& Eccles. Pos.)	Natural Law
Normative Approach	Physicalism	Personalism	Personalism
Conclusions	Traditional	Unchanged	Changed

draw new practical conclusions in medical ethics. They would have seen changes of theory and method as less directly opposed to papal teaching.

Now there are very difficult theological problems in this issue. There is no doubt at all but that God's will must certainly be obeyed. No Christian, indeed no theist—no one who believes in an active God—could hold differently. The problem is not in obeying or disobeying God's will. Rather, the theoretical problem—as we saw our discussion of supernatural metaethical absolutism and then again in our discussion of natural law—is how we find out what God's will is.[3] Supernatural metaethical absolutists tend to limit the expression of God's will to one or two specific sources. They read the scriptures, perhaps in a fundamentalist or literal manner, for example, and see there the specific answers to moral questions. This is a kind of biblical positivism. Or they look to specific members of a church hierarchy for the same answers. This is ecclesiastical positivism. Catholic natural law moral theologians, on the other hand, claim that what God wills can be discovered by examination of God's creation, including the scriptures and the Church and revelation in all its modalities.[4] The nuances of how the teaching of the magisterium fits into a natural law metaethics will not be examined here (Kelly 1979, 311–20, 429–36). We will say only that a natural law metaethics does not admit that there are judgments concerning actual material norms that are in principle available only to members of one religion or to the leaders of one religion. To admit this is to deny the basic idea of a *natural* law, that it is possible to discover right and wrong using reason (and life experience) to examine God's creation. There may be some exceptions to this in areas dealing with specific religious practice. If one accepts Jesus Christ as God and Savior, for example, it becomes morally obligatory to worship Him. This norm is, in principle, not available to members of other religions. But this kind of norm has never really been said to belong to the natural law. Thus, the first reason for the delay in changing conclusions was a respect for Church authority as a source of moral knowledge, even perhaps a touch of ecclesiastical positivism.

Fear

Fear is easier to understand, though we might wish it were not a factor. Most Catholic moral theologians of the 1960s worked in Catholic seminaries, and most were priests. They feared that they might lose their jobs and even their priesthood if they were too forthright in saying what they thought. This fear continues even today, but there has been a declericalization of Catholic moralists and medical ethicists, and many now teach in universities, not all of them Catholic. In any case, it seems that gradually medical ethicists spoke their minds despite worries about losing jobs.

Clerical Arrogance

Clerical arrogance is also easy to understand, though surely not defensible. This is the idea that only the elite (clerics with deep knowledge and proper discipline) can "handle the truth." Others might go amok without the old rules to guide them. It is not clear how much if any of this was present, but, at least tacitly, it is likely that there was some.

Humility

There was an understandable and quite valid sense that the wisdom of the past ought not to be jettisoned. Specifically, there was a sense that even if the (physicalist) reasoning process for arriving at traditional conclusions was inadequate, and even misleading, there was still the possibility that the conclusions were of value and quite possibly right. This is always a great difficulty in times of change. For example, even though the physicalist method had arrived at the conclusion that contraception is always wrong is to be rejected, it is quite possible that contraception is wrong for another reason. Janssens thought this way for a time. Today, official church teaching often claims that contraception is wrong because it separates the unitive aspect of sexuality (as promoting love between spouses) from the procreative aspect. We will see in the next chapter why this reason, though valid in itself, cannot lead to the conclusion that pills and condoms are wrong while natural family planning is right. It is certainly possible, however, that there is some reason other than physicalism why the traditional conclusions in medical ethics might be the correct ones. Humility requires that we not move too quickly into proposing new judgments in matters as important as ethics.

Conclusion

This chapter describes the shift in Catholic medical (and sexual) ethics from physicalism to personalism, from deontology to proportionalism/intrinsic consequentialism, from natural law according to nature to natural law according to reason. This methodological revision has not, of course, been accepted by all Catholic scholars.[5] Many remain convinced by the older approaches and the conclusions reached through them. This becomes apparent as we move to more directly practical issues in studying the method of Catholic medical ethics. Controversy continues concerning method and its application.

Notes

1. See chapter 8.
2. Janssens himself actually wanted that term to mean the intended end rightly chosen by the agent (Selling 2002, 7).
3. Jack Mahoney puts it this way: "Where do these moral values come from? . . . One reply is that we respect them because God, through the Bible and the Church, so commands. Another reply that represents a strong philosophical current within the Catholic tradition of Christian reflection is because it is a properly human way to behave. If one reflects on what it is to be human, one can conclude that the importance of . . . moral values arises simply from human nature as created so by God" (Mahoney 2003, 720).
4. For an inquiry into the relationship of supernatural and natural influences on magisterial teaching, see O'Meara 2003.
5. Opponents of proportionalism, who defend the idea of intrinsically evil acts, often point to the 1993 encyclical letter of Pope John Paul II, *Veritatis spendor* (*The Spendor of Truth*). In it the pope rejects proportionalism. Whether the proportionalism he rejected is what its proponents actually claim has been debated (Ashley and O'Rourke 1997, 159–64; Ashley, deBlois, and O'Rourke 2006, 16).

CHAPTER 11

CATHOLIC METHOD AND BIRTH CONTROL

THIS CHAPTER ON CONTRACEPTION is included here in the section on method in Catholic medical ethics because the birth control debate was the issue around which the shift in method that we described in the last chapter took place, and because "the key to unlocking this seemingly intractable controversy is actually a question of *method* in moral theology" (Selling 2012, 149, emphasis his). Birth control was the center of the controversy, the issue that led to the questioning of physicalism and the shift to personalism and proportionalism. Richard McCormick, one of the most influential Catholic moral theologians of the second half of the twentieth century, said of the contraception question that he could think of "no moral issue or event in this century that has impacted so profoundly on the discipline of moral theology" (McCormick 1994, 11).

Historical Development of the Catholic Position on Contraception

The present official Catholic position on contraception is that nothing may be done to keep any individual (voluntary) act of sexual intercourse from attaining its possible goal of conceiving a child. That conclusion, in itself, has been held consistently throughout the centuries of Catholic moral theology. When it was first declared, however, it was coupled with other conclusions as well. It was equally wrong for a married couple to have sex after menopause or during pregnancy. And what we now know as natural family planning (NFP)—the deliberate limitation of conjugal intercourse to the wife's infertile period—was also said to be seriously wrong. Thus, while in one sense the official position has been consistent, in another more important sense it has been radically altered because the reasons for the condemnation of contraception have totally changed. Today's official teaching on contraception is a conclusion in search of a reason. That was not the case in the beginning. Reviewing the important events in the development of the church's position on contraception sheds considerable light on how the official Catholic position became what it now is.

Augustine

Augustine (AD 354–430) condemned all forms of contraception and birth control, including what we now call rhythm, periodic continence, or natural family planning (Augustine 1901, 65; Noonan 1967, 152). For Augustine, it was gravely wrong (a mortal sin) if married people had sex when they knew they could not have a child. Thus, sexual intercourse was forbidden during pregnancy and after menopause (Augustine 1998, sec. 3, ch. 21, sub. 43). For Augustine, sexual intercourse is permitted to married couples only when they specifically intend to have children. Even if they are capable of conceiving a child and do not actually do anything to prevent conception, conjugal intercourse is at least slightly wrong (a venial or pardonable sin) unless married people have sex for the specific motive of conceiving a child. Sex for any other reason, even if the act in fact turns out to be fertile, is a venial or slight sin (Augustine 1887c, 1:17).

There is some controversy about his reason for this, but in much of what Augustine wrote it is clear that he considered sexual pleasure, or at least male orgasm, to be the result of original sin (Kelly 1983, 101–8). He writes that before their sin, Adam and Eve would not have had sex with the kind of pleasure we experience (Augustine 1887d, 40). It would have been calmer (he compares it to urination and to menstrual flow), easily following the mandate of their wills (Augustine 1887c, 1:6, 2:20, 2:53; 1903, 16–18, 23–26). Augustine rejected any notion that sexual intercourse might itself be a help for the spiritual love of married people (Noonan 1967, 159). For him, the conjugal embrace "is by reason of this body of death . . . impracticable without a certain amount of bestial motion which makes human nature blush" (Augustine 1887d, 43). He speaks of the "union of the sexes, which cannot even accomplish its own honourable function [procreation] without the incident of shameful lust" (Augustine 1887c, 2, 15). For Augustine, sexual intercourse in a Christian marriage for the explicit purpose of procreating Christian children is not a sin, but even here there is a "good use of an evil thing" (Augustine 1887d, 1, 57). Augustine does claim that marriage is good, and he speaks of the three "goods" of marriage: the good of offspring, the good of fidelity, and the good of the sacrament. But only the first of these is for him a positive good. The others are negative, at least when it comes to sex. The good of fidelity means there is no adultery; weak people who cannot stay virgins at least limit sexual intercourse to the married state. And the good of the sacrament, or bond, means there is no divorce. The only role sexual intercourse plays in these latter two goods is that it keeps the married couple from greater evils like adultery and divorce. It "allays concupiscence," as later Catholic authors put it (Davis 1946, III, 247).

This position (that sexual pleasure is somehow in itself evil) is no longer held in the teaching of the magisterium (the pope and the bishops, hence "official Catholic teaching"). Recent popes and bishops have spoken of sexual pleasure very differently, as a good willed by God in creating us that we might love one another more closely in marriage and be drawn to procreate the species. It is from this newer, and far better, theological anthropology that the magisterium now speaks about the unitive purpose as well as the procreative purpose of marriage and of sexual intercourse. But Augustine's position has been of great influence in determining later church teaching on sexuality and specifically on contraception (Noonan 1967, 174–75). Today, when Augustine's theological reasons for insisting that procreation be the only motivation for conjugal intercourse have been in effect rejected by magisterial teaching, his conclusion about contraception is still maintained. This leaves a conclusion in search of a reason.

Thomas Aquinas

Thomas (1225–74) accepted Augustine's position. Even though he did not himself emphasize sexual pleasure as evil to the degree that Augustine did, he supported the practical conclusions Augustine set down. When married couples had sex, it was a venial sin unless their explicit motive was procreation (Noonan 1967, 303). There was some debate during the medieval period about whether intercourse during pregnancy was a mortal sin, as Augustine had held, or a venial sin (because procreation could not be the motive), or a sin only if there was danger to the fetus—Thomas seems to have held this last position (ibid., 342–43). But he continued to hold that sex during menstruation was mortally sinful (ibid., 340). And of course any use of contraception was seriously wrong (ibid., 285, 300). Thus, for much of Catholic history, sex when procreation was not possible was forbidden (as gravely wrong by some and as slightly wrong by others), and sex for "secondary purposes" (love, sexual release) was considered slightly wrong (a venial sin) even if procreation was possible. And there was no change in Augustine's teaching that engaging in sex during the woman's infertile period for the deliberate purpose of avoiding children was seriously wrong.

Nineteenth-Century Opening toward Natural Family Planning

The first hesitant change in this traditional official position came in the nineteenth century when Louvain theologian Auguste Lecomte wrote a book proposing that the newly discovered ovulatory cycle might be used by couples wishing to avoid pregnancy (Noonan 1967, 523–24). Here was a deliberate use of sexual intercourse in such a way that procreation could be avoided. This was precisely what the official tradition had until then rejected as seriously wrong. But Lecomte had the backing of some European bishops. A debate ensued, and in 1880 the Vatican Penitentiary, speaking officially, responded to a question submitted to Rome asking what to do about married couples who deliberately limited intercourse to the times of the woman's cycle when she was known (or hoped) to be infertile. The Vatican answered: "Spouses using the aforesaid way of marriage are not to be disturbed, and a confessor may, though cautiously, insinuate the opinion in question to those spouses whom he has vainly tried with other reasons to lead from the detestable crime of onanism [withdrawal]" (Noonan 1967, 525).

Now this rather oracular response can mean either of two things. It can mean that such behavior is wrong, but since some of the people who do it are ignorant of its wrongness (invincible ignorance), they do not sin. Since they will go on doing it anyway, or, worse, use withdrawal instead, it is better not to turn a materially wrong act into a formally blameworthy sin. So leave them alone. Or it can mean that "rhythm" is indeed not wrong, which would be a clear change in the received tradition. This was one of the first indications that the older position might be changing.

On Christian Marriage *by Pope Pius XI*

In 1930 Pope Pius XI wrote an encyclical letter titled *On Christian Marriage* (*Casti connubii*) to the whole church. In it he speaks of the practice of having sex during infertile times. He says that such actions are not "against nature" (Pius XI 1939, 93–94). This is, of course, a direct contradiction of Augustine's teaching, which condemned such actions as mortal sins. But it is not clear that Pius XI meant to include persons who deliberately *limit* their sexual activity to those infertile times. In other words, though Pius XI clearly permitted conjugal intercourse after menopause, during pregnancy, for infertile persons, and during times of periodic infertility, he may or may not have meant to include the deliberate avoidance of fertile times, that is, rhythm or periodic abstinence (ibid.). In the same encyclical, he insisted on what has become over the centuries the central teaching about conjugal intercourse: "For in matrimony as well as in the use of the matrimonial rights [sex] there are also secondary ends, such as mutual love, and the quieting of concupiscence which husband and wife are not forbidden to consider so long as they are subordinated to the primary end and so long as the intrinsic nature of the act is preserved" (ibid., 93–94). Forgotten, rejected really, is Augustine's insistence that the only proper motive for sex is procreation. Now other motives, the so-called secondary ends, are acceptable, provided they are properly subordinated to procreation and provided nothing is done to the act-in-itself that thwarts its physical purpose of begetting a child.

And one of these secondary ends is now called "mutual love." We have seen that for Augustine sex did not enhance love; it merely kept the married couple from sinning outside the marriage. So this is a significant change for the better in theological anthropology, in how we ought to understand the human person. But this change leads to inevitable questions about why contraception is wrong. For Augustine, it was easy: sex is tainted and has to be avoided except when married couples want children, since there is no other way to conceive a child. Thus, to have sex and not want to have a child is wrong. But now for Pius XI, and for all the popes since him, conjugal intercourse is seen as good, as a way to increase love as well as to propagate the species. *Now* why is contraception wrong? The reason is not as clear as it used to be.

Pope Pius XII

When Pius XI stated, in *On Christian Marriage*, that it was permitted to married couples to have sex even when they knew they could not conceive, he suggested the possibility that the deliberate limitation of intercourse to infertile periods might also be right, but this was not clear. Pius XII ended the confusion on October 29, 1951, in his speech to a group of Italian midwives and in another talk a month later that added some further clarifying remarks by explicitly permitting the deliberate limitation of conjugal intercourse to infertile periods as long as there was a serious reason for postponing or avoiding children (McFadden 1955, 128). He included medical, economic, genetic, and other reasons as ones that would permit a couple to practice the rhythm method. This was permitted not only for a time but even for the entire length of a marriage so long as the reasons for doing this were serious ones. What had been absolutely condemned was now explicitly permitted.

Other means of preventing pregnancy were still forbidden, however. These were considered artificial contraception and were forbidden because they prevented individual acts of intercourse from achieving their procreative goal. The rhythm method, or natural family planning, was permitted because it did not attack the act in itself. The purpose for using rhythm might be exactly the same as the purpose for using condoms: a desire, for a good reason, not to have children. The difference could now be found only in the structure of the act itself. Clearly repudiated here are all of Augustine's original reasons for condemning birth control. What is left is the physicalist notion that each sex act must be allowed to achieve its primary (physical) purpose, the conception of a child.

Moralists during this period had also arrived at a change in another conclusion of the received official teaching. No longer would sex in marriage motivated by the desire for pleasure be considered wrong at all, not even slightly or venially wrong, as had been held from the time of Augustine through the Middle Ages, with some suggestion of change beginning in the fifteenth century (Chauvet 1977, 242). John Ford and Gerald Kelly wrote in 1963: "If sexual pleasure is to serve as an inducement to propagate, then God must want men to choose the act because of the pleasure, not the other way round. . . . The older authors seemed oblivious of this psychological aspect of the matter" (192–93).

The Birth Control Commission

In the 1960s, just before and during the Second Vatican Council, Pope John XXIII and then Pope Paul VI established a commission to look into the issue of the regulation of births, which had by then become an issue of some contention. The Pontifical Commission for the Study of Population, Family, and Births originally consisted largely of clerics, but later married people and physicians were included. When the bishops who gathered at the Second Vatican Council suggested that the council consider the topic, the pope told them that he was reserving this issue to himself (Noonan [1966] 1969, 3). The Pontifical Commission finally submitted its report to Pope Paul VI in 1966, recommending that the received tradition be changed. Contraception should not be considered an intrinsically evil act. If married couples had the kind of serious reasons that Pope Pius XII had said were enough to allow deliberate periodic abstinence, then these reasons ought to be enough to allow other methods as well (Pontifical Commission [1966] 1978, 305–7). The commission pointed explicitly to the decision of Pius XII, which had changed previous tradition: "The acceptance of a lawful application of the calculated sterile periods of the woman—that the application is legitimate presupposes right motives—makes a separation between the sexual act which is explicitly intended and its reproductive effect which is intentionally excluded" (ibid., 305). This is the exact opposite of what the tradition received from Augustine had insisted on: that the reproductive effect of marital sex must never be excluded. The commission noted that artificiality cannot of itself make something wrong. Thus, the commission concluded that other means of birth control than periodic continence cannot be a priori forbidden.

But this official report was not agreed to unanimously in the commission. Some members, together with theologians who supported the position of Pius XII that only periodic continence could be allowed, submitted their own second report, authored mainly by American moral theologians John Ford and Germain Grisez, to Pope Paul VI. This second, unofficial report became known as the "minority report"; as a result, the original official report of the Pontifical Commission became known as the "majority report," even though only one report, not two, had been officially submitted by the commission. The minority report gives a great deal of emphasis to the role of the magisterium, so much so that it appears to be perhaps the strongest reason proposed against changing the teaching ("Minority Papal Commission Report" [1967] 1969, 187-92, 109-11). This report also worries about how a change in this teaching might lead to changes in sexual morality of a wider nature (ibid., 203). It concludes that contraception, defined as "any physical intervention in the generative process which, before or after the proper placing of generative acts, causes these acts to be deprived of their natural power for the procreation of life by the industry of man," is always wrong (ibid., 174-75). Note again the emphasis on the physical structure of the act. Whereas for Augustine it was the intention of the married couple not to procreate that made all forms of birth control including periodic continence wrong, according to this minority report it is the intentional physical intervention in the act itself that is wrong.

On Human Life *by Pope Paul VI*

In the summer of 1968 Pope Paul VI issued an encyclical titled *On Human Life* (*Humanae vitae*). In this letter he concluded that the received tradition (received at least since Pius XII a decade and a half earlier) would stand. Any deliberate attempt to interfere in the act itself of sexual intercourse or to interfere in the reproductive faculty by direct sterilization was forbidden. (We discuss direct and indirect sterilization when we consider the principle of double effect in the next chapter.) *Humanae vitae* is written largely in language that upholds the beauty of sexuality and its importance in a loving marriage. In keeping with what the Second Vatican Council said about marriage and sex—the bishops explicitly refused to repeat the older formula (Vatican Council II 1966, 50)—there is no reference to procreation as the "primary end" and to other purposes of marital sex, such as fostering love or avoiding sexual sin ("allaying concupiscence") as "secondary ends." Pope Paul introduces in this encyclical the idea of "the inseparable connection, willed by God and unable to be broken by man on his own initiative, between the two meanings of the conjugal act: the unitive meaning and the procreative meaning" (Paul VI 1969, 220-21). In other words, the letter is largely "personalist" in the sense we have given this term. But the beauty of what Pope Paul says about marriage and sexuality has been largely overshadowed because of the importance given to his conclusion that "each and every marriage act must remain open to procreation" (ibid., 220). This seems to many moral theologians to be at least implicitly physicalist (McCormick [1989] 1993, 102-9). Each *act* of sexual intercourse must be open to procreation. Nothing can be done to hinder each *act* from being procreative. Both meanings of marriage and sexuality—the unitive and the procreative—have to be present in each *act*. This physicalist foundation for the condemnation of contraception has not been persuasive. Many Catholic moral theologians and priests, and almost certainly a majority of Catholic laypersons, have not been persuaded that contraception is always wrong.

A Conclusion in Search of a Reason

The current official Catholic position on contraception is hotly contested. It is impossible to find a consistent position. Augustine's position was consistent, but it was based on bad theology (that human sexual pleasure was the evil result of sin) and possibly on bad biology (that the male ejaculate contained a "homunculus" or "little man," and thus that unprocreative ejaculation was abortive). No Catholic theologian or bishop today supports either of these ideas. Nor are Augustine's conclusions about sex accepted any longer. Pope Pius XII and Pope Paul VI, among others, have explicitly taught the moral rightness of periodic abstinence, which Augustine said was seriously sinful.

Augustine's position was theologically and psychologically flawed, but at least it was consistent. The present teaching permits and indeed encourages periodic abstinence in the form of a natural family planning method that uses signals in the woman's body (primarily temperature and consistency of cervical mucus) to determine the exact time when ovulation occurs. This logically implies permission for a deliberately intended attempt to avoid procreation and still have intercourse. As John Noonan puts it in his exhaustive study of the history of the Catholic positions on contraception, "Use of the sterile period, once attacked by Augustine when used to avoid all procreation, approved in 1880 for cautious suggestion to onanists, guardedly popularized between 1930 and 1951, was now fully sanctioned. The substantial split between sexual intercourse and procreation, already achieved by the rejection of Augustinian theory, was confirmed in practice" (Noonan 1967, 532). Thus, when Paul VI enunciates the principle now most often used to defend the official position, that there is an "inseparable connection, willed by God and unable to be broken by man on his own initiative, between the two meanings of the conjugal act: the unitive meaning and the procreative meaning" (Paul VI 1969, 220–21), that reasoning stands contradicted by the very official position it claims to defend. Permission to limit sex to the sterile period has already officially broken the "inseparable connection."

The only difference between the permitted method and other forbidden methods, such as condoms, would have to be found in the act itself. Surely the couple's intention is the same in both procedures: to have sex and to avoid having children. Thus, *both* procedures would seem equally to "separate the unitive and the pro-creative aspects of married sexuality," which recent documents forbid and propose as the basis for the condemnation of direct contraception. Nor does it seem plausible that only direct contraception (condoms, the pill, and so on) and not natural family planning involves the couple in making a "contra-life intention," as some moralists who defend the position, such as Germain Grisez, propose (Grisez et al. 1998, 91–92; Grisez 1993, 511; 1964, 98). The reason for both kinds of birth control—natural family planning and contraceptive devices such as condoms and the pill—would be equally "contra-life" in the restricted sense of not wanting children from this act of intercourse; the contraceptor does something to prevent it and so does the natural family planner. And neither would necessarily be contra-life in the more formally wrong sense of opposing life, wanting death, being selfish, subscribing to a "contraceptive mentality," and so on. Despite Grisez's lengthy argument to the contrary (Grisez 1964, 155–67), the only difference between the permitted and the proscribed methods of birth regulation is found in the nature of the act in itself. And that is what is meant by "physicalism."

There are, of course, certain bad effects for some couples from the various methods of birth control. The pill can cause hormonal harm to the woman and may possibly at rare times be abortifacient, working to prevent implantation—though this is not clear after the first cycle on the pill, once the woman's ovulation has presumably stopped, and some scientists claim there is no evidence that hormonal contraception has any anti-implantational abortifacient effect at all (Hamel 2003).[1] But natural family planning may possibly itself be abortifacient if a couple misjudges the timing and an embryo is formed from an egg at the end of its life cycle (NFP tries to miss the fertile period, but a slight miscalculation could increase the likelihood of having sex just before the woman has entered a certainly infertile stage; embryos formed at this time are more likely to miscarry). In any case, condoms would seem not to be subject to any of these disadvantages.

Several advantages for couples have been proposed for natural family planning, including a more disciplined sexual life, greater anticipation, deeper communication, and so on. This may well be true for some couples. Others may find that the process of timing and the resulting lack of spontaneity hinder communication and hurt the human quality of this expression of love. And in the hectic lives of many married couples, periodic continence effectively practiced (intercourse has to be limited to less than two weeks out of each monthly cycle) may well reduce the frequency of conjugal sex to the point where both the procreative and the unitive dimensions of sexual inter-course are thwarted, the former deliberately and the latter inevitably. In any case, the possible advantages of NFP are insufficient to lead to the conclusion that all methods other than NFP are intrinsically evil acts and absolutely forbidden.

There is one other area of possible inconsistency in the teaching on contraception. We have seen that the intrinsically evil act of contraception seems to be "any physical intervention in the generative process which, before or after the proper placing of gener-ative acts, causes these acts to be deprived of their natural power for the procreation of life by the industry of man" (Minority Papal Commission Report [1967] 1969, 174–75). This seems precise enough. But there are at least two cases in which official permission has been given to deprive sexual acts of their power to procreate. It is widely known that Catholic nuns in situations in which rape is a very real risk are allowed to take the contraceptive pill. And official policy permits American Catholic hospitals to use birth control pills immediately after rape, as long as steps have been taken to make sure the victim is not already pregnant, presumably from some previous sexual encounter (USCCB 2009a, 18–19, dir. 36). This seems to mean that the "intrinsically evil act" of contraception is not just the stopping of a sex act from achieving its proper physical purpose but a more complex combination of two acts, one sexual and the other contra-ceptive. The sexual act must be consensual. The combination and complexity of this dual act is an unusual way to define an intrinsically evil act. Perhaps this is what the Minority Papal Commission Report meant when it included the phrase "proper placing," but that is not clear.

Germain Grisez defends the use of contraceptives in the case of threatened rape by arguing that the woman's intention is not "contra-life" but is rather a "defense against violence" (Grisez 1964, 216). And this is certainly true. But few if any persons make a "contra-life" intention when they use contraception. Just like those using NFP, they make a "pro-health" or "pro-educating the other children" or "pro-waiting till we get out of graduate school" or "pro-not having children with our genetic disease" intention. So the problem here is that Grisez thinks that couples who use contraception must make a contra-life intention whereas those who use NFP need not. This makes Grisez's notion of intention hard to comprehend. Why should the married woman who uses contraceptives fearing a serious medical crisis if she gets pregnant be accused of a contra-life intention, whereas the nun fearing rape may use contraceptives and not intend to be contra-life? Both do exactly the same thing in taking the pill. Both have exactly the same intention: they do not want to get pregnant. The sexual acts themselves are radically different, of course. The married woman makes love; the nun is violently attacked. The former action is morally noble; the latter (on the part of the rapist) is a heinous crime. But the intention of both women relative to the taking of the pill is the same: no baby. The very act that many authors claim is intrinsically evil is permitted in cases of rape and threatened rape. This adds even more confusion. The official Catholic teaching on contraception as it is now proposed by the magisterium is a conclusion in search of a reason.[2]

Notes

1. Even if there is a possible abortifacient effect in rare cases, the claim can be made that, according to traditional double effect reasoning, the abortion would be indirect. We will examine the principle of double effect in detail in the next chapter. Peter Cataldo argues this way in an article on what Catholic hospitals should do if state laws mandate worker insurance coverage for contraception (Cataldo 2004, 111–13). For Cataldo all contraception is wrong, but he claims that Catholic hospitals may materially cooperate with this by offering contraception in their workers' insurance policies if the alternative is closing the hospital or something similarly hurtful. In this context, he distances contraceptives from the abortion issue by arguing that any possible abortion caused by the anovulant pill would be indirect as long as the woman intended to stop ovulation and not to stop implantation. He likens this to the procedures permitted by official Catholic medical ethics, the kinds of indirect abortion we discuss in the next chapter. Cataldo lists a number of disagreeing sources on the likelihood that the anovulant pill might be anti-implantational and thus abortifacient (ibid., 111n9). On this, see also Yavarone 2004.

2. For a convincing refutation of the claim that the general moral method of Thomas Aquinas provides a nonphysicalist basis for the condemnation of contraception, see Selling 2012. Selling concludes his essay this way, and we agree: "Perhaps when the discussion shifts away from focusing on mere physical acts (in themselves) and moves in the direction of determining what might be a proportionate manner for reaching the admirable end of being responsible parents, we may begin to address the impasse that has plagued moral theology for over 40 years" (ibid., 150).

CHAPTER 12

THE PRINCIPLE OF DOUBLE EFFECT

T HE PRINCIPLE OF DOUBLE EFFECT (PDE) was the primary operational principle in pre–Vatican II Catholic medical ethics. The kinds of topics Catholic medical ethics dealt with from around the turn of the century to the 1960s were the ones doctors and nurses were actually meeting in their daily professional practice. Unlike the discipline of pastoral medicine, which had addressed a wider array of topics, Catholic medical ethics limited itself to the actual professional practice of medical personnel. That meant that most of the topics concerned physical interventions for physical ailments. For this kind of topic, the principle of double effect claimed to be able to give precise and definitive answers. The PDE is still widely used, not only in Catholic medical ethics but for some issues in secular bioethics as well. We see the primary example of this in the opening chapters of part III, when we discuss end-of-life issues. Even those who have serious problems with the PDE, as proportionalists do, may defend its use in certain issue areas. The PDE was the operative principle for applying physicalism to medical procedures. This becomes clear later in the chapter, when we see how the PDE was used.

Definition of the Principle of Double Effect

The principle of double effect is a principle that purports to answer the following question: Is it right to perform an action from which two or more effects result, some of which are good and may rightly be intended and some of which are bad and may not rightly be intended? In a sense, this is the basic question of normative ethics (at least of question 2, which deals with judging right and wrong). If an action produces only good for all involved, no one, whether deontologist or consequentialist, is likely to have any problem with it. And if an act produces only evil, again there is not likely to be any dispute. It is wrong to do it. Indeed, persons are unlikely to be tempted to such an action, since it produces nothing good for anyone. The actions that normative ethics discusses, actions where there is some controversy or disagreement, are those actions that do some good as well as some evil, acts with both good and bad effects. Whatever one's stand, say, on abortion, it is clear that this is a controverted action because it does, or at least is perceived as doing, both good and bad. It kills the fetus, but it saves the life (or the economic well-being, or the reputation) of the woman. Similarly, euthanasia does, or at least is perceived as doing, both good and bad. It stops pain, saves money, ends the dying process; but it kills, it hurts the doctor–patient relationship, it threatens the poor and the disabled. Not everyone would accept all of these goods or all of these ills as being in fact caused by the acts in question. But reasonable people do claim these effects, and that is what makes the actions morally controversial. The PDE, then, asks about acts that have both good and bad (evil) effects. The PDE has had a controverted history, but we need not concern ourselves with that (Kelly 1979, 244–74). We will discuss it only as it is currently used in official "traditional" Catholic medical ethics.

The Four Conditions of the Principle of Double Effect

The principle of double effect proposes that an action with both good and bad effects is right (licit, permissible) if and only if all four of the following conditions are met. The following order is the most helpful, but sometimes conditions 2 and 3 are reversed (Kelly 1979, 250–51n13): (1) The act in itself must not be morally wrong. (2) The bad effect must not cause the good effect. (3) The agent must not intend the bad effect (as an end to be sought). (4) The bad effect must not outweigh the good effect. We will discuss these conditions one at a time.

1. The Act in Itself Must Not Be Morally Wrong

The first condition is clearly deontological, and, in Catholic medical ethics, it was and often is interpreted in a physicalist manner. The act in itself must not be morally wrong. This condition is in fact sometimes stated as: "The act-in-itself, considered apart from its circumstances and consequences, must not be morally wrong." In one sense, this condition begs the question; it is a petitio principii. The PDE is asking whether an act with plural effects is right or wrong, and the first condition says: "If it's wrong, it's wrong!" From the perspective of a deontologist, however, in the definition we have been using for deontology, the first condition simply asks whether the act in itself is one of those acts determined to be absolutely wrong in and of itself. If it is, then one need go no further. The answer is clear; the action is wrong regardless of circumstances, situations, or consequences.

For example, suppose a married couple has been unable to conceive a child and they go to a fertility specialist. After taking their history, the physician will probably want a sperm sample to check on male-factor infertility. The usual way to acquire the sperm is to ask the man to masturbate. But masturbation is considered one of the "intrinsically evil acts" forbidden by traditional Catholic moral theology. It is an act outside of the marriage act and cannot of itself be procreative. So, even here in a context where the man's intention is to find out whether (and how) he can have children, this act remains evil in itself and is forbidden. The same applies, of course, to actions that many would find more objectionable: abortion, active euthanasia, artificial insemination by a third-party donor, and so on. Since the acts in themselves are wrong, nothing can justify them.

2. The Bad Effect Must Not Cause the Good Effect

The second condition requires that the causal chain from act to effects must not include a causal link where the bad effect causes the good effect. There are three possibilities: (a) the act might cause the good effect, which then in turn causes the bad effect—this passes the PDE's second condition; (b) the act might cause the good effect and the bad effect without either effect causing the other—this also passes the second condition; and (c) the act might cause the bad effect, which then in turn causes the good effect—this fails the second condition, and the act is thus considered wrong.

This second condition is in fact the equivalent of the first (Kelly 1979, 252–54). Whether the first or the second condition is said to apply depends in many cases on how the act in itself is specified. If it is specified in one way, the term used to name an act might indicate an action considered to be intrinsically evil. Then it would fail the first condition. On the other hand, the same act might be called something else. It would then pass the first condition but fail the second. Both conditions are intended to make sure that neither the end (the consequences) nor the intention might be used to justify the physically specified means (the act in itself) if that act is considered wrong in itself.

The same example we used for the first condition is helpful here. We have seen that a man may not masturbate to obtain sperm for sterility testing. But what if we decided not to call this masturbation? What if we called it "touching the genitals"? Now this seems silly, but Catholic sexual ethics in fact did this (and presumably still does, though seldom is this any longer spoken about) in the case of a young man who finds that his self-touching in the shower to get himself clean leads to sexual arousal and possibly even orgasm. Now the action is not called masturbation. And so it gets by the first condition. It also gets by the second, since the bad effect, the "pollution" or extramarital sexual pleasure, does not cause the good effect, the cleanliness. In the case of acquiring sperm, however, the bad effect, the "pollution" or the extramarital sexual pleasure, does cause the good effect. Hence, the second condition is violated and the act is judged wrong.

Over the years, of course, terms used to name actions came to be determined. But there is not always clarity about why one term rather than another is used. Nor is there always clarity about what exactly constitutes the act in itself. Is it masturbation (the touching and the pleasure), or is it just the touching, such that the pleasure is the effect and not part of the act itself? The first and second conditions of the PDE were developed in combination and used to cover various specifications of acts in themselves. Together they ensured that the end (the intended consequences) would not be used to justify the physically specified means (the act in itself).

Now no Catholic moralist has ever argued that the end justifies the means in the usual sense that this is given: that a good end justifies virtually any means, regardless of other consequences or of intentionality. Nor has any Catholic moralist ever held that a good end can justify an immoral, wrong means. Wrongs acts are never justifiable. What proportionalists do say, in rejecting deontology, is that one cannot know for sure that an act is wrong without examining it in its circumstances, including its effects and the intention of the agent.

3. The Agent Must Not Intend the Bad Effect (as an End to Be Sought)

The third condition is one that all Catholic moralists accept, proportionalists and deontologists alike. The agent must not intend the bad effect as an end to be sought. There is no need to go into detail here on the complex problem of intentionality. We spoke of it in the chapter on contraception and discuss it again in chapter 14 on the distinction between killing and allowing to die. It is better, however, to understand the third condition as meaning "intend as an end to be sought," as some Catholic medical ethicists interpret it (Kelly 1958, 14; McFadden 1961, 28–30), and not "intend either as a means or as an end," as others have put it (Finney and O'Brien 1956, 102; Healy 1956, 96). This is controverted, but if the third condition is interpreted as saying "The agent may not intend the bad effect either as an end or as a means to that end," this makes the PDE useless in some cases where the Catholic tradition has insisted on its useful-ness, especially in the forgoing of life-sustaining treatment (we return to this in chapter 14). Moreover, it reduces the third condition to another form of the first two. The "intention of the agent" (*finis operantis*) is reduced to the "end of the act" (*finis operis*). This, it seems, is what Germain Grisez does when he argues that a woman taking the birth control pill must make a contra-life choice or intention, whereas a woman taking her temperature so that she can limit her sexual activity to infertile times does not necessarily make such an intention (Grisez 1964, 155–67). Grisez makes the mistake of reducing the intention (or end) of the agent to the end of the act. But the third condi-tion is not a restatement of the first two. It is best interpreted to mean "The agent may not intend the bad effect as an end to be sought." Thus interpreted, the third condition makes perfect sense. People ought not to want evil.

We can return here to the example of the infertile married man who wants to have children. We assume for the sake of the argument that extramarital sexual pleasure, or self-pleasuring, is morally wrong if done for its own sake, something the Catholic tradi-tion accepts but many proportionalists question. What is the man's intention here? Surely he would not choose to "pleasure himself" in the doctor's office! His intention here (the end he seeks) is to have children. He may well intend the act as a means to that end, but his intention, in the human moral sense of that term, is not self-pleasuring. The meaning of intentionality in the third condition is best understood in this way, as what the agent intends as an end to be sought.

4. The Bad Effect Must Not Outweigh the Good Effect

Proportionalists have no difficulty with the fourth condition either, since they think it an essential part of coming to conclusions about rightness and wrongness. About it we need only note that the fact that this condition is here in the traditional PDE means that those Catholic ethicists who claim that weighing good and bad effects is impos-sible are rejecting what has been a basic part of their tradition for a long time.

Direct and Indirect

Before moving on to medical ethical examples, we need to introduce the terms "direct" and "indirect." These adjectives are applied to actions after they have been analyzed by the principle of double effect. If they pass, they are "indirect" and permitted. If they do not, they are "direct" and are forbidden. This will make more sense when we get to examples. For now, it is enough to say that the PDE enables the distinction between direct abortion, direct euthanasia, direct sterilization, and so on, which are considered always wrong, and their indirect counterparts, which are, or at least may be, right. Whether they may be right or are right depends on whether the direct/indirect distinction is based on just the first two conditions of the PDE, which is the usual way it is done, or on all four, which is sometimes done. If an abortion is found to be indirect on the basis of the first two conditions, then it may be right, depending on whether it passes the last two. But if it is found to be indirect by passing all four, then it has been shown to be right. The more usual way is to make the distinction on the basis of the first two conditions, since the terms "direct" and "indirect" are usually used to refer to acts in themselves.

For example, a direct abortion is one where the act itself is, physically, the actual act of aborting (this would violate the first condition), or where the act itself immediately brings about an abortion, which in turn leads to something else (this would violate the second condition). On the other hand, an indirect abortion is one where the act itself is something else than aborting—chemotherapy or a hysterectomy for a pregnant woman with cervical cancer, for example—and where the act does not directly produce an abortion in order to bring about some other end. That is, the hysterectomy does not abort the fetus in order to cure the cancer; rather, it cures the cancer while also bringing about the unintended but foreseen side effect of aborting the fetus. This abortion is, therefore, indirect and, assuming the woman does not intend (want, desire) her fetus's death (the third condition) and assuming the hysterectomy is necessary to save the woman's life (the fourth condition of proportionality), the procedure is considered morally right. Now we can turn to the application of the principle of double effect in Catholic medical ethics.

Application of the Principle of Double Effect

The principle of double effect is applied to many issues in Catholic medical ethics. The most important are described here.

Abortion

The first application of the principle of double effect, and one of the most consistently important issues in medical ethics, is that of abortion.[1] Roman Catholic medical ethicists gradually arrived at a consensus as to the exact application of double-effect physicalist criteria, which enabled them to make clear and precise judgments in each kind of abortion situation. These distinctions and judgments are now questioned in part by some proportionalist–revisionist Catholic scholars, but they remain the basis for official Catholic teaching (USCCB 2009a, dir. 45–50). Direct abortions are those in which the act in itself is the removal of the fetus "directly" from the body of the woman, or the "direct" killing of the fetus by any other means while still within the mother's body. These acts are never permitted and are considered gravely immoral, identical to murder.

Indirect abortions are, however, permitted according to the principle of double effect. Here the act in itself is specified as an operation or other procedure whose directly intended effect is the preservation or restoration of the mother's health. The foreseen but unintended death of the fetus is "indirect." The two classic cases are the removal of a pregnant cancerous uterus and the removal of a fallopian tube in the case of ectopic pregnancy. Other cases are the use of certain medications or operations where there is some danger that the fetus may die as a result but where the procedure is directed at some other effect. Thus, for example, an appendectomy may be performed on a pregnant woman, even though some (perhaps even great) danger exists of a consequent abortion (miscarriage).

It is clear in official teaching, however, that the fetus itself can never be "directly" attacked. Thus, although the cancerous uterus may be removed with the fetus inside, the fetus can never be removed from the womb if its presence is itself the cause of a woman's dangerous ailment (severe vomiting, eclampsia, hemorrhage, etc.) (Kelly 1979, 265-66). There has been some discussion as to whether the use of contraceptive agents for a woman who has been raped—we discuss this in chapter 11—constitutes a danger of direct abortion, but the fact that the latest *Ethical and Religious Directives* permit this use of contraceptive agents (USCCB 2009a, dir. 36) suggests that those who oppose them as always abortive are too restrictive (Slosar and O'Brien 2003).

Ectopic Pregnancy

Similarly, in cases of tubal ectopic pregnancy, the fallopian tube may be removed with the fetus inside. This is accepted as an indirect abortion. Whether the fetus may be removed from the tube or medically aborted is now disputed. For a time it was clear that the official position was to forbid these as direct abortions violating the first two conditions of the PDE. This is probably still the official teaching although this is no longer as clear as it was. It might be of interest to go into detail on how this decision was reached, especially since this "traditional" judgment is now causing some serious problems.

Prior to 1933 Catholic medical ethicists permitted surgery only on an already ruptured fallopian tube. Their reasoning was essentially that prior to that time the cause of danger was the fetus, not the tube. Hence, any attempt to intervene would be a direct abortion, aimed at the fetus, and thus an intrinsically evil act. Some authors specifically mentioned the possibility of removing the tube with the fetus inside but forbade this as a direct abortion (Kelly 1979, 303; Finney 1922, 135). A retired Catholic hospital chaplain spoke to one of the authors of this book and recalled his anguish at having to allow women to die from ectopic pregnancies; often the surgery, which had to be postponed until after tubal rupture, was too late.

In 1933 Jesuit canon lawyer T. Lincoln Bouscaren, who had been an assistant district attorney in Oklahoma, wrote a dissertation for his doctorate in theology at the Gregorian University in Rome (Bouscaren 1933). It was he who argued for the first time that a salpingectomy (removal of the tube with the fetus inside) was an indirect abortion. To do so, he had to specify the act in itself as the removal of a pathological tube, which causes with equal causal immediacy both the good effect (removal of the pathology) and the bad effect (death of the fetus). Since the first two conditions of the

PDE were passed, the abortion was indirect and hence lawful. He answered the objection of earlier authors that one must wait till the tube ruptured, since otherwise the cause of the problem would be the fetus and the abortion direct, by stating that the tube rupturing was not the causal chain that mattered. The cause of the problem (fetus or tube) was irrelevant. What counted was the causal chain of the act to intervene. And this causal chain did not contain a link where the bad effect caused the good effect. Hence, he argued, salpingectomy, even before the tube ruptured, was morally right. The chaplain mentioned earlier considered Bouscaren a lifesaver, which he was.

But Bouscaren was explicit in rejecting any "direct" attack on the fetus, as in salpingostomy, where the tube is slit open and the fetus removed. But because this was not possible when he wrote this, the rejection of salpingostomies was of no real practical import.

This opinion quickly came to be accepted by the tradition, and the tradition changed to include it. When in 1971 the United States Catholic bishops published a revised edition of the *Ethical and Religious Directives for Catholic Health Facilities*, they included a directive that explicitly and in detail required that Bouscaren's thesis be accepted. They allowed salpingectomies and rejected salpingostomies, spelling out each surgery precisely (US Catholic Conference Department of Health Affairs 1971, dir. 16).

But medicine's advance has now brought us to the point where laparoscopic salpingostomies are often possible and medical abortion by methotrexate is another option. Morbidity is significantly decreased, hospital time greatly reduced, costs cut, and sometimes the tube can be saved for future attempts at procreation. These procedures, which have become the standard of medical care in many cases, would seem to be forbidden by the received (physicalist) tradition of Catholic medical ethics. Proportionalists, of course, are not caught in this bind. We would simply say that we should do the procedure that causes the most good and the least harm. The fetus is lost whatever we do, even if we do nothing. Therefore, we should do the salpingostomy (or do a medical abortion by methotrexate); do whatever is best. That is the morally right thing to do (Kelly 1998).

When the American bishops came to revise the *Ethical and Religious Directives* once again in the early 1990s, they ran up against this problem. An early draft available in December 1993 included a blank directive 53 stating that the issue of ectopic pregnancy was under study. This was the only place in that draft where such a remark was made; it is apparent that the drafting committee was having some difficulty with this.

Another draft, early in 1994, said simply: "In extrauterine pregnancy, if the embryo cannot be moved safely to the uterine cavity [this is never or almost never possible] the embryo may be removed in order to protect the mother's life and fertility, only if the means employed do not constitute a direct abortion." An astute undergraduate student in medical ethics at Duquesne University, having just finished studying the PDE, said that this meant it's OK to do a direct abortion as long as it's not a direct abortion! And given the tradition's definition of "direct abortion," that is indeed what it says; "removing" the embryo had been considered a direct attack on it, and hence forbidden.

The final document, promulgated in late 1994 and revised in 2001 and again in 2009, simply reiterates the proscription of direct abortions: "In case of extrauterine pregnancy, no intervention is morally licit which constitutes a direct abortion" (National Conference of Catholic Bishops 1995, dir. 48; USCCB 2001, dir. 48; 2009a, dir. 48). There is a footnote reference to directive 45 that defines direct abortion in the traditional (physicalist) manner. The detail about procedures that was in the 1971 edition is gone. It seems, therefore, that official Catholic teaching requires doctors to perform procedures that are likely to cause harm to women when other procedures are available that are less risky. Physicians who do this may well face legal jeopardy.

John Tuohey made a suggestion in 1995, however, that parallels in many ways Bouscaren's opinion some sixty years earlier (Tuohey 1995). Tuohey begins by saying that he would not make his proposal if the American bishops had repeated in 1994 what they said in 1971 in their explicit condemnation of salpingostomy. But they did not and so have opened the door. Note here how Tuohey suggests an ecclesiastically positivist metaethics rather than one based on the natural law. If his argument is valid that salpingostomies are morally right, then a natural law metaethics would propose that he say so.

Tuohey argues that since what we call the embryo or fetus in fact consists of two sets of tissues, both defined and separated early in the gestational process, it may be right to attack one of these even though we can never rightly attack the other. The trophoblast is the outer layer of cells and tissue that will develop into the placenta; the cytoblast is the inner layer that will be the embryo and fetus itself. Since it is the trophoblast (the placenta) and not the cytoblast (the fetus) that attaches to the tube, it is the trophoblast that is directly removed in a salpingostomy (and in a methotrexate abortion, too). Thus, just as Bouscaren argued that it is always wrong to remove the embryo from the tube but right to remove the tube with the embryo inside, Tuohey argues that though it is wrong to remove the cytoblast directly, it is right to remove the trophoblast with the cytoblast inside. For those who accept the PDE in its physicalist specifications, this may provide a way out of the dilemma.[2]

There has not yet been any magisterial response to Tuohey's suggestion. One can wonder, however, what accepting his position would mean to the official teaching on other instances of abortion. Presumably conditions three and four of the PDE would reject abortions done for trivial reasons; perhaps they would be seen as rejecting all abortions where the woman's life is not in real danger. But what would become of an abortion, traditionally considered "direct" and therefore always wrong, where a woman takes methotrexate to remove a pregnancy that threatens her life, as for example when a pregnancy threatens her heart? This is clearly said to be a direct abortion and therefore wrong by the received tradition. But Tuohey's approach might move this from a direct to an indirect abortion—the entity physically attacked seems to be the trophoblast and not the cytoblast. If this means the first two (physicalist) conditions are met, surely in this case the third and fourth would be easily met as well. Thus, Tuohey's proposal would seem to change all abortions using methotrexate or removing fetuses intact from direct to indirect, leaving the judgment to be made by proportionalist criteria. I doubt that the magisterium is ready for such a move. On the other hand, bishops surely will be slow to reiterate their earlier condemnation of salpingostomies now that physicians doing salpingectomies instead (where the less intrusive salpingostomy or methotrexate abortion is possible) might run the risk of having their licenses taken away. What we have here is another example of the absurdity of using the PDE in this physicalist kind of way. As Peter Knauer once put it, "Who can understand this?" (Knauer [1967] 1979, 149).

Ashley, deBlois, and O'Rourke also permit salpingostomy and methotrexate, though it is not entirely clear how they can do so and remain consistent with the received (physicalist) tradition of the earlier Directives, which the latest edition does not seem to change. They claim that "while it would be wrong to detach a fertilized ovum from its normal site of implantation, to detach it from an abnormal site that constitutes a serious pathological condition in the woman's body would seem to be licit" (Ashley, deBlois, and O'Rourke 2006, 82). They go on to say that the "direct intrinsic intention (*finis operis*) . . . seems to be to protect the health of the mother, and the death of [the] conceptus is not intended." But could not the same be said about *any* abortion to save the woman's life, that the intention is the treatment of a pathological condition? And is not the means used in a salpingostomy or a methotrexate abortion the removal of the fetus, which has traditionally been said to be wrong in itself? The fact that the fetus will die soon anyway is not supposed to count in determining whether the abortion is direct according to the first two conditions of the PDE, nor is the gravity of the consequences of doing nothing. So while the conclusion that the authors reach is without question the correct one, it seems to demand a rejection of intrinsically evil acts and an acceptance of proportionalism.[3] That is, it cannot be held consistently without also changing the conditions of the PDE and thus questioning other conclusions reached from them. This is the claim made by Benedict Guevin, who insists that Ashley and O'Rourke are wrong (Guevin 2007). Guevin uses the (physicalist) PDE and refers to the Directives to support his position.

The debate continues. A number of Catholic moralists who are considered "faithful" (Anderson et al. 2011, 66n1) or "respected" (ibid., 2011, 65)—that is, who are viewed as defenders of official church teaching on such issues as opposition to proportionalism and prohibition of direct contraception—are trying to explain how salpingostomy and methotrexate abortions (and even possibly craniotomy) are morally right when used to save the woman's life. They rightly wish to avoid the apparently outrageous judgment that women be subjected to an operation (salpingectomy) that significantly increases morbidity and risk of mortality and does nothing to benefit the fetus. These authors make various attempts to show that in these circumstances such procedures are not direct but indirect abortions (Rhonheimer 2011a).

They are opposed by others who argue, convincingly it seems, that once one rejects proportionalism and accepts "intrinsically evil acts" and the four-condition PDE, one is compelled as well to forbid salpingostomy and methotrexate, as these are indeed "direct" abortions according to that method.[4] Consistency requires such a conclusion. Rejecting the conclusion, as seems only proper to protect women, demands as well revision of the method.

The Phoenix Case

A widely publicized event in Phoenix, Arizona, in November 2009 can serve as a further illustration of the application of the PDE to the analysis of abortion. A Catholic nun in a Catholic hospital authorized an emergency dilation and curettage procedure to save the life of a woman with pulmonary arterial hypertension whose pregnancy was threatening to kill her. The fetus would have died in any case, even if nothing was done to save the mother's life, and immediate action was required. Subsequently, the Bishop of Phoenix announced publicly that the nun had been automatically excommunicated for authorizing a direct abortion.

Scholars in canon law quickly pointed out that automatic (*latae sententiae*) excommunications have requirements attached to them that almost certainly were not met in this case; there almost certainly was never any automatic excommunication. And a number of Catholic moral theologians and philosophers added their own analyses, proposing in various ways that this was not a direct abortion and was the morally right thing to do (Magill 2011; Lysaught 2011; [by implication] Rhonheimer 2011b). The Catholic Health Association sided with the hospital against the decision of the bishop (Furton 2011b). But others came to the bishop's defense, arguing that the PDE forbids procedures like these because the act saved the woman's life by directly killing the fetus (Furton 2011a; Cavanaugh 2011; Austriaco 2011b). The act caused the bad effect, which then caused the good effect. Like all direct abortions, this one was immoral.

One interesting point in this debate parallels what we have just noted in the discussion of ectopic pregnancy procedures concerning the suggestion of John Tuohey in distinguishing trophoblast (placenta) from cytoblast (fetus). Gerard Magill (2011, 878) suggests that the procedure used in Phoenix was directly aimed at removing the placenta, as a shared organ between the mother and fetus, and not the fetus itself. The abortion was indirect and hence licit in this sense: removing the placenta (as the offending organ that threatened the mother's life) occurred by extracting the amniotic membranes containing the embryo, akin to the justified removal of a cancerous uterus containing a fetus. In contrast, Nicanor Austriaco argues that the placentectomy was a direct abortion: removing the placenta, which he interprets as the child's placenta, means removing a vital organ of an innocent human being, thereby killing the embryo (Austriaco 2011b, 516, 518). Another attempt to resolve this case using the principle of double effect is suggested by Kevin L. Flannery, who makes an argument along the lines of the removal of the cancerous gravid uterus. He argues that it may be possible to detach the placenta at the maternal portion of the placenta (the *desidua basalis*). This would eliminate the pulmonary hypertension and the embryo would die due to lack of blood supply. Then the contents of the uterus could be evacuated (Flannery 2011).

The decision by the Bishop of Phoenix and its defense by those who agree that the procedure was immoral is based on an interpretation of the traditional four conditions of the PDE, assuming the intervention involved a direct assault on the embryo. Other aspects—the saving of a life, the intention of the people who did it, the fact that the fetus would have died in any case—cannot overcome the fact that this is a direct abortion, an intrinsically evil act. However, another approach to the case (Magill 2011) using the traditional four conditions of PDE reaches the opposite conclusion. The intervention was ethically justified because there was no direct assault on the embryo. The pathology was caused by the woman's placenta, and its removal resolved the imminent threat of her death, despite the foreseen and unavoidable but unintended death of the embryo. Nonetheless, in either case, it is this kind of PDE analysis with its physicalist deontology that proportionalists and intrinsic consequentialists reject.

Euthanasia

Direct (active) euthanasia is forbidden by the PDE. That is, any act that of itself brings about or hastens the death of a dying person is forbidden. On the other hand, drugs can be given that lessen pain, as long as these drugs do not "directly" hasten death. Likewise "negative" euthanasia is permitted. That is, extraordinary means are not required to preserve or prolong life, and such means, once begun, may be stopped. In this latter case, the distinction between ordinary and extraordinary means is not at all physicalistically restricted, and this provides a flexible principle in the care of the dying. It is applied, however, only within the double-effect framework. Any direct killing or direct hastening of death must be avoided. Similarly, direct suicide is forbidden whereas indirect suicide is permitted. We examine this in greater detail starting in the next chapter.

Mutilation

The case of mutilation presents a complex set of issues. Distinctions have been made between nonsterilizing mutilations (amputations of limbs, lobotomies, appendectomies, etc.) and sterilizing mutilations (hysterectomies, vasectomies, etc.). Further complications arise when the purpose of the "mutilation" is for organ transplantation to another person or for medical experimentation.

Nonsterilizing mutilations were for a time judged explicitly according to the PDE. When they were, the act in itself had to be specified in such a way as to exclude the (bad) mutilating aspect from the cause, and to relegate it to the (indirect) effect so that the mutilation could be said to be only indirect. The act in itself was thus specified as a cutting, or some similar procedure that resulted both in a mutilation and in the health of the patient, or both in the removal of a leg and in the removal of gangrene, for example. Thus, the first two conditions of the PDE were said to be met. There was much confusion here, however. Seldom if ever was there any understandable explanation of how an operation to remove a limb, for example, was only "indirectly" a physical (first two conditions) mutilation.

Most authors ultimately accepted the fact that all mutilations were direct in the physical sense. Since such mutilations were generally thought to be good, Catholic scholars needed a different principle to justify them. This was the principle of totality, which holds that a part of a physical body may be sacrificed if it is necessary for the physical health of the whole individual physical organism.[5] The restriction of this principle to the good of the same physical body was necessary to avoid giving approval to castration for boy singers or for men hoping thus to escape sexual temptation. Here the mutilation would not be for the physical good of the same body (Kelly 1979, 267–68).

Sterilizing mutilations were and are permitted only if indirect. Here the act in itself has to be specified in such a way that, although the mutilating aspect can be a part of the act in itself, and the mutilation direct and justified by the principle of totality, the sterilizing aspect has to be excluded from the act in itself and the sterilization indirect. Thus, a direct mutilation for removal of the uterus would only be an indirect sterilization, providing that the good effect is not the result of the sterilization but only of the mutilation. A woman is thus permitted to have her uterus removed if it is cancerous or otherwise diseased. The removal (a direct mutilation) causes with equal immediacy the good effect (removal of the cancer) and the bad effect (sterility). Thus, the second condition is met. On the other hand, a woman with a series of caesarean sections whose womb is dangerously weak is not permitted a hysterectomy since in this case only future pregnancy will bring about any difficulty, and the good effect (the preservation of health or the avoidance of danger) is caused by means of the bad effect (sterility), and thus the second condition of the PDE is violated. Similarly, a woman with a heart condition who might be put at risk by pregnancy is refused hysterectomy, tubal ligation, or other sterilizing operation since the good effect (avoidance of heart strain) is caused by the bad effect (sterility). Her health is preserved by keeping her from being pregnant, which makes the procedure a direct sterilization. A man can be castrated if his testicles are diseased (indirect sterilization), but castration for his spiritual good, to remove the danger of sexual sin, is forbidden, since the sterilization is the cause of the decrease in temptation and is thus direct (Kelly 1979, 267–70).

It is clear that sterilization has been seen to constitute a special case of mutilation, to which the normal rules do not apply. Traditional moralists have insisted that the direct and primary end of the sex act, and of marriage itself, is the biological procreation of children. No individual sex act may be posited that would directly thwart that end. Nor can any operation be performed that would directly thwart that particular faculty of a man or a woman. The generative faculty has thus been given a special set of controls that are not applied to other faculties. Some moralists have explained that the reproductive faculty is "social," for the good of the whole race, and not just individual. Yet despite this argument, they have been consistent in rejecting any "social" arguments for sterilization or other forms of birth control, such as eugenic or demographic arguments. Regardless of the social effects, the generative faculty may not be directly thwarted.

As we saw in chapter 11, the various (nonsterilizing) methods of contraception are included in this context. With the exception of total or periodic abstinence (rhythm or natural family planning), all methods of contraception are considered direct attacks upon the operation of the generative faculty. Although oral contraceptives may be used when their contraceptive or sterilizing effects are indirect, they can never be used for the purpose of avoiding pregnancy, with a possible exception granted to women who are threatened by or who have been the victims of rape. Thus, drugs that are usually used for contraceptive purposes may be used for other reasons than contraception even though sterility results as an indirect, unintended side effect. For example, a woman may use birth control pills if these are prescribed to correct or to palliate seriously irregular cycles or to correct other pathologies, provided the woman does not intend the sterility and provided the bad effects of the pills (sterility and other risks) do not outweigh the good effects for which they are taken.

This approval of indirect contraception applies as well to HIV-positive persons who use condoms as a prophylactic against the transmission of AIDS (Kelly 2002, 204–8). For them, the direct effect of the condom is to inhibit the transmission of the virus. The indirect effect is the prevention of possible pregnancy. So, prescinding from the question of effectiveness, which itself has ethical implications, even those who oppose all contraception as intrinsically evil ought to permit the use of condoms by married couples when one spouse has contracted HIV. Some have disputed this position, however (Johnson 1993). Others have arrived at the same conclusion using the principle of material cooperation, or the principle of toleration (Keenan 2000, 21–29), which we will discuss later in this chapter. The bishops themselves seem divided on the question (ibid., 21–23).

Organ transplants added yet a further complication to the developing position on mutilation. At first, all organ transplants were forbidden since they were direct mutilations of one person's body for the sake of another person's body, which was not allowed by the physicalistically limited principle of totality. In 1944 Bert Cunningham proposed that the principle of totality not be restricted to one physical body, but that it be extended to apply to all members of the Mystical Body of Christ, among whom he included all persons. Cunningham insisted that sterilizing transplants would always be wrong since direct sterilization was always forbidden. He even allowed that a donor might accept total blindness in giving both eyes to another, but he forbade a donor to sterilize himself or herself to give another fertility (Cunningham 1944).

There was much debate about Cunningham's opinion, and some medical ethicists continued for a time to maintain the earlier prohibition. Ultimately, however, his basic conclusion—that living-donor organ transplants can be morally right, even heroic—has been accepted. His reasoning process (that the principle of totality should be extended to all humanity) was later rejected largely because of an understandable fear of ideologies (Nazism and Communism) that claimed that individuals were merely part of the collective. Since then, various attempts have been made to support the conclusion, and no real clarity has been given as to why organ donation might be right. It is likely that most Catholic scholars accept it on the basis of Christian self-giving love. This does not mean that living-donor transplants are without ethical problems. It simply means that the Catholic tradition no longer forbids them (Kelly 1979, 270–71).

Sterility Issues

We have already noted the use of the PDE in questions of sterility testing. If masturbation is used to obtain sperm for the testing, the procedure is forbidden since masturbation is a directly immoral act in itself. The intrinsic immorality of masturbation is in turn supported by arguing that this is a direct misuse of the generative faculty. Sperm for sterility testing can be acquired only by removing some semen from the wife's vagina some time after conjugal intercourse—this was sometimes forbidden (O'Donnell 1959, 306)—or by removing sperm from the testes with a needle. The use of a perforated condom is also allowed by some, and there has been dispute as to the number and size of the holes required so that the sex act is not directly thwarted in its biological end (McFadden 1956, 96–97). Some authors have forbidden even this practice, arguing—not without some internal consistency—that it is intrinsically evil to keep *any* sperm from having a chance to get to the egg (Glover 1948, 73–74; McFadden 1956, 95). But generally this technique is currently considered acceptable.

Artificial insemination, at least as it is usually practiced, is forbidden for similar reasons, even when the husband's sperm is used (artificial insemination by husband, AIH). The 1987 *Instruction on Respect for Human Life in Its Origins and on the Dignity of Procreation* (*Donum vitae*) from the Congregation for the Doctrine of the Faith, quoting from *On Human Life* (*Humanae Vitae*), insists on the "inseparable connection, willed by God and unable to be broken by man on his own initiative, between the two meanings of the conjugal act: the unitive meaning and the procreative meaning" (CDF 1987, 705). Thus, "artificial insemination as a substitute for the conjugal act is prohibited" (707). If a donor other than the husband is used (artificial insemination by donor, AID), the procedure is considered adulterous in addition to the other difficulties. Masturbation cannot be used to gather the husband's sperm. Thus, only the use of a cervical spoon to inject the husband's semen more deeply into the wife's reproductive tract in the context of sexual intercourse is permitted. All other methods are seen as direct misuses of the generative faculty. Even if sperm is gathered from the husband by the use of a perforated condom and then placed in the wife's reproductive tract, since the sperm has been removed from the immediate context of the sexual act, some now claim that this also violates the principle that the unitive and procreative meanings of each sexual act cannot be separated, though many earlier authors permitted this. This conclusion is rejected by those who reject its physicalist premise.

In vitro (in glass) fertilization of any type is forbidden for the same reason (CDF 1987, 706–7). TOTS (tubal ovarian transfer with sperm) and GIFT (gamete intrafallopian transfer), which allow the actual fertilization to occur in the woman's body (in vivo) rather than in a laboratory dish (in vitro), seem to be forbidden as well in light of *Donum vitae*, even though they had been supported by some interpreters of official Catholic teaching as not contradicting earlier Vatican and papal pronouncements (Kubat 2002). Some claim that GIFT may still be permitted since it is not explicitly forbidden by *Dignitatis personae*, a document promulgated by the Congregation for the Doctrine of the Faith in 2008 that largely repeats the teaching of *Donum vitae* (CDF 2008). Some authors permit it; others forbid it (O'Rourke 2010, 721–22). *Dignitatis personae* permits fertility procedures as long as "the married couple is able to engage in conjugal acts resulting in procreation without the physician's action directly interfering in that act itself" (CDF 2008, no. 13). In GIFT, the ova are taken surgically from the woman and as long as the sperm are collected after sexual intercourse by the use of a perforated condom, some claim that this does not directly interfere in the act. Others say that it does, since the sperm must be separated from the woman's body and then transferred with the eggs into the fallopian tube. Catholic scholars who are not concerned with these physical details do not see any reason to prohibit GIFT or TOTS. The same negative judgment applies to such techniques as human reproductive cloning and surrogate motherhood, and here many—probably most—Catholic ethicists agree that these are morally wrong, though many do so for other reasons than that they violate the inseparability principle and the integrity of the individual sexual act.

Mental Reservation

All of the cases cited thus far involve some kind of surgery or at least medicinal therapeutic intervention. The other issues of medical ethics generally have not been solved by the use of the PDE. Thus, for example, there is no application of physicalism or the PDE to the problem of an ignorant or greedy physician, or to the question of the medical secret, or to the complex problems of justice in our health care system.

One exception, however, is the case of truth-telling. Here Catholic moralists had a traditional concept drawn from the double-effect framework: mental reservation. Although all "direct" lies were forbidden, it was allowed to posit an act in itself consisting of the physical utterance of a series of words that would be misunderstood by the hearer but that in themselves were not directly untruthful. Thus, a nurse could say to a patient, "The doctor is not in," even though the doctor was in the office, since the physical words might (by an astute listener) be correctly understood as meaning "The doctor is not in for you," or "The doctor is not in this reception room." Similar evasion techniques could be applied to questions that a physician might not wish to answer. Thus, a doctor might say, "I don't know," even though he did know, since the words could mean "I don't know anything I can tell you about." Or the doctor might say, "Your temperature is normal," mentally reserving "for a person dying of infection." The speaker would mentally withhold or reserve the explanatory clause, and the listener would presumably misunderstand. Moralists insisted that the speaker drop enough of a hint as to what he or she was reserving so that there was at least a decent chance for the listener to understand "correctly," that is, to grasp the factual truth. This attempt to justify mental reservations as "indirect lies" by means of the PDE was never even internally consistent. They never got by the third condition, where the agent must not intend the bad effect (presumably the listener misunderstanding), since that is exactly what the agent does intend, or even the second condition, since the bad effect, the misunderstanding, is the cause of the good effect, for example, the doctor not having to talk to the caller. In any case, the idea of mental reservation is seldom proposed anymore (Kelly 1979, 272).

It is interesting to note that there was an attempt in the first edition of the *Catechism of the Catholic Church*, the official Vatican publication approved by Pope John Paul II and written by a commission appointed by him and chaired by Joseph Cardinal Ratzinger, prefect of the Congregation for the Doctrine of the Faith, now Pope Benedict XVI, and thus a compendium of official Catholic teaching, to suggest that a lie might be defined in other than physicalist ways. "To lie," said the catechism, "is to speak or act against the truth in order to lead into error someone who has the right to know the truth" (*Catechism* 1994, 2482, p. 595). Now this is a formal norm. We ought not to deceive those who have a right to the truth. But we can and should deceive the Nazi at the door who asks if there are any Jews living in our building. Unfortunately, Cardinal Ratzinger asked that the definition be changed to read: "To lie is to speak or act against the truth in order to lead someone into error" (Ratzinger 1997, 262). Surely the cardinal does not mean to apply his definition in such a way, but it appears that this more physicalist definition might mean that we would have to tell the Gestapo about the Jewish family in the attic.

Cooperation in an Evil Act

One final application of the principle of double effect is in the case of cooperation in an evil procedure. For example, what part can a nurse take in the care of a patient who is to undergo or has undergone a direct abortion or other immoral operation? To what degree can she or he be a part of the procedure itself?

The principle of cooperation, typically credited to St. Alphonse Liguori, is different from the principle of toleration, which was developed from the time of St. Augustine in the Catholic tradition. The principle of toleration typically refers to the power of the nation or state when it has the means to overcome a serious evil but opts to "tolerate" the evil for the sake of accomplishing a much greater good for society, such as maintaining public order. Pope John Paul II recognized this general principle in his 1995 encyclical, *Evangelium vitae*, explaining that "public authority can sometimes choose not to put a stop to something which—were it prohibited—would cause more harm" (no. 71). In contrast, the principle of cooperation deals with individuals and organizations whose actions are necessarily involved with the evil actions of others. The encyclical also explains the use of this principle of cooperation in the Catholic tradition (nos. 73–74).

To explain the principle of cooperation, moralists have distinguished between direct (or formal) and indirect (or material) cooperation. Direct or formal participation in the immoral act, where the cooperator agrees with and intends the procedure, is forbidden. Indirect or material cooperation is permitted if there is a proportionate reason and the danger of scandal is eliminated. However, there is a form of material cooperation that is not permitted. It is called immediate material cooperation with evil. What is meant is that an act of cooperation is so closely connected with the evil action that there is no other explanation for the cooperation than intending the wrongdoing. Thomas O'Donnell defines it as follows: "Immediate material cooperation is had when one person actually performs the sinful action in cooperation with another person" (O'Donnell 1959, 45). He gives the example of an assistant surgeon who incises the fallopian tube after the chief surgeon has clamped it off.

The example of a bank robber might clarify these abstract concepts. The getaway driver does not rob the bank but formally cooperates with the bank robbery and intends the wrongdoing: this is formal cooperation. In contrast, if a bank robber hijacks an innocent passerby to drive the getaway car, the passerby materially cooperates with the robbery but is not morally complicit. There is a legitimate material cooperation: the passerby does not intend the wrongdoing. But if the father of the bank robber is coincidentally passing by, sees his child fall over and incur a serious injury while running from the bank, and stops his car to drive the child to a hospital, the father does not intend the original robbery but seeks only to assist his injured child. Thus far there is no cooperation, just paternal assistance. If, however, after discovering that a robbery has occurred (perhaps by innocently opening the child's backpack), the father does not report his child to the authorities, the father is now so immediately involved with the wrongdoing as to be morally complicit. This would be immediate material cooperation, which is implicitly equivalent to formal cooperation and therefore wrong. When the principle of material cooperation is used to justify a cooperating action, the action is referred to as mediate material cooperation to distinguish it from illicit immediate cooperation.

In turn, licit mediate material cooperation can be either remote or proximate, depending on the distance between that act of cooperation and the wrongdoing. This is important for ethical dilemmas in organizational ethics as well as clinical ethics, and we return to it in chapter 24. Simply stated, the more remote the material cooperation, the more likely it is to be right. Thus, a cleaner would be permitted to clean a surgical room used for abortions, or a nurse might be allowed to set up abortion utensils if this is a small part of the job but would probably not be permitted to work at an abortion clinic.

Often this concept of cooperation was applied to participation in (evil) non-Catholic worship. Prior to the Second Vatican Council, some Catholic medical moralists forbade the calling of a non-Catholic minister by a Catholic nurse or in a Catholic hospital, though this practice was probably common and the rule was likely often ignored. Later, most writers accepted this as indirect cooperation at worst. Today such an approach is never proposed. Protestant and Jewish chaplains are always welcome at Catholic hospitals and are often hired to work in their pastoral care departments (Kelly 1979, 273).

The most common application of the principle of material cooperation is in the context of abortion and sterilization, often in cases where Catholic hospitals merge with other institutions where these procedures have been a part of those institutions' practice. But the 1994 *Ethical and Religious Directives* explicitly forbid the use of this principle with respect to abortion (National Conference of Catholic Bishops 1995, dir. 45), and in 2000 the Vatican Congregation for the Doctrine of the Faith ordered the American bishops to change the directives on mergers to include a statement about the principle of material cooperation and sterilizations (Place 2000). The latest edition of the Directives explains that "Catholic health care organizations are not permitted to engage in immediate material cooperation in actions that are intrinsically immoral, such as abortion, euthanasia, assisted suicide, and direct sterilization" (USCCB 2009a, dir. 70). It is important to note that what is forbidden here is immediate material cooperation with proscribed services but not mediate material cooperation. It would seem that since the principle of material cooperation has been considered a principle of the natural law rather than a law posited by the Catholic Church (a part of canon law), its interpretation and application are subject to the right use of reason and not to ecclesiastical decree. But perhaps the intention here is to enforce a disciplinary rule in Catholic hospitals rather than to suggest a change in the underlying moral teaching about material cooperation. We return in chapter 24 to the complex issue of the use of the principle of cooperation.

Conclusion

We have analyzed the traditional principle of double effect and have shown how physicalist criteria are applied according to its first two conditions. We have enumerated and described the most important of the medical ethical issues to which double-effect physicalism was applied, and in doing so have illustrated how the received tradition of Catholic medical ethics has answered and does still answer a number of important issues.

This section has been critical of much of this approach, and has included reasons for the criticism. In the third and final part of this book, we will see that Catholic medical ethics has been of great benefit to many issues in American health care ethics, including but not limited to the end-of-life issues that will concern us for the next several chapters and the issues of justice in the American health care system. Fortunately, the conclusions reached by Catholic medical ethics in the question of treatment for dying patients have been largely accepted in American law and in secular American bioethics. Here the Catholic tradition has been at its best, allowing its theological and anthropological insights to influence its own and the nation's developing ethics and law. Unfortunately, the Catholic insistence that the provision of health care to all is a basic obligation of justice has been largely ignored.

Notes

1. This section is substantially revised from Dr. Kelly's book *The Emergence of Roman Catholic Medical Ethics in North America.* Details and more substantiation, primary sources, and so on can be found there (Kelly 1979, 264–73, and generally 274–309, 321–99).

2. Christopher Kaczor has recently adopted Tuohey's position on salpingostomy (Anderson et al. 2011, 73), but whether the same argument can be made about methotrexate is disputed. Some argue that "methotrexate attacks both the trophoblast and the embryo proper" (ibid., 73).

3. In the 1997 edition of their work, Ashley and O'Rourke explicitly and at length reject proportionalism and affirm intrinsically evil acts (Ashley and O'Rourke 1997, 159–64). In the latest edition this rejection is less explicit and the analysis given to the issue much less detailed (Ashley, deBlois, and O'Rourke 2006, 15–16). In both editions the authors uphold the moral rightness of salpingostomy (and methotrexate) in ectopic pregnancy (1997, 253–54; 2006, 82).

4. For a description of analyses defending salpingostomy and methotrexate by Christopher Kaczor and Martin Rhonheimer, together with a refutation of their position and a defense of the claim that Catholic teaching requires they be forbidden as direct abortion, see Anderson et al. 2011. The authors conclude their article by asking the Holy See to end debate on the issue by making a final judgment about it. If Catholic moral theology is indeed based on a natural law metaethic, such a judgment ought not to end the debate, but, as we saw in chapter 10, ecclesiastical positivism has been and still is an operative force in some aspects of Catholic ethics. For a defense of his position, see Rhonheimer 2011b. Like proportionalists, Rhonheimer rejects physicalism, and like them he accepts the moral rightness of certain abortion procedures (craniotomy in certain emergency cases when the mother's life is in immediate peril and salpingostomy in ectopic pregnancies) that the traditional (physicalist) approach to the PDE would reject. Yet he consistently rejects proportionalism as opposed to Church teaching, claiming that only his nonphysicalist approach to the PDE can defend the PDE from its proportionalist critics. Rhonheimer's critics in turn accuse him of rejecting Church teaching by accepting these abortion procedures as moral, and use largely physicalist arguments in doing so (Guevin 2011; Flannery 2011).

5. The principle of totality is sometimes given greater prominence than it is given here. This is because its specific application in Catholic medical ethics has been largely limited to the question of nonsterilizing mutilation. In a wider sense, it can be said to apply generally to medical ethics in the same way that the fourth condition of the PDE is applied, requiring that the whole be served by any negative effects that are foreseen as inevitable. Finally, there is a sense in which the principle of totality is similar to proportionalism or intrinsic consequentialism. Those procedures are right when their consequences, considered in the context of the human person adequately considered, are properly proportionate. But the principle of totality as it developed in Catholic medical ethics has indeed been subordinated to the PDE, and that is the way we have presented it here. Ashley and O'Rourke call it "the principle of totality and integrity" and claim that it sets priorities among human values, though it is clear that this cannot for them permit an action forbidden as intrinsically evil. See Ashley and O'Rourke 1997, 219–21. For a more traditional interpretation of the principle of totality, see O'Donnell 1959, 127.

PART III

Application

CHAPTER 13

FORGOING TREATMENT, PILLAR ONE

Ordinary and Extraordinary Means

THE ISSUE OF FORGOING life-sustaining treatment constitutes perhaps the central ethical issue for American hospitals, nursing homes, and health care providers. It occupies our attention for the next eight chapters.[1] Five chapters (13–17) present and discuss the three main ideas that provide the basic "pillars" of support for what has become the general American agreement on this issue. The next three chapters (18–20) defend each in turn from certain attacks.

The American Consensus

From the 1960s to the 1980s, Americans were unable to reach a consensus on the morality and legality of forgoing medical treatment. Scholars disagreed about many of the issues—this continues today, as we will see—the basic stance of American law had not been determined, the medical profession was largely unsure of what to do, and hospital policies varied widely. To the degree that there was a general approach, it was usually that the physician decided what to do in each individual case, and often that choice would be to insist on ongoing aggressive treatment even when there was little human benefit. In the 1960s and 1970s, the growing field of bioethics in America reacted against this approach, against what came to be called "medical paternalism" (Veatch 1973b). This criticism and other factors resulted in a radical change, so that by the beginning of the 1990s it was possible to speak, at least in some sense, of an American consensus. This consensus emerged from bioethical scholarship and showed itself in a number of significant court cases, starting with the *Quinlan* case in 1976 and continuing through the US Supreme Court cases on physician-assisted suicide (PAS) in 1997; it was also the result of a number of important decisions reached by governmental committees and commissions. It is true, of course, that the consensus has never achieved universal agreement. Today it is under attack from those who would insist that certain treatments, especially medically assisted nutrition and hydration, are obligatory; from those who would legalize euthanasia or physician-assisted suicide; and to a lesser extent from those who would use "medical futility" to reduce the decision-making authority of patients and surrogates and return it in some degree to physicians. Yet despite these areas of controversy, it is possible to speak of a general agreement or consensus in American law, medicine, and ethics about the legal and ethical rightness of forgoing life-sustaining treatment.

The Three Pillars of the Consensus

The best way to understand the current consensus is to see it as based on three pillars of support. The first is the recognition that not all treatments that prolong biological life are humanly beneficial to the patient. In the Catholic tradition, this concept is expressed in the distinction between ordinary and extraordinary means of preserving life, which is the topic of this chapter. The attack against this pillar comes mainly from those who insist that medical nutrition is obligatory even for those who would seem not to benefit from it. That issue is the subject of chapter 18.

The second pillar is the agreement that there is a moral difference—and that there ought to be a legal difference—between killing (active euthanasia) and allowing to die. This is the topic of chapter 14. The attack against this pillar comes from those who support euthanasia and physician-assisted suicide, which is the topic of chapter 19.

In the US legal system, these two ethical bases have been combined with a basis in law, the legal concept of the right to autonomy, privacy, and liberty to decide for oneself. This is the third pillar, which is developed in chapters 15, 16, and 17. Attacks against this pillar come in part from those who would expand physician authority by expanding the notion of medical futility, which is the topic of chapter 20. Taken together, these three pillars provide the foundation on which the present consensus concerning the moral and legal rightness of forgoing treatment has been built.

The first two of these pillars are well established within the Roman Catholic tradition, which had already developed prior to the arrival of the so-called American bioethics in the 1960s and 1970s, a detailed and complexly argued system of medical ethics. The only other tradition to have done this, religious or secular, was Jewish medical ethics; and that tradition, for reasons to which we have already alluded, has had a lesser impact on American secular medical ethics and American law than has the Catholic tradition. Indeed, it is probable that the American consensus would have been impossible had these concepts not already been developed in Catholic moral theology.

Ordinary and Extraordinary Treatment

The first pillar on which the current American consensus is based is the general agreement that not all medical treatment that prolongs biological life is of human benefit to the patient. Thus, some life-sustaining treatment can be forgone.

The ethical distinction between mandatory and optional treatment has been provided by the Catholic tradition in its centuries-old distinction between ordinary and extraordinary means of preserving life, terms often used even in secular conversation and policies. The distinction goes back at least to the sixteenth century, was included in the important work of Alphonse Liguori in the eighteenth century, and was emphasized and made popular by the teaching of Pope Pius XII in the 1950s (Paris 1986,

31–32; Pius XII 1958, 395–96). It is essential to recognize that this is a moral distinction, not a medical one, and it relies on theological and philosophical understandings of the meaning of human life of which the practical implications, if not the theological bases, have largely been accepted in the American consensus. It is mostly a question of human benefit versus human burden.

There is no need to go into detail about the history of the distinction. It is important to note, however, that there have been two different approaches among the moralists who have proposed it (Shannon and Walter 1988, 638). The more restrictive approach looked only to the burdens of the treatment itself. A treatment was said to be extraordinary if it was painful, caused great hardship, or was expensive. But the likely outcome, that is, the state of the patient after treatment, was not considered. The other approach, most often used today, weighs both the burdens and benefits of treatment. Here, even if the treatment itself may be inexpensive and not cause any great discomfort, it is extraordinary and therefore optional if the benefits it promises are slight or nonexistent when seen in the context of the patient's overall condition. This second approach is the one used by Gerald Kelly, arguably the most important Catholic medical ethicist prior to the Second Vatican Council (Kelly 1958, 129). His definition, quoted by others (McFadden 1961, 227), is given clear approval in the Declaration on Euthanasia, an official document issued by the Vatican in 1980. The declaration states that "a correct judgment can be made regarding means, if the type of treatment, its degree of difficulty and danger, its expense, and the possibility of applying it are weighed against the results that can be expected, all this in the light of the sick person's condition and resources of body and spirit" (CDF [1980] 1998, 653). Precisely. The latest version of the *Ethical and Religious Directives* quotes this as its source in adopting the same approach (USCCB 2009a, dir. 56, 57). The *Catechism of the Catholic Church* says in a similar vein: "Discontinuing medical procedures that are burdensome, dangerous, extraordinary, or disproportionate to the expected outcome can be legitimate" (*Catechism* 1994, 2278, p. 549). Recent debate about feeding tubes has reopened this question. We return to this in chapter 18.

Vitalism

The distinction between morally ordinary and morally extraordinary means of preserving life proposes a reasonable middle ground between vitalism and subjectivism, two extreme positions that are sometimes advocated. The first of these, an absolute vitalism, permits no cessation of efforts to prolong life. This position claims that life itself is the greatest possible value, and is to be sustained at all costs. We mentioned this in chapter 6 as one answer to the third question of normative ethics.

Those with clinical experience can give examples of this. A nurse once told Dr. Kelly that she finally refused a physician's fifty-second order for cardiopulmonary resuscitation (CPR) on the same patient within forty-eight hours. Here is vitalism in the worst possible sense of the term. Perhaps it was the doctor's orders, or perhaps a surrogate was insisting that everything be done to keep the patient alive. Many hospital professionals have encountered situations where a dying person's relatives insist that everything be done to keep their loved one alive, perhaps out of guilt, or fear of being left alone, or a belief that Jesus may perform a miracle. In this last case, it is often helpful to suggest, gently, that Jesus—or God—does not need ventilators and defibrillators for miracles, but there are persons who are sure they have an obligation to keep a dying loved one alive as long as possible to give God time. No theological explanation that God does not need more time, that the ventilator and the defibrillator have already been shown to be inadequate, and so on, seems to help in these cases. We speak in detail of this kind of case in chapter 20 on medical futility.

Catholic medical ethics has never considered this kind of prolongation of dying as morally required or even as a particularly good option. Theologically, Catholic faith in the Resurrection has a good deal to do with this. The present life is to be treasured, but it is not all there is. Biological life need not be prolonged by extraordinary means.

Subjectivism

The other extreme position is a totally lax subjectivism that permits cessation of treatment, and even active killing, based only on the subjective choice of an individual. Here the idea that human life is of intrinsic value is rejected. Life is of value only if the individual gives value to it. There is too much of this in the United States, too much individualism, too much insistence on absolute subjective choice. This does not suggest a preference for a totalitarian or authoritarian system where government would ordain our values. But we are, after all, social beings. We owe help to others precisely because they are of value, even if for some reason they have lost a sense of this value themselves. And American law has not moved all the way to the subjectivist extreme. Attempted suicide, for example, while not a crime, is still a reason for insisting on treatment, even for involuntary commitment. While this can in some cases be ill-advised, even hurtful, it is good for us to maintain the sense that human life is valuable even if an individual rejects that value. Human life, while not of absolute value, is always intrinsically valuable. American law does recognize that the state has an interest in preserving life, an interest in avoiding subjectivism.

Roman Catholic tradition has rejected both vitalism and subjectivism. It has recognized both the sanctity of life (life is sacred) and the ethical import of at least some aspects of the quality of life (life need not be prolonged under all circumstances). That is, at some point a lack of the ability to carry out humanly meaningful purposes, which some would term a lack of quality of life, means that life can be let go (Sulmasy 2011, 192–95). This does not mean that a person's life therefore loses its worth, that it ceases to be of intrinsic value. But it does mean that when, in an individual case, the benefits of continued living truly are outweighed by the burdens of the kind of life that is likely to result from life-sustaining treatment or by the burdens of the treatment itself, the treatment may be forgone. And the American consensus, including American law, has come to agree with this. There are times when enough is enough.

The distinction between ordinary and extraordinary means of preserving life, as we have noted, goes back several centuries. According to this tradition, one is not obliged to preserve one's life by using measures that are morally extraordinary. The terms "ordinary" and "extraordinary" are useful and should not be abandoned even in the face of some recent criticism. Critics do have a point, however, when they argue that the words "ordinary" and "extraordinary" are open to misinterpretation if the distinction is understood as a medical one (CDF [1980] 1998, 653). It is, rather, a moral distinction, and there are no simple technical or statistical criteria for determining the difference. Means that are usually thought of as medically ordinary (no longer experimental, normal hospital procedures in some cases, not requiring Institutional Review Board protocol approval) may be morally extraordinary. Thus, what would be an ordinary or reasonable means when used in caring for a person whose chance of renewed health is great would become extraordinary in the care of a patient who has little or no chance of recovery.

Other terms have been suggested and are in general usage, but there is no pair that exactly replaces the nuances of "ordinary" and "extraordinary." "Reasonable" and "unreasonable" work in some cases but not in others. "Unreasonable" means that the treatment is irrational. This implies that it should not be given, whereas "extraordinary" means that the patient may choose to reject the treatment, not that it must be rejected. The treatment is optional, not necessarily wrong. "Proportionate" and "disproportionate" suffer from the same problem, as well as from the difficulty of implying a methodology about which there is considerable disagreement. "Heroic" treatment might work, but "nonheroic" is awkward, and these terms suffer from the same problem as do the more traditional "ordinary" and "extraordinary" because they might imply that medical criteria determine the difference.

Some wish to avoid pair-terms altogether and speak only of the right of autonomy as this is guaranteed by American law—we return to this issue in detail later. But this is to restrict the issue to the legal aspects and to the ethics of the law, ignoring what the Catholic tradition has properly included and what has been important in the general American consensus, the moral rightness and wrongness of the decision itself. It is wrong to forgo ordinary means of preserving our lives. We describe in detail in part I the theological basis for this judgment. Briefly put, the dignity of human life means that we owe it to ourselves, to others, and in a very different way to God not to reject the gift of life. Because we have responsibilities to self, to others, and to God to take basic good care of ourselves, some (morally ordinary) treatments are obligatory whereas others (morally extraordinary) are optional. This is not just a decision that we make up (posit). It is a moral decision we make on the basis of what we discover objectively in the actual clinical situation.

Illustrative Examples

Some examples will help clarify the claim that the distinction between ordinary and extraordinary is a moral one, not medical. When one of this book's authors (Kelly) gives a lecture on this topic, he often asks his listeners what they would do if right then and there he should happen to grab his chest, groan, and fall over on the floor. Sometimes there is silence! But someone will finally say that she or he would check for a pulse, and if there is none, start CPR. And someone else will volunteer to call 911 (or, if we are in a hospital, to call a code). These are ordinary means of prolonging life. In his present physical condition, Dr. Kelly would have a moral obligation to accept this treatment, to go to the emergency room and then the cardiac care unit, to take the thrombolytic agents to dissolve the blood clots, and so on. These are likely to be of real benefit, and this seems objectively to outweigh the burdens. On the other hand, if Kelly and his listeners were all to come back in fifty years for an anniversary of the lecture, and he, at a very advanced age, with a multitude of diseases and previous insults, were to fall off his stretcher, gasp, and stop breathing, it would be morally right of him to have "DNR" (do not resuscitate) written on his forehead. The treatment for the cardiac arrest would be the same as before (or even more advanced), but humanly the circumstances have changed. What was morally ordinary treatment for a person with a good chance for recovery has become morally extraordinary for one with little chance. The (human) benefits no longer outweigh the (human) burdens.

Another example is the use of antibiotics for pneumonia, surely a medically ordinary treatment. Yet they may be "morally extraordinary" for a person dying of cancer or some other similar condition. A person diagnosed with terminal cancer with only a few weeks to live might rightly see pneumonia as "the old man's friend." Of course, the medication might be morally ordinary, too—if, for example, the dying person still had work to do to help his or her family by preparing a will or some similar task.

The criteria for distinguishing between morally ordinary and morally extraordinary means of prolonging life are not clean or precise. Though the distinction is an objective one in the sense that it is based on real situations, on real conditions, real prognoses, and so on, subjective elements come into play here—not subjectivism but subjective elements. For example, a person who truly is terrified of surgery can rightly consider that fear in determining whether or not the burdens outweigh the benefits. Here terror is a real burden.

There is, then, no moral obligation to preserve life at all costs. Many factors must be weighed in this decision: the chance of success; the degree of invasiveness, pain, and patient fear; the likely outcome; the social cost (this can be quite risky, of course, and demands caution, especially in a health care system that refuses to recognize the right of all to basic care); the needs of others; the patient's readiness for death; the patient's likely condition after successful treatment and after partial success. And a person may rightly consider financial costs among the burdens. The Catholic tradition is quite clear about this. The sick need not sacrifice the financial survival of their families to prolong life, certainly not when the treatment is of questionable benefit and perhaps not even when the treatment is almost surely a cure. In earlier centuries, even the sense of shame or modesty a woman might feel when being examined by a male physician was sometimes said to be sufficient reason for calling the treatment extraordinary. Of course, in those days doctors were unlikely to cure, so there was far less likelihood that the treatment would do any good. The point, however, is that the distinction, as developed in Catholic medical ethics, is a flexible one.

Drawing the Line

In this context, one can describe various treatments as though they were located along a spectrum. On one end are clearly ordinary means of prolonging life, treatments such as antibiotics for pneumonia in otherwise healthy people, or appendectomies, or even other behaviors such as eating habits, exercise, sleep, and so on. Then there are means that most would consider ordinary but that might be extraordinary for some conditions or for some persons. Then come morally extraordinary treatments that people would be likely to consider reasonable but not obligatory—a third round of chemotherapy, for example, that might offer a small but still real hope of remission for some months. A person might choose it or reject it; it really is morally optional. Then, further along on the spectrum, there are some treatments most of us would consider not only extraordinary but also unreasonable, even silly or stupid. Feeding tubes for the irreversibly comatose in this category; yet some people, even some Catholic bishops, claim they are morally required (as many people did in the case of Terri Schiavo, the Florida woman said to be in a persistent vegetative state). We return to this in chapter 18. Finally, at the extreme end of the spectrum are those procedures that are "medically futile" in the strict sense. We examine this in detail in chapter 20.

With the exception of this last category, medical futility, the lines between the others cannot really be clearly drawn. There are often conflicts among those involved—patients, families, physicians, and others—a topic to which we return in chapters 15, 16, and 17, when we examine who has the authority to make the decision. Supposedly we might either try to avoid all risk of undertreatment by imposing all possible life-extending technologies on everyone, or try to avoid all risk of overtreatment by doing nothing for anyone seriously ill. But we cannot do both, and in any case these options are each clearly unacceptable. Thus, despite the difficulty of drawing precise lines, the general agreement that some treatments are morally obligatory and others morally optional remains of great significance in supporting the present consensus. If the United States were basically vitalist, our laws would doubtless require that no life-sustaining treatment ever be withheld or withdrawn. If we were completely subjectivist, our laws would put no restrictions of any kind on decision making. Yet, as we see in chapter 16, the law does restrict surrogate decision making. Thus, this first pillar, "fuzzy" as its lines may be, is an essential support for the present American consensus on forgoing treatment.

Summary and Conclusion

The distinction between ordinary and extraordinary means as developed and applied within the Catholic tradition is thus very wide and very flexible. Ordinary means, which are morally obligatory, are those that offer the patient a significant human benefit without imposing a disproportionate burden. Extraordinary means, which are optional, are those that promise little significant human benefit or those that impose burdens disproportionate to the likely benefit.

The moral obligation to which this principle speaks is, of course, that of the patient. The patient is morally obliged to use ordinary or reasonable means of preserving life and is not morally obliged to use extraordinary ones. But it clearly has implications for hospital policy and for the law. If a patient is not obliged to use every possible means of preserving life, then hospitals and health care practitioners may not impose them on patients. The fact that such a distinction had been developed within Catholic medical ethics was important in support of the consensus we have reached, however tentatively, in the United States.

Note

1. An earlier version of these eight chapters has been published as Kelly 2006.

CHAPTER 14

FORGOING TREATMENT, PILLAR TWO

Killing and Allowing to Die

THE SECOND PILLAR on which the American consensus on the issue of forgoing treatment is based is the distinction between killing and allowing to die, which has been provided by the Catholic tradition in its analysis through the principle of double effect. According to this distinction, as we have seen already in detail, the direct killing of an innocent person is never morally right, but allowing a person to die is sometimes morally right. Some would now question the absoluteness of this distinction; that is, some now argue that direct killing (active euthanasia or assisted suicide) may be morally right in some cases. And some wish to legalize the practice. We return to this question in chapter 19. But the acceptance of this basic distinction has helped form both American medical practice and American law.

The word "euthanasia," which comes from the Greek and means "good death" or "dying well," generally means doing something that brings about this "good" death in a person who is hopelessly ill or who is suffering pain or other burdens from an illness. The Catholic tradition uses terms such as "direct" and "indirect" or "active" and "passive" euthanasia. Direct and active mean killing and are claimed to be always wrong; indirect and passive mean allowing to die and are sometimes right. But it is better to avoid confusion and use the word "euthanasia" only to refer to the actual killing of a patient.

The best way to state the second pillar for the present American consensus is to state it as the Catholic tradition has done: It is always morally wrong directly to kill an innocent person, but it is sometimes morally right to allow a person to die. Two simple words here are at times overlooked: "always" and "sometimes." The norm is not that it is always wrong to kill and always right to allow to die; dismissing the norm on the basis that it is not always right to allow people to die misses the basic point. Clearly, it is sometimes wrong to allow people to die of their illnesses. If someone arrives at an emergency room (ER) at a full-service hospital in the United States with acute appendicitis and is denied an appendectomy because of lack of insurance and dies in the ER, the hospital has not in fact killed that person. No one has shot a gun or injected a lethal dose of medication. It has (only) allowed the person to die. But in doing so, it has done a great injustice. It has also broken the law. It is clear that a consistent under-standing of the distinction between killing and allowing to die requires this insistence that some incidents of allowing to die, even though they are not killings in the sense of what physically causes death, may nonetheless be morally wrong.

Five Types of Actions

There are five different kinds of actions to be considered in a discussion of the distinc-tion between killing and allowing to die.

Withholding Life-Sustaining Treatment

First, one may decide not to use certain medical means that would prolong life (not to use a ventilator for a terminally ill patient, or not to resuscitate a patient who suffers from some severe illness). This withholding of treatment is not the killing of a person. It is an allowing to die. It is not always morally right, but it is sometimes—indeed, it is often—morally right. If the means in question are "morally extraordinary," the act (the decision not to use the means) is generally accepted as moral.

Withdrawing Life-Sustaining Treatment

Second, one may decide to stop the use of a means that has already been begun (to withdraw a treatment, to turn off the ventilator, to "pull the plug," to "do a terminal wean"). Catholic moral tradition considers this action to be the equivalent of with-holding life-sustaining treatment. Morally, assuming the burdens outweigh the benefits, it is the nonuse of extraordinary means and is normal procedure in American hospitals. Until the American consensus was achieved, this second kind of action was sometimes considered legally more dangerous, more open to legal repercussion or at least to mal-practice litigation because it is physically the actual doing of something rather than the simple nondoing of it. But recent court decisions, especially the Supreme Court decisions in the *Cruzan* case (*Cruzan v. Director* 1990) and on physician-assisted suicide (*Vacco v. Quill* 1997; *Washington v. Glucksberg*, 1997), have made it clear that the second action, withdrawing treatment, is legally the equivalent of the first, withholding treatment.

Thus, it can now be stated that if it is morally right and legal to withhold treatment *X* in circumstances *ABC*, then it is morally right and legal to withdraw treatment *X* in the same circumstances. The circumstances may change, of course, as when patients or surrogates state they would have withheld treatment but are unwilling to withdraw it. But that is a question of who decides. There is no ethical or legal difference as such between withholding and withdrawing.

This is important for a number of reasons. The most obvious is that otherwise we would be forced to maintain useless and unwanted treatment. And we would be forced to use scarce resources in doing so. But there is a danger of undertreatment as well. If patients and their families were to fear that certain procedures, such as ventilators, could never be discontinued, they might be overly hesitant to authorize them in the first place. Families often need assurance that a ventilator is not a sentence to permanent medical imprisonment. They may remember earlier occasions when patients were refused permission to turn them off even when they were doing no human good. Sometimes early discussion with patients and their families can result in withholding unwanted and nonbeneficial treatment so that the emotionally more difficult later decision to withdraw is not necessary. In many cases, however, this is not possible because the prognosis is not yet clear. Families need to be assured that, after a time-limited trial, medical procedures that turn out to be ineffective can be discontinued. Additionally, if withdrawal of treatment were not allowed, people might insist in their advance directives that they never want certain procedures (intubation seems the most common fear) regardless of the outcome. And ER physicians might be overly hesitant to begin emergency care, fearing that later diagnostic tests could show such treatments to be unwarranted. The moral and legal identity of withholding and withdrawing, which has its origins in Catholic ethics, is thus essential to good ethics, good law, and good medicine.

Although moralists of earlier times often used the terms "negative" or "passive" euthanasia (or, more technically within Roman Catholic moral theology, "indirect" euthanasia) to refer either to withholding or withdrawal, it seems far better, as we have already seen, not to use the word "euthanasia" to apply to either of them. It is less confusing if we reserve this word for the actual killing of patients. Neither withholding nor withdrawing medical treatments are acts of killing. Rather, they allow the patient to die of the underlying condition. They are not always morally right. But "allowing to die" is morally right when it is the forgoing of morally extraordinary treatment. Withholding and withdrawing may feel different, but ethically and legally there is no reason to distinguish them.

Pain Relief That Hastens ("Co-Causes") Death

Third, one may take positive means aimed at relieving the patient's suffering but not directly intended to cause death, even though the drug one administers may indeed "co-cause" or hasten death. This is rare, but it does happen in some instances when pain medication must be increased to relieve pain at the very end of life (Quill 2008, 18). For example, in some rare cases a patient builds up such a tolerance to a drug that the dose needed to eliminate pain suppresses respiration and thus is a causal factor in the person's death. In such cases it is morally right and legal to use that needed dosage. It is certainly a moral act to relieve pain, and this sort of medication cannot be considered ethically wrong as long as consideration is given to the patient's wishes.

The Catholic tradition would tend to call this third kind of action "indirect killing." It meets the four conditions of the principle of double effect. Indeed, this is sometimes called "double-effect euthanasia," a term that is better not used because of the confusion it causes. Pain relief that hastens death meets the first condition because the act itself is not a killing but a giving of medication that relieves pain. It meets the second because the bad effect, death, is not caused by the good effect, pain relief. Rather the "act in itself" causes both with equal causal immediacy. Third, the intention of the agent in the sense of "end to be sought" is not that the patient should die but that the patient should be pain-free. And fourth, in the case of a dying patient, the bad effect, a slightly earlier death, is outweighed by the good effect, the relief of pain. Thus this action, like the first two, may well be morally right according to the Catholic moral tradition. And in the American legal and ethical consensus the same judgment is made.

This means that it is always medically possible, and, assuming the proper decision maker agrees, it is always morally right and always legal to eliminate physical pain in the imminently dying patient. It is extremely important to stress this because it is not always recognized. The claim is sometimes made that there are exceptions, that is, that there are cases in which complete pain relief is not possible even for an imminently dying person. But if we look more closely at the reasons sometimes given for this claim, we find that none of them are valid.

Three reasons are sometimes given to explain why elimination of pain in a dying patient is not possible in some cases. First is fear of addiction. Happily, when this is now mentioned as a reason to withhold pain relief, medical professionals laugh at it. And it is indeed laughable. Addiction is certainly an important problem for persons whose unwarranted use of drugs causes harm to their lives and the lives of others. Heroin, cocaine, alcohol, nicotine, and other agents, including drugs such as morphine used by doctors for pain relief, can cause great damage when they are improperly used. For an imminently dying patient, however, pain medication is not addictive in this sense. The term "addiction" indicates both a description of a physical condition (withdrawal causes physical symptoms) and a social condition. In this latter sense, addiction is a social construct. It connotes crime, violence, the need for rehabilitation, and so on. None of these are present in the imminently dying patient. A person dying of cancer on a morphine drip is unlikely to go out and rob a liquor store for a fix! Recent medical literature has claimed that even physical addiction is very rare in people who need opiates for pain relief. Even the nondying person is unlikely to become physically addicted to a drug given for relief of pain. Usually, when the source of the pain is ended, the drugs are ended, too, without symptoms of withdrawal. In any case, even if there is some physical "addiction," it is irrelevant in the case of dying patients who need pain relief as they die.

The second reason sometimes given for why it may be impossible to eliminate pain in some dying patients is that an increase in the drug will cause death. But we have just seen why this is not a problem. As long as the amount of drug given is what is needed to relieve pain, and as long as no one intends the patient's death as an end to be sought (we discuss this in chapter 12), the drug increase is morally right and legal. Concerning the amount of drug given and the way it is administered, physicians need simply to follow the standard range suggested for this patient's condition in these circumstances. The standard of medical care clearly permits using enough drug to eliminate pain in these patients. Doctors need to be sure they do not give an amount so clearly beyond what is needed that the only reason for doing so would be to kill the patient.

Concerning the intention of the physician or the family in doing this, it is understandable and even praiseworthy that they may see the earlier death, if it occurs, as a blessing. They may be glad that the patient's long illness and dying process are over. The family may even be relieved to get back to their lives and their families. None of this means they "intended" the patient's death in the sense meant by the Catholic tradition or by American law. As long as they know that they would have wanted the patient cured and back with them alive and well, they can be sure that they did not "want him dead." Especially in the case of a "terminal wean"—an unhappy phrase but we may be stuck with it; a "terminal wean" is the withdrawal of a ventilator even though the doctors know the patient will not be able to breathe unassisted—physicians should make sure they avoid using phrases such as "Let's give the patient enough morphine to prevent any attempt at breathing." This can be used as legal evidence that the doctor indeed intended to kill the patient.

The third reason given for why it is sometimes not possible to alleviate a dying patient's pain is that the amount of drug needed to do so will render the person unconscious as he or she dies. This is sometimes called "terminal sedation," another unhappy term because it can easily be taken to mean active euthanasia. A preferable term is "palliative sedation," as suggested by James Walter (2002, 6), or "sedation to unconsciousness" (Quill 2008, 19). This is indeed a case where pain relief "fails," but only insofar as it fails to do what is the ideal. It fails to eliminate the pain while leaving the person alert and capable of interaction. But surely this is no reason to reject pain relief in the dying patient if the patient or surrogate asks for it. If the patient decides it is better to stop the pain than to be conscious in constant agony, surely that wish must be followed. The directly intended effect is to relieve pain, not to cause unconsciousness; care should be taken to use only enough sedation as is necessary to eliminate the pain. This practice has been approved by the American Medical Association and other professional medical groups (Quill 2008, 22). And there is a general agreement that surrogates may not legally or morally reject pain medication for dying persons.

There are cases, of course, where dying persons themselves choose to suffer pain rather than lose their capacity to complete tasks they wish to do before dying. In these cases, the wishes of competent persons should be followed. Cases where persons have written in their advance treatment directives that they refuse pain relief (perhaps out of guilt, or fear of God) are very rare, if they exist at all. It seems right to try to override such directives for now-incompetent persons, following a surrogate's decision to relieve pain or seeking legal relief from the directive if necessary.

However, while it is right and legal to eliminate physical pain, the same does not necessarily apply to other kinds of human suffering. James Walter makes a helpful distinction between "neurophysiological suffering" and what he calls "agent narrative suffering" (Walter 2002, 6). The former is what we usually mean by "pain" and includes the kind of physiological distress that comes from the experienced inability to breathe. This pain can and ought to be eliminated. But the other kind of human suffering is sometimes a human reality that persons have to deal with. Worries about dying, guilt for past sins, concern for family, and a sense of hopelessness might be examples of this. These kinds of sufferings should not be ignored by physicians and others involved with the dying patient. Dying persons often reach out to others for conversation, therapy, prayer, and other kinds of human interaction. And when these anxieties threaten to overwhelm, there is nothing that forbids alleviating them by medication. But often they call more for compassion and communication than for sedation. They are, in any case, not the "physical pain" that can be "eliminated."

(Physician)-Assisted Suicide

Fourth, one may act in conjunction with the patient by assisting in active euthanasia. The patient wishes to die and makes this known to the health care practitioner, asking the practitioner to provide the necessary means. The patient actually consumes the drug or initiates the suicide. This is assisted suicide in the strict sense. It is a direct self-killing. In the Catholic tradition and, until recently, in the American moral consensus, it is judged to be wrong. In addition, assisting in suicide is illegal in most, though not in all, American jurisdictions. We return to this issue in chapter 19.

(Active) Euthanasia

Fifth, the health care practitioner may take action that directly causes the patient's death. Like the fourth action, this is referred to as positive euthanasia, active euthanasia, or, within the Catholic tradition, direct euthanasia. It is a direct killing according to the principle of double effect and is considered first degree murder in all American jurisdictions. Apparently, however, until the conviction of Dr. Jack Kevorkian in Michigan, no physician was ever convicted of the crime of killing a dying patient, although family members have been. We come back to the question of physician-assisted suicide and euthanasia in chapter 19.

The Complex Problem of Intentionality: Is the PDE Useless?

In an important article by physician Timothy Quill, attorney Rebecca Dresser, and philosopher Dan Brock, the authors object that it is not possible to use the principle of double effect to distinguish killing from allowing to die (Quill, Dresser, and Brock 1997). That is, the first three of the acts discussed earlier, especially the third—alleviating pain—are not always distinguishable from the last two. The authors say this is because when a family elects, for example, to use pain-relieving opiates that render a patient unconscious until the moment of death—"terminal sedation" or, as we have suggested, "palliative sedation"—and at the same time elects to withhold medically induced means of hydration and nutrition, it is not clear what the intention is (ibid., 1769). The authors argue that in this case—and presumably this would apply also in some other cases of forgoing treatment—"life-prolonging therapies are withdrawn with the intention of hastening death" (ibid., 1769). This, they say, is the same as the intention of many who choose physician-assisted suicide. In both cases the intention is to bring peace to the patient through death. And this, they say, is precisely what the PDE's third condition forbids: "the agent may not intend the bad effect." The bad effect is death, and in both cases the agents intend it. So the PDE would logically prohibit "terminal/palliative sedation" for pain relief as the patient dies without nutrition and hydration and would prohibit giving the lethal overdose. The authors also question how physicians are supposed to know the intentions of patients and family members.

It is important to underline the significance of this claim—at least one article has already been written trying to answer it (Sulmasy 1999), and it has been cited by scholars who conflate active euthanasia and terminal/palliative sedation (Battin 2008, 29; Berger 2010, 34). Here we have a well-known physician (Quill is the Quill in the physician-assisted suicide case decided ultimately by the US Supreme Court), a well-published legal scholar, and a prominent bioethicist writing in an important medical journal that the entire American consensus depending on a difference between killing and allowing to die is worthless. Since, according to Quill, Dresser, and Brock, the PDE rejects both some instances of pain relief and physician-assisted suicide, it is useless at distinguishing between them. Yet the Catholic tradition has for centuries made precisely that distinction. Although "terminal sedation" is a new term, the decision to sedate a dying patient to eliminate pain at the cost of unconsciousness, when this is necessary, is not considered killing and is (often) permitted by the PDE. And the decision not to use medical means of nutrition and hydration is, in many cases, the decision to withhold extraordinary treatment (we return to this in detail in chapter 18) and is (often) permitted by the PDE. Traditionally, then, the PDE does not reject these actions. Yet Quill, Dresser, and Brock say it does. What is going on here?

We will begin with a needed distinction. The PDE actually plays two interrelated but distinct roles. The PDE is both a moral principle of justification and an empirical principle of differentiation. It is usually seen as a way to decide which actions are right and which are wrong. That is the way we discuss it in chapter 12. But before it can be a moral principle, there has to be an empirical means of differentiating between the act of killing and the act of allowing to die. Otherwise, there is no way to distinguish them and therefore no way to judge the ones (actions one through three) that are sometimes right and the other (actions four and five) that are always wrong, as official Catholic medical ethics does. It should be clear by now that the authors of this book do not accept the use of the traditional (physicalist) PDE as a moral principle of justification. We are not deontologists or physicalists in the meanings we gave to these terms in chapters 5, 8, 10, and 12; we do not think that acts in themselves or causal chains from act to effect determine rightness and wrongness. Yet we do distinguish between acts of killing and acts of allowing to die, and are quite sure that this can be done on the basis of the PDE as an empirical principle of differentiation. Even if one rejects the (physicalist) PDE as a moral principle, one can accept it as a way to tell the difference between killing and allowing to die. Clinicians do this all the time in hospitals and nursing homes. American law presupposes that this is possible. Yet this is exactly what Quill, Dresser, and Brock say cannot be done. And that poses a problem.

The answer is found in chapter 12 where we examine the PDE and its third condition and say that there is a complex issue about the meaning of intentionality. The third condition really means that the agent must not intend the bad effect (death) as an end to be sought. Thus, this third condition (the intention of the agent—*finis operantis*) does not forbid either terminal sedation (or withdrawing a ventilator) or giving a lethal overdose, assuming that in neither case does the agent want the patient dead (never liked him, would not cure him were that possible, wants him dead to get his money). These nefarious intentions are forbidden by the third condition. But the third condition does not distinguish between killing and allowing to die. The first two (physicalist) conditions make that distinction.

On the other hand, if we accept the alternative proposal for what the third condition means, that it does not mean "intend as an end to be sought" but means "intend either as an end or as a means," then Quill, Dresser, and Brock are right. In these cases many families do see death as a way for the patient to end suffering; they do in a sense "intend death as a means." But they do not intend it "as an end to be sought." As Alison McIntyre puts it, "the attitudinal defect that we condemn in such cases need not be present when harm is intended regretfully as a means to a good end" (McIntyre

2001, 229). So if the "intending" forbidden by the third condition includes "intend as a means," the PDE may well forbid terminal sedation, as the authors claim, and probably also terminal weans and many other instances of forgoing treatment and relieving pain in dying patients.

And this is, in fact, the way they understand the third condition: "Neither the patient nor the physician intends the patient to die, either as a means or as an end" (Quill, Dresser, and Brock 1997, 1768). They put the second and third conditions together: "the second and third conditions are used to determine whether the potentially inflicted harm is intentional or unintentional, as either a means or an end" (ibid., 1768). Seen this way, the third condition would forbid many instances of terminal weaning and other such actions. The patient "wants to get it over with," "wants to be at peace," "wants to be with God," and in a real sense death is the means to accomplish this. But this is not the way the PDE has traditionally been used in Catholic ethics. The PDE has always been interpreted by the Catholic tradition as allowing such actions in at least many cases. So those Catholic theologians who argue for the "means or end" meaning of intentionality in the third condition of the PDE are wrong, and thus Quill, Dresser, and Brock are also wrong when they claim that the PDE forbids terminal sedation and, at least by implication, that it forbids at least some other cases of forgoing treatment.

This same "intention" motivates those who, like Quill, Dresser, and Brock, support physician-assisted suicide. They do not "want the patient dead" any more than do those who act to relieve the patient's pain. This is what is so often misunderstood in this whole debate. The intention of the agent (*finis operantis*) of any good physician who performs euthanasia or who supplies the means for physician-assisted suicide is the same as that of those who relieve pain with the knowledge that that relief may hasten death. The difference is not in the intention of the agent. The difference is in the means to bring about this intended end. And there are three possible analyses that can be made about these means. First, Roman Catholic tradition claims that euthanasia is intrinsically evil; the first two (physicalist) PDE conditions (the act in itself must not be morally wrong; the bad effect must not cause the good effect) rule out such actions. The end of the act in itself (*finis operis*) is said to be morally wrong; it directly causes the good effect intended by the agent. Thus these means are forbidden, though the end intended by the agent may well be a good one (peace, freedom from suffering). Killing is always wrong; letting die is sometimes right. Second, Quill, Dresser, and Brock, along with other supporters of physician-assisted suicide (or euthanasia), argue that the difference of means is morally irrelevant. It makes no difference whether we kill or allow to die in situations of the imminently dying person. Killing (or helping to provide the means for self-killing) is often the morally better choice. Third, we—along with many others—hold that there is a moral difference between killing and letting die, a difference based not on differences in the acts in themselves but on significantly different outcomes for health care in our society. The argument for this third position is presented in detail in chapter 19. So the answer to the authors' objection is that the PDE does indeed allow us to distinguish killing from allowing to die. It is a perfectly useful principle of differentiation. It does that in its first two conditions, the ones that argue from physical causality. These distinguish withholding, withdrawing, and pain relief from physician-assisted suicide and euthanasia.

As to the authors' worry that physicians cannot be expected to know the patient's or the family's intention, that is sometimes true but is usually beside the point. Once intention is seen as "intend as an end to be sought" and not "intend as an end or as a means," there are surely far fewer cases when physicians will need to worry about this. If physicians do suspect that a family is intending to let a patient die early to get the person's money or from some similarly criminal motive, then they ought to get legal advice. There are standards of surrogate decision making that we come to in chapter 16, and if the family violates these standards, physicians should not do what the family says. But this kind of evil intention is almost never the case.

There are practical implications of this question of intentionality that occur often in hospitals where families may feel guilty about withholding or withdrawing treatment or about pain relief where this may hasten death. Some family members worry that somehow they "intend" their loved one's death since they will say "let him die a natural death," or "let him die with dignity," or "let him be at peace with God," or "his death was (or will be) a blessing." They may even be grateful that their own long ordeal will now be over, and they fear this means they intend their loved one's death. There is a simple way to alleviate such anxiety, and it is by asking them if they would want their loved one with them if a cure were possible. Of course they say yes! This means they do not intend death. They do not want their loved one dead. So the question to ask in deciding whether family members intend death is, if there were an alternative (a cure) that would cause the good effect (freedom from the dying process) and not cause the bad effect (death), would you choose that alternative? Families inevitably say yes. And this relieves them from at least some of the worry that so often accompanies this kind of decision.

Finally, it may be helpful in this context to point out a possible source of confusion in the definition of euthanasia given in the official 1980 "Declaration on Euthanasia" from the Congregation of the Doctrine of the Faith: "Euthanasia here means an action or omission that by its nature or by intention causes death with the purpose of putting an end to all suffering. Euthanasia is, therefore, a matter of intention and method" (CDF [1980] 1998, 652). This definition is not a problem if properly understood. But, at first glance, the word "omission" might be confusing. Omitting extraordinary means of preserving life is permitted, not prohibited. Does the Declaration wish to consider this euthanasia? The answer is clearly no. Omitting life-sustaining treatment is euthanasia only when the means omitted are morally ordinary or when the agent intends death. And this means "intend as an end to be sought." Actions one through three are not forbidden by the Declaration.

CHAPTER 15

FORGOING TREATMENT, PILLAR THREE

Decisions by Competent Patients

Summary Introduction to Decision-Making Authority

WE HAVE NOW FINISHED the survey of the first two pillars that support the present American consensus on forgoing treatment, the two that are based in Catholic medical ethics. The third pillar is that of the legal concepts of privacy, autonomy, and liberty. This has been interpreted to mean that patients capable of making decisions of this type may refuse treatment even against the advice of their physicians. The patient has the rights of autonomy to choose and of privacy to be left alone. The June 1990 *Cruzan* decision of the Supreme Court, relying on common law liberties, established this right of competent patients to refuse treatment as the law of the land (*Cruzan v. Director*, 1990). Similarly, the courts in most cases have decided that patients not capable of making decisions may also refuse through surrogate decision makers.

The precise relationship between this third pillar (the right of privacy, autonomy, and liberty) and the first pillar (the difference between mandatory and optional treatment) is not yet theoretically clear, though in most jurisdictions the practical judgments rendered have led to consistent outcomes. Not theoretically clear is the question of what legal implications follow from the distinction between reasonable and unreasonable (or ordinary and extraordinary) treatment. Although we cannot here explore the complex theoretical issues, we will look closely at their practical implications. We have seen that the moral obligation to use reasonable or morally ordinary means to preserve life falls primarily on the patient. What if a patient deemed capable of making such decisions chooses to forgo a means of treatment that, in any reasonable judgment, is "ordinary," beneficial, inexpensive, and of little burden? I go to the hospital with a pain that is diagnosed as acute appendicitis, but, after admission, I refuse permission for surgery. What moral obligation does this bring to the health care institution and practitioner? Should this have any bearing on the courts' decisions or on the legality of forgoing treatment?

In practical terms, courts have tended to resolve such questions by upholding the right of patients to refuse for themselves with little or no insistence on the distinction between reasonable and unreasonable treatments. Of course, the fact that a person refuses a treatment that seems reasonable might be an indication that the person lacks capacity to decide. But it might not be—for example, in the case of a person who refuses treatment for religious reasons. The treatment is generally considered to be reasonable or "ordinary," but it is unreasonable, even repugnant for the patient. The right of autonomy and privacy has prevailed in those cases where the patient is presently capable of deciding.

Legal Basis

American law comes from three sources. Statutory laws are passed by legislatures on the federal, state, and sometimes local level. The American Constitution and interpretations of that document in state and federal courts and ultimately by the United States Supreme Court are a second source of American law. The third source of law is known as "common law," which is the totality of court cases that have resolved certain issues, and which becomes a kind of unwritten and universally accepted complex of laws and codes of conduct. Part of common law was adapted from English law before the American Revolution, so we sometimes refer to "Anglo-Saxon common law."

Legal scholars have looked at this third pillar and have identified several possible sources for the generally accepted legal conclusion that patients have the authority to decide about treatment. Some suggest that it comes from the rights to privacy and autonomy found in the Constitution. Others argue that a better source is the common law liberty to refuse unwanted treatment, which is part of the common law liberty to refuse unwanted touching. This source is the clearest, the oldest, and the least controversial basis for the right to refuse treatment. The right to privacy has been found in the Constitution only recently and has been applied in the context of abortion and birth control, controversial issues in their own right.[1] All agree that no one has an absolute right to privacy or autonomy; only a few claim that the state has no right to tax us, and the Constitution gives us only a freedom from unreasonable search and seizure, not from all search and seizure.

The common law basis does not suffer as much from controversy or ambiguity of this kind. No one may touch us without our consent. Admittedly, there are times when we must give consent, as to customs officials who search our persons or police officers who arrest us, but these are rare exceptions and they are rather clear. The common law liberty to refuse unwanted touching is really common sense. States do not need statutes that forbid one person from hitting or beating another, or statutes that forbid unwanted sexual touching. It is simply clear that people have the right to refuse such attacks. And the same applies to unwanted medical treatment. Individuals have the right to choose or decline such interventions.

The Ace of Trump: The Contemporaneous Refusal of a Competent Person

In a sense, this right of refusal by competent patients is the only ace of trump in this context—"competent" really is not the right word here, as it refers technically to a court decision, but "decision-making-capable" is so awkward that "competent" has usually replaced it. If a person who is clearly capable of making the decision refuses treatment, the physician may not treat. Treating in this case is criminal assault and battery. Even the threat to treat is already assault. If a competent patient says, "I do not want any more chemotherapy," and the doctor replies, "You're going to get it anyway, if I have to hold you down and make you take it," that physician has already criminally assaulted the patient, even if he has no intention of following through on the threat and says it just to get the patient to acquiesce. And if the nurses, following the physician's orders, come in and begin to restrain the patient, they and the doctor have both assaulted and battered the patient.

Exceptions That Seldom Trump the Ace of Trump

There are theoretically two exceptions in law to the right of competent persons to refuse treatment: first, the exception sometimes made for pregnant women, and second, the exception sometimes made for parents, usually mothers, of small children. But the first of these hardly ever occurs and the second, although courts used to impose it on occasion, has to our knowledge not been imposed in recent American court decisions.

First Rare Exception: Pregnant Women

Some courts and some state laws have made an exception for a pregnant woman, but this issue is very controversial, and courts often allow the woman and the fetus to die if the woman refuses treatment (Meisel 1989, 110–12; 1995, 1:645–53; 2003, 258). Some advance directive statutes, such as Pennsylvania's Advance Directive for Health Care Act, include an exception for a woman whose fetus might be brought to the stage of viability. But advance directive acts do not apply to presently competent patients, so they do not affect the contemporaneous decision of a competent woman. And, of course, the woman may choose an abortion, which would render the whole issue moot. Indeed, the exception clause for pregnant women clearly stands in tension with the abortion decisions in *Roe v. Wade* (1973) and *Doe v. Bolton* (1973). It is inconsistent on the one hand to allow abortions at the pure choice of the woman and on the other to insist that she cannot refuse life-sustaining treatment for herself if she is pregnant and the fetus can be saved. The right to refuse treatment is far better based in ethics and in law than in the right to abort.

Second Rare Exception: Parents (Mothers) of Small Children

In the past, courts have sometimes required reasonable ("ordinary") treatment to save the lives of parents whose children would otherwise be left orphans, but they have recently stopped doing this (Meisel 1989, 102–3; 1995, 1:516–24; 2003, 229). The exception was more often imposed on mothers than on fathers, and therefore has been perceived as sexist. In addition, American law has been moving further in the direction of the defense of the rights of individuals, and of each person's right to control his or her body regardless of other factors. Thus, parents are usually now given the same right as nonparents to refuse life-sustaining treatment, even if that treatment seems medically indicated or "morally ordinary."

Still the Ace of Trump

So the distinction between kinds of treatment has generally not been a major factor. Even though we might wish to say that we have a moral obligation to take reasonable care of ourselves, to use morally ordinary means to preserve our lives, the law does not recognize this as a legal obligation for competent persons. If a person capable of making this kind of decision decides to refuse life-sustaining treatment, that decision stands.

Illustrative Case: The Anti-Appendectomist

A man comes to the hospital's emergency room with a pain in his lower abdomen, which is quickly diagnosed as acute appendicitis. He is otherwise healthy. The doctor tells him he needs an appendectomy. He says, "No! Take anything else out, but not my appendix." The doctor says, "What are you talking about? Appendectomies are common. Without one, you will almost certainly die." The man says, "I'm terribly sorry, but I belong to the Anti-Appendectomy Sect of the Old Irish Catholic Church. We believe that the appendix is where God keeps our souls. If you take it out, I can never get to heaven to meet St. Patrick." The doctor, if he knows the man well, might even say, "That's the silliest thing I've ever heard." But the man asks, "Do you believe in God?" "Yes," the doctor says, "I'm even Catholic. But I never heard of this Old Irish thing." The man then asks, "Does God act stupidly?" "No, of course not" is the answer. "Then what is the appendix for?" The doctor admits to having no idea. The patient says that the Old Irish know what it's for, since St. Patrick left a hidden message telling us that our souls are in our appendices, and we should never let go of them. He takes out his Old Irish wallet card that says "In an emergency, call an Old Irish priest, but never ever take out my appendix." The doctor, to make sure this is a real church, calls the number on the card, and it is answered by the headquarters of the Old Irish Anti-Appendectomy Church, and they confirm this, even providing their tax exemption number, which the doctor confirms with the IRS. The doctor tries once more. "Once your appendix ruptures, your soul gets loose anyhow." The man says that's irrelevant, because God will keep the soul in a small part of the appendix that will not rupture.

All these seemingly silly details are included as a way of making it perfectly clear that this is a competent person with a perfectly consistent belief on which he is willing to risk his life. He tells the doctor that he will accept the use of antibiotics and other treatments, but not an appendectomy. And that is that. If the surgery is done despite his refusal, it is criminal assault and battery. There is no possible reason to think that he is deluded by sepsis (he has the card and the phone number; his belief is not new). There is no internal inconsistency in that belief; he has thought it out well. He is aware of his condition as it now is. He is aware that he may well die because of his refusal. He is aware that the operation itself is common and will doubtless save his life. He still refuses. Game over. Ace of trump wins. Supreme Court decisions have established this as the law of the land.

Persuasion

None of this means that health care professionals are reduced to silence when a patient refuses a treatment that will offer clear benefit, a treatment that will "fix" the problem.

They are the experts in medicine, and they should try to convince patients to accept beneficial treatments. They serve life when medicine can truly be lifesaving, and it is quite correct to "err on the side of life," as long as this often-used phrase is properly interpreted and applied. When it is clear that "life" cannot be served, that is, when the proposed treatment is morally extraordinary, then "to err on its side" is wrongheaded at best and possibly immoral and illegal. But health care professionals ought to try to persuade patients to accept treatments with a reasonable chance of success for a good outcome. Physicians are not merely "providers" of procedures to "consumers" who choose them and pay for them. The relationship is much more than that. It includes trust and is a covenant between persons seeking a common goal (May 1983). Health professionals are quite right to try to persuade their patients to do what is in the patients' best interests (Groll 2011; Garrett and Lantos 2011). They rightly tell patients to stop smoking, to change diet, to use this medicine. They rightly argue and try to convince, just as the fictional doctor did in the strange appendix case. But the final decision rests with the competent patient.

Demand for Treatment Is Not an Ace of Trump

Competent patients do not have a similar legal right to demand treatment. Although the contemporaneous decision of a competent person to refuse treatment is legally definitive (with the two possible but unlikely exceptions we have noted), the same cannot be said for the decision to request a treatment. Persons cannot ask for treatments that are contrary to the standard of medical care. They cannot pick and choose which treatments they want from a list. They cannot demand treatment A and reject B if B is necessary for A to work. We return to this point in chapter 20.

Waiver of Decision-Making Authority by Competent Patients

The fact that competent patients have the legal right to decide about their treatment, to accept or reject the treatment that the physician recommends, does not mean that they need to exercise that right by making the decisions themselves. They can and sometimes do delegate that authority to someone else. This is most likely to happen when patients feel that someone else, usually a close family member, will understand the medical complexities better than they could themselves. In some cases this may indicate that the patient is really not fully able to make these decisions, but in other cases it is really more a matter of preference.

Some of the most difficult cases involve patients from cultures where custom dictates that other family members, often the oldest male, make these decisions. Here it is not enough to know that the patient wants her son to decide, for example. Doctors, or social workers or chaplains, should try gently to find out why this is the patient's wish. Perhaps she does not agree with the custom but is being forced to comply. Or perhaps the custom itself is so unjust that the physician may decide not to honor it. Insoo Hyun argues that "to be autonomous, a person must also have authentic moral values. She must act on her own values, not on values that were improperly impressed upon her" (Hyun 2002, 14). Yet it is hard to know exactly what "improperly impressed" means. These are difficult cases, and there is no single norm for solving them. In any case, a physician should never simply accept the family's word that they, not the patient, should be informed and should give consent. At the very least, such patients must be informed that in America it is the law that they be allowed to make their own decisions if they wish to do so. Then they should be asked if they want to keep or waive their right to do this.

What Is Competence?

The issue of determining capacity to make decisions of this kind is so complex that we will not attempt here to go into detail (Grisso and Applebaum 1998). The basic idea is that persons have the right to give "free and informed consent" to medical treatment, or to freely and understandingly refuse that consent. To do this, they need to have the capacity to choose freely and to understand what is being asked of them. The factors that might reduce or eliminate freedom and understanding are so many and so controversial that no exhaustive treatment is possible. Indeed, if "free and informed consent" is taken to mean "free from all outside influence whatsoever and informed at the level of medical experts," then true consent is seldom if ever possible. But to conceive it this way is wrong. The human person is not an isolated individual, free from all social influence and interaction. So perfectly "competent" patients will quite rightly take into account the wishes of their families and others who may be influencing their decisions, and such influence does not mean that the consent is not free.

There are some general criteria used in determining that a patient has decision-making capacity. Many are found in the Anti-Appendectomist case. The patient must be free from all openly coercive influence. If a physician suspects this may be present, the patient should be questioned alone. The patient must be able to understand in basic human terms the diagnosis and prognosis and the risks and benefits of the treatment as well as any reasonable alternative approaches. The physician is legally required to give whatever information the patient reasonably needs to make an informed judgment (Meisel 1989, 28–29; 1995, 1:95–97). Heather Gert suggests that it is better to give more than this, to give enough so that the patient "will not be surprised by whatever happens—unless the physician is also surprised" (Gert 2002, 23). And the physician should explain this in language the patient can understand. Hospital ethicists find that this is the key issue in many consults. Patients (or, if the patient is not competent, surrogate decision makers) are all too often given medical jargon, and in the often overwhelming context of the modern hospital, they may well nod and say they understand. But how is a patient or a family to know that a total bilateral occipital infarct means permanent blindness unless the doctor takes the time to say that? The patient should be able to answer the doctor's well-worded questions. "Do you understand that you will be blind?" "Yes." "What will that mean for you?" "It will mean that I will need help because I won't be able to see."

The competent patient's decisions will exhibit consistency. This means two things. First, the decisions reached on Monday should not differ seriously from those reached on Wednesday unless the patient's condition has changed or unless she is able to articulate why she has changed her mind. Second, the decisions reached should be consistent with the patient's own articulated values. If a patient says that he wants to be allowed to die in peace and then insists on CPR after cardiac arrest, it may be that he does not understand what CPR is, so that the doctor should tell him, or it may be that he is not able to understand. Usually conversation will disclose which is the case. In any case, competent patients will be able to articulate to some degree a consistent sense of what their goals are, as well as to understand how suggested treatments would impact those goals.

It is important to note that competence in this sense is relative to the kind of decision that is to be made. Decision-making capacity should be seen more as a sliding scale than as an either/or judgment. Patients who cannot balance their checkbooks or do their own taxes may be perfectly able to understand their diagnosis and prognosis and the treatment options available to them. On the other hand, deciding about life-sustaining treatment requires more capacity than deciding what to order for supper. And it is often the case that patients are more capable at certain times of the day than at others, or more capable just before, or just after, a medication is administered. Effort needs to be taken to accommodate these differences.

It is quite proper to worry more about capacity in patients who reject ordinary means of getting better than in those who reject extraordinary ones. The decision to reject a truly beneficial treatment is simply less "reasonable," as most "reasonable people" would accept this kind of treatment. This does not mean that the value system of the physician, or even that of "reasonable people," should trump the values of the patient. The Anti-Appendectomist case has made that clear. But decisions to reject clearly beneficial treatments call for greater attention to patient capacity than is the case when patients accept them.

In most cases it is easy to tell whether a patient is competent to make treatment decisions. There is no legal requirement that a neurologist or psychiatrist must be consulted; in most cases the attending physician knows and can make the decision (Meisel 1989, 211–13; 1995, 1:174–79). But in some cases a psychological or neurological consult may help. Experience tells us, however, that these are far more helpful when the consulting specialists are aware of what the context is than when they are merely called to do a general work-up. The fact that a patient is "oriented times three" (is able to give his or her name, location, and the date) is seldom very helpful in this context.

One issue that often arises is the problem of depression.[2] Sometimes a clinical depression does mean that a patient lacks capacity to decide about treatment. But sadness and hopelessness are not the same as clinical depression, and not all depressions impede this kind of decision-making capacity, as we are starting to learn. Feeling hopeless is not at all irrational when faced with a terminal diagnosis. We need to understand this and not assume that depressed patients cannot make a free and informed consent about treatment (Grisso and Applebaum 1998, 9, 57).

A second question now being raised more formally is the question of competence in adolescents. State laws are often of little help here because they simply determine an age of majority—often eighteen—and then make some statutory exceptions to it for so-called emancipated minors. These may include married teenagers, or military personnel, or girls seeking abortions or contraceptives. Legal investigations by Rhonda Gay Hartman have disclosed that there is significant legal precedent for heeding the wishes of adolescents (Hartman 2000, 2001). The general principle is in any case clear, at least in theory. The contemporaneous decision to forgo treatment made by a person capable of making it must be followed. The question thus is whether a particular adolescent is capable of making this kind of decision. In many cases adolescents are quite capable of doing this. All the same restrictions and concerns that we have been describing that apply to adults apply also, of course, to adolescents. And there is reason to be even more cautious according to the age and experience of the adolescent; twelve-year-olds and seventeen-year-olds may have very different capacities. There is no clear line here. And there is no reason for keeping adolescents out of the conversation.

Catholic Hospitals and Competent Patients Rejecting Ordinary Means

We began this chapter by noting that the relationship between the first pillar (ordinary and extraordinary means) and the third pillar (the legal right of a patient to refuse treatment) is not theoretically clear. Yet, it has become clear in practice, at least regarding patients with decision-making capacity. They may legally reject any and all treatment, even if to most of us such treatment would appear morally ordinary. What is the ethical obligation of Catholic hospitals when faced with a decision by a capable patient to refuse morally ordinary treatment? What should a Catholic hospital do if the Anti-Appendectomist arrives at its ER? Or what should it do if a Jehovah's Witness comes with an easily treatable but potentially fatal loss of blood?

The *Ethical and Religious Directives*, a set of policies for Catholic health care institutions issued by the American Catholic bishops, are not particularly helpful here. Directive 59 concerns the decision of a competent patient to forgo life-sustaining treatment. It states: "The free and informed judgment made by a competent adult patient concerning the use or withdrawal of life-sustaining procedures should always be respected and normally complied with, unless it is contrary to Catholic moral teaching" (USCCB 2009a, dir. 59). But the rejection of morally ordinary treatment is, presumably, "contrary to Catholic moral teaching." Yet American law is quite clear that judgments of competent adults to refuse treatment must always be complied with, whether they are in keeping with Catholic moral teaching or not. Are Catholic hospitals obliged to violate the law against assault and battery by forcing life-sustaining procedures on competent persons?

This situation can perhaps be answered by arguing that for these patients the treatments are morally extraordinary—the ordinary/extraordinary distinction does admit of a good deal of subjective variation—but in some cases this approach gives a more relativist or subjectivist twist to that distinction than it is good for it to bear. For example, do we want to say that appendectomies for acute appendicitis in otherwise healthy individuals become morally extraordinary when the sick person is an Anti-Appendectomist? If we say this, then it becomes morally right for him to reject it. Or we might prefer to say that the treatment is objectively morally ordinary, so that his rejection is ethically wrong but that he is not personally blameworthy (or guilty of sinning) because he does not understand his obligation to have the appendectomy because of his religious beliefs. Saying that the treatment is for him morally ordinary is the more irenic way of approaching this—we might well do that for the Jehovah's Witness who refuses blood—yet it is somehow a bit puzzling to call this treatment "morally extraordinary" and still maintain that this distinction is basically an objective one, as we clearly have to do.[3]

In any case, it is quite clear that Catholic hospitals are not expected to assault their patients. Unlike certain procedures that Catholic hospitals are told to avoid (direct abortion, direct sterilization), this would be a case of requiring them to violate the basic right of a person not to be treated against his or her will. Catholic hospitals could ask competent patients who refuse morally ordinary means to seek help elsewhere, but this would surely not be a common practice.

Is the Law Morally Right?

We have seen that there is an ethical obligation to use ordinary means, and we have found that the law grants competent patients the right to refuse this very treatment. What are we to say about the ethical rightness or wrongness of the law here? Is the law contrary to Catholic ethics? Is it contrary to bioethics in general? Should we try to change it so that competent patients are legally obliged to do what they are ethically obliged to do: take basically decent care of themselves?

It is helpful in this context to distinguish three levels of judgment: (1) the moral rightness or wrongness of the action (the decision to forgo ordinary treatment); (2) the legal status of the action; and (3) the moral rightness and wrongness of the law establishing the legal status. In the case in which someone chooses to reject a morally ordinary means of preserving her life, the answer to (1) is that she acts wrongly, though she may or may not be morally blameworthy in doing so—that depends on subjective factors like knowledge and consent. The answer to (2) is that the law says no one can force her to have the treatment. And the answer to (3) seems to be that the law upholding the right of competent persons to refuse treatment is a morally right or just law.

Reasonable people might dispute this claim. It is important to take seriously the state's interest in preserving life. Yet we need also to worry about the state's imposing its power against the free decisions of clearly competent persons concerning their own health and the treatment they do or do not want. There is something wholesome about the tendency in American law not to intervene in personal decisions. It seems that in the final analysis we are, when considering the contemporaneous decision of a competent person, better off running the risk of a bad decision than running the risk of governmental interference in this kind of decision. The distinction between ordinary and extraordinary, while basically an objective one, includes subjective elements. When competent patients decide for themselves, they are better able than others to take account of these elements. It would be difficult for the courts or other outsiders to determine which treatments should be imposed and which should not. But this difficulty, great as it is, cannot excuse the law from trying to make similar judgments when surrogates decide to forgo treatment for incompetent patients—we turn to this complex question in the next chapter. When surrogates decide, the state simply must require that certain standards be followed.

Conclusion

The right of a patient capable of making free and informed consent to refuse any and all medical treatment is firmly established in American law. The contemporaneous decision of a competent patient to refuse treatment is the "ace of trump" or the "gold standard" as far as American law is concerned. We can now turn to more complicated matters. What happens when we cannot get the contemporaneous decision of a competent person? Here the law tries to get as close as it can to the "gold standard." This sometimes leads to considerable difficulties.

Notes

1. The right to privacy was first articulated by the Supreme Court in *Griswold v. Connecticut* (1965), the case that struck down a statute forbidding contraception, and was repeated in *Roe v. Wade* (1973), the decision legalizing abortion, then in the Quinlan case (*In re Quinlan*, 1976), and often since then. An excellent review of this is found in a paper by David S. Pollock and Todd M. Begg (1990). The *Cruzan* decision (1990) did indeed base itself on this sort of liberty rather than on the right to privacy, and in this the decision was correct. The liberty was claimed on the basis of the Fourteenth Amendment.

2. The ethical issues pertaining to mental health are many, and they are complex. Although much of what is treated in this book can be applied to mental health care, no attempt has been made to investigate those issues in detail. For one approach to a Catholic ethic of mental health care, see Ashley and O'Rourke 1997, 355–94; and Ashley, deBlois, and O'Rourke 2006, 125–61. For an investigation of mental health issues in the context of managed care, see J. L. Nelson 2003.

3. For a Catholic defense of the right of Jehovah's Witnesses to refuse blood, see Devine 1989.

CHAPTER 16

FORGOING TREATMENT, PILLAR THREE

Decisions for Incompetent Patients

Surrogate Decision Making

THUS FAR IN OUR DISCUSSION of the third pillar, we have examined the decisions of a competent person, where the problems are not as difficult as those concerning incompetent patients. The "gold standard" or the "ace of trump" in these matters is the contemporaneous decision of a competent patient. When the patient is not able to make decisions, this ace of trump is not possible. But American law, with its emphasis on individual autonomy, wants to get as close as it can to this gold standard. So the question is, how can we try to follow the wishes of a person who cannot now tell us what he or she wants?

The brief answer is that the treatment decisions will be made by a surrogate, who is a substitute decision maker for the patient. Surrogate decision makers, however, do not have the same total authority as the presently competent person. There is only one ace of trump (the contemporaneous decision of a competent patient). Surrogates are legally and ethically held to certain standards.

A good basic rule to follow when faced with surrogate decision making is this: Ordinarily, surrogates may not choose to forgo (withhold or withdraw) treatment when that treatment is in the objective best interests of the patient. There may be an exception to this when an advance directive specifically rejects a treatment. But even here we need to be very careful before we reject a treatment that has a good chance of success. Advance directives, as we see in the next chapter, always require interpretation. Experience tells us that persons almost never mean to reject truly beneficial treatment in their advance directives. They may say they never want CPR after their heart stops, but they do not mean they would reject CPR if they were electrocuted and could recover. They may say they never want a ventilator, but they mean they would not want to be tethered to it if they have little or no hope of ever getting off ventilation. They would not reject it for a few days in an acute case of pneumonia that would probably respond to antibiotics. And in the rare cases where persons really do mean to reject what most of us think of as morally ordinary or reasonable treatment, it is usually convincingly clear why they do so—for example, when a Jehovah's Witness writes an advance directive rejecting blood transfusion.

This position is not idiosyncratic. In *Principles of Biomedical Ethics*, Beauchamp and Childress write:

> We believe the best interests standard . . . can in some circumstances validly override advance directives executed by autonomous patients who have now become incompetent, refusals by minors, and refusals by other incompetent patients. This overriding can occur, for example, in a case in which a person has designated another by durable power of attorney to make medical decisions on his or her behalf. If the designated surrogate makes a decision that clearly threatens the patient's best interests, the decision should be overridden unless there is a clearly worded, second document executed by the patient that specifically supports the surrogate's decision (2001, 102).

Courts have been increasingly clear that most decisions made by surrogates should be made in the clinical context, "at the bedside," and not by the courts, and in most states a court decision is seldom necessary (Meisel 1989, 238–48; 1995, 1:237–64). Judges realize that they do not have any special competence to make this kind of decision, and that usually it should be made by the family or by some other surrogate decision maker. But the law also recognizes that when this happens, there are certain standards to follow. We will find that the law has tried to make sure that the surrogate makes the decisions the patient would have made. That is, the law tries to get as close as possible to the gold standard, to the competent person's own decision. But since the patient cannot tell us *now* what he or she wants, it is often hard, indeed it is sometimes impossible, to know what that would be.

Standards of Surrogate Decision Making: The *Conroy* Case

Since the 1985 *Conroy* case in New Jersey (*In re Conroy*), three standards—or, as Alan Meisel puts it, "a single standard with three hierarchical parts" (Meisel 1989, 279; 1995, 1:433)—have been applied to cases when surrogates are to decide for the now incompetent patient (Meisel 1989, 277–84; 1995, 1:432–42). *Conroy* referred to a subjective standard, to a limited objective standard, and to a pure objective standard. In the language often preferred by ethicists, these standards are called, respectively, "substituted judgment," "substituted judgment mixed with best interests," and "best interests."

The approach usually preferred by the courts is that the first of these (pure substituted judgment) should be used if possible, then the second, and then, only in default, comes the third (best interests) (Meisel 1989, 268; 1995, 1:345). Although this hierarchy is understandable, it seldom works in the hospital setting. And it is often wrong.

The First Standard: The Subjective or Substituted Judgment Standard

The first standard, the subjective standard, is based *only* on the subjective preferences of the patient. This presumes clear evidence of what a patient actually said she would want under specific circumstances. In a real sense, then, the more widely used term, "substituted judgment," is misleading (Meisel 1989, 278–79; 1995, 1:433). The surrogate's own judgment is not supposed to "substitute" for that of the patient. The surrogate is rather to decide as he or she *knows* the patient would have decided. That is what

Conroy meant by the "pure subjective standard." It was supposed to be purely subjective, based only on the patient's known wishes. And the substituted judgment standard has come to mean this in its usual usage.

The law consistently claims a preference for this standard. This is understandable since the only legal ace of trump in deciding what treatment to give and what to forgo is the contemporaneous clear decision of a clearly competent patient. A decision-capable competent patient tells the doctors that he or she knows that, without this treatment, death will be the result. The patient chooses to forgo the treatment. Game over.

We understandably tend to think that the closest we can get to this ace of trump, when a patient is now not able to decide, is what that person said beforehand. As we criticize the adequacy of this standard, we in no way suggest that the wishes of a competent patient should be ignored after competency is lost. For example, it is sometimes suggested in cases where a competent patient freely rejects a treatment that doctors or family members think should be accepted that perhaps we might wait until the patient loses consciousness and then let the family (the surrogate decision maker) impose the treatment. Clearly this is wrong. Legally and ethically, what we have here is the contemporaneous decision of a competent patient, rejecting this treatment in this illness, knowing that the decision will almost certainly result in death. No one has the right to make any "surrogate" decision for this patient, who does not need a surrogate. But when there is a need for surrogate decision making, this clarity about what the patient would want is often not available. And so there are difficulties connected with the substituted judgment or pure subjective standard.

Problems with Substituted Judgment

The substituted judgment (or pure subjective) standard applies only to now incompetent patients who were previously competent and who expressed something about their treatment preferences. This standard cannot apply to persons who were never capable of making this kind of decision, such as very young children, since they never had wishes about their treatment. But knowing the exact wishes even of a previously competent person presumes some significant amount of evidence. What is not well understood until we have experience with this kind of case is that the availability of this evidence in the kind of precise way that is sometimes (but not always) required almost never happens. Sometimes, of course, this kind of clarity is not needed. Physicians tell the family that nothing useful or curative can be done, and the family can turn to a general treatment directive that asks that nothing be done if there is no realistic hope of a cure. In effect, the advance directive says "Please don't do stupid stuff to me." In this kind of case, the treatment directive can be of great help in assuaging family guilt. The ethicist or the chaplain can explain to the family that they need not worry that they are doing too little to help the dying patient or failing in their responsibilities because this is what the patient would have wanted and is the best way to help him. In these cases, the general treatment directive is very helpful. But it is not the precision of the directive that is essential. It is that the directive helps the family deal with the very real emotional difficulty of letting go. We discuss advance directives in the next chapter.

In other cases, we would like to know the precise wishes of the patient. There is a variable probability of success of a treatment; there is a variable scale of quality-of-life outcomes after a treatment, and this is overlaid with the varying probability of success; and there is some disagreement among the physicians as to either or both of these. One doctor thinks there is a 10 percent chance of full recovery to the patient's base state; another says 30 percent; a third says the treatment can actually improve on the base state but that there is a 50 percent chance treatment will not work at all and another 35 percent chance that it will keep the patient alive in a reduced base state. What to do now?

Very few of us can anticipate what disease we will get, what treatment modalities are available to us, what prognosis and probabilities physicians will present to our surrogates, or, as a matter of fact, what we ourselves would actually decide in that precise unanticipatable situation. Empirical research is now being done to support these claims (Fagerlin and Schneider 2004, 33–35). We may think we know what we would want if we were to be given the choice of a nursing home or death, but when actually faced with this kind of decision, many of us change our minds (for a case similar to this, see Neher 2004). We may think we know that we would not like to go on living if we could not recognize our relatives, but when we see happy people in nursing homes in precisely this state, interacting with their environment in an admittedly reduced way but still quite interested in living, we are perhaps not so sure we would want to die in this condition if we had some easily curable disease.

So the first standard, the one given legal preference, is often far less helpful than we might want it to be. Even when patients have a written treatment directive, it will need to be interpreted, and there is no simple way to make sure it will be interpreted as the patient would want if he or she were able to make the decision in the present circumstances. Indeed, for this and other reasons, some bioethicists are now claiming that treatment directives are not worth the cost and should be abandoned except in situations where clarity is possible (Fagerlin and Schneider 2004). As we have noted, treatment directives can help families make these decisions, especially by alleviating guilt, and thus the claim that they should be abandoned altogether is not valid. But treatment directives are not exact blueprints and need interpretation.

The Second Standard: Mixed Subjective and Objective (Best Interests) Standard

The second standard from *Conroy*, the so-called limited-objective standard, presumes that there is some evidence about what a patient would want but not sufficient evidence on which alone to base a decision. Thus, objective criteria concerning the best interests of the patient have to be used as well.

The Third Standard: Pure Objective or Best-Interests Standard

The third standard, the so-called pure objective standard, assumes that there is no evidence at all about what an incompetent patient would want. The decision is made according to the patient's best interests.

Conclusion to the Standards of Surrogate Decision Making

The legal standards suggested in *Conroy* have been referred to and applied in varying ways by different courts. However, there has been a general preference for ranking them in the order proposed in *Conroy*. We are supposed to look first at the purely subjective wishes of the patient as these are known from previous evidence. Only if this test fails are we to turn to the objective best interests of the patient. As we have noted, this pure subjective standard is seldom available in daily hospital practice. It is therefore clear that in almost all cases the objective best interests of the patient must be considered. This means that the first pillar, the distinction between morally ordinary and morally extraordinary treatments, does indeed come into play when surrogates make decisions for incompetent patients.

Thus, in almost all cases, surrogates may not legally or ethically choose to reject treatment that is in the objective best interests of the patient. The Anti-Appendectomist (introduced in chapter 15) may have the legal right to reject the appendectomy. But his family cannot reject it for him unless they have exceptionally strong, overwhelming evidence that he would have made that fateful choice for himself. It is probably not enough for them to know that he is a member of the Old Irish Anti-Appendectomists. They have to present clear, perhaps even overwhelming evidence that he would have made this judgment in this case, faced now with the real likelihood of dying for his beliefs. And if hospital experience is any basis for judging, this kind of evidence is seldom available.

Courts have been trying to deal with this question. What weight of evidence is needed if a surrogate is to decide to reject a treatment? Is there any difference if the treatment is "objectively" beneficial to the patient? Do we need more evidence of the patient's wishes if the treatment is beneficial—that is, it will probably make the patient better—than we do if it is not? Suppose a time-limited trial on a ventilator will keep a patient alive as doctors try to determine what has caused an illness; it may well be reversible and the patient will go home cured. But the family tells the doctor that the patient told them never to use a breathing machine. Is this enough evidence to let this person die? It should be clear by now that it is not enough evidence. But if we require too much evidence in the other kind of case—the more usual case where families agree with doctors that further treatment is not humanly beneficial to the patient—then we face the opposite problem and we impose too much unreasonable treatment on dying patients.

Thus, there are problems as to how much evidence the law requires and as to whether the objective diagnosis and prognosis count. We will turn now to how the courts are dealing with these problems. We will look first, and in depth, at the *Cruzan* decision, the first case of this kind to be heard by the US Supreme Court, where the proposed treatment was, by any reasonable standard, morally extraordinary. How much evidence of the patient's wishes must surrogates have before they can get the treatment stopped? Second, we will look more briefly at two cases of the other type, where state courts ordered treatment continued because it was considered beneficial to the patient even though the surrogates wanted it stopped. And third, we will turn to the case of Theresa Marie Schiavo, which caused so much controversy. It seems that courts are coming to recognize that when surrogates make the decision, the objective best interests of the patient really do count.

The *Cruzan* Decision

Nancy Cruzan was in her early thirties when her case was decided by the US Supreme Court in 1990 (*Cruzan v. Director,* 1990). For more than six years, she had been in a persistent vegetative state as a result of an automobile accident. She was in a state hospital in Mount Vernon, Missouri, hooked up to a feeding tube that kept her alive. Her parents asked for permission to remove the tube. In most states this could have been done at the bedside without a court order. But in Missouri, disagreement resulted in a court hearing.

The circuit court granted the parents' request. But the state of Missouri appealed to the Missouri Supreme Court, which in a four-to-three split decision overturned the lower court and ruled that because Missouri was a right-to-life state, Nancy Cruzan could not be taken off the feeding treatment. Her parents, with the support of many amicus curiae briefs, appealed to the US Supreme Court. The case was decided on June 25, 1990.

What Might Have Happened

When the case was appealed to the Supreme Court, there were a number of possible directions the Court might have taken. One helpful way to show the importance of this case is to speculate on what the Court might have decided, and to assess the implications of those possible rulings. *Cruzan* is now established in law. But when it was being heard, there was considerable worry among health care providers that the decision might do great harm to the way decisions about forgoing treatment are made.

The worst outcome would have occurred had the Court connected this case with the abortion issue and used it as a way to establish an extreme constitutional interest in defense of life by misapplying to this issue a right-to-life interpretation of the Constitution. To do this, the Court might have insisted that no life-sustaining treatment could ever be forgone. Or it might have allowed the forgoing of treatment only for competent persons and might have refused it for all others. This move toward a more vitalistic posture would have been possible in *Cruzan* without directly overturning *Roe v. Wade*, the 1973 abortion decision with which the *Cruzan* case has often been unfortunately linked. Courts are usually slow to overturn their prior decisions directly, and this might have offered the Court a chance to move in this direction without a direct repudiation of its earlier ruling.

Missouri decided as it did in *Cruzan* because of its stand as a right-to-life state. It was also Missouri that sent the Supreme Court the *Webster* case (*Webster v. Reproductive Health Services,* 1989); there the Supreme Court did move in a more conservative direction away from some previous interpretations of *Roe v. Wade*. In addition, some among the right-to-life movement, though by no means all, have tied the two issues together, insisting that states have an absolute interest in preserving life, an interest that requires them to have laws against all or almost all abortion and against all or almost all cessation of life-sustaining medical treatment.

That the Court did not choose this direction is probably due to a number of reasons. First, the abortion controversy concerns two beings, the pregnant woman and the fetus. All recognize the woman to be a human person, and many claim personhood for the fetus. In *Cruzan* there is no question of a second person being harmed. Second, Nancy Cruzan, like all patients with her condition, could never be conscious, whereas in most cases the fetus, if not aborted, would grow to live a sapient, sentient, meaningful human life. Third, and perhaps most importantly from the Catholic perspective, the tradition of the Roman Catholic Church is best understood as permitting the forgoing of Cruzan's treatment. We return to the specific issue of feeding tubes in chapter 18, but from what we have already seen we can say that a treatment that causes no real human benefit is morally extraordinary. The official position of Catholic moral theology should thus have been in favor of overturning the Missouri Supreme Court's decision and permitting withdrawal of treatment, though some bishops and theologians, misinterpreting their tradition, disagreed. In the abortion issue, the official teaching of the Catholic Church is quite clear that all direct abortions are morally wrong, though many Catholics, including a number of Catholic moral theologians, hold that this judgment cannot be absolute.

The difference between these two judgments in Catholic ethics is based on the distinction between killing and allowing to die, discussed in chapter 14. Abortion, when it is a killing, that is, when it is a direct abortion, is always wrong according to traditional Catholic moral theology. But when abortion is an allowing to die, as in so-called indirect abortions (for example, in hysterectomies as cure for uterine cancer of pregnant women, or in some procedures as treatment of ectopic pregnancy), it is permitted. In the *Cruzan* case, since there is no question of killing, forgoing treatment is not contrary to Catholic tradition. For all these reasons, and doubtless for its own reasons as well, the US Supreme Court did not choose to rule that life-sustaining medical treatment must always be maintained in cases such as Cruzan's.

A second possible outcome, one with equally disastrous potential, was that the Court might have thrown the issue back to the states for state-by-state regulation. Some states might then have ruled that nutrition and hydration might never be forgone, even by competent patients; or that no life-sustaining treatment at all might be forgone; or that surrogates might never choose to forgo such treatment; or that, although such treatment might be withheld, it might not be withdrawn; or states might have passed other similar restrictions. As we have already seen, most states have decided that there is no need for laws on this issue, that decisions can be made by the patient or the surrogate; state legislatures need not design detailed legislation. The Supreme Court did not open the door to the chaos that such a decision might well have brought.

The best decision would arguably have been for the Court to overturn the Missouri decision and with it the Missouri law, thus upholding the right of surrogates to refuse morally extraordinary treatment. Unfortunately, the Court rejected this direction as well. But although it did not make that decision, it did avoid the worst of its possible options.

The Decision

The *Cruzan* decision is a complicated one. There is both good and bad news. This doubtless accounts for the varied reactions the decision received in the media and from ethicists, jurists, and health care professionals. Those who feared a disaster were pleased; those who hoped for the right decision were disappointed.

First the good news. The Court upheld the right of competent persons to refuse medical treatment and based this on the liberty guarantee of the Fourteenth Amendment to the US Constitution. The Court ruled that medical nutrition and hydration are indeed medical treatment and may rightly be forgone. It ruled that withdrawing does not differ from withholding. It pointed to the right of competent persons to write living wills and implied that these directives must be followed when they provide clear and convincing evidence of a patient's wishes. And it suggested the importance of durable power of attorney laws, such that a competent person might hand over decision-making authority to another.

In thus ruling, the Court established for the first time a nationwide legal right to forgo treatment. Eight of the nine justices, with the exception of Antonin Scalia, who claimed that refusing treatment is suicide (Annas 1996, 187), concurred in this, establishing the likelihood that this will not be overturned by a later decision. This is in keeping with the emerging American consensus. It is good law and good ethics.

But there is bad news as well. In a narrow five-to-four decision, the Court ruled that states may require clear and convincing evidence that patients had wished life-sustaining treatment to be forgone before surrogates may choose to forgo it. This applies not only in cases where the treatment can be argued to be in the objective best interests of the patient, but in all cases. On this basis, the Supreme Court upheld the Missouri decision refusing to allow Cruzan's nutrition to be stopped, and it upheld as well the Missouri law requiring clear and convincing evidence of a patient's wishes.

This part of the decision is misguided. The dissenting opinions of Justices William Brennan and John Paul Stevens accurately demonstrate the potential for harm that this decision could bring if other states were to join Missouri in requiring clear and convincing evidence of patient wishes. In this respect the majority opinion, written by Justice William Rehnquist, is seriously flawed. And the opinion of Justice Scalia, who equated refusal of treatment with suicide and who would have had our nation reverse the emerging consensus in radical ways, is quite simply outrageous.

But what is so problematic about allowing states to require "clear and convincing evidence"? It certainly seems reasonable. As Justice Rehnquist points out, decisions to forgo treatment are not reversible. If the requirement for clear and convincing evidence can be met by advance directives such as living wills and durable powers of attorney, why is this such a problem?

The problem is twofold. First, "clear and convincing evidence" is the highest standard of evidence that the law can require in civil matters. If states were to move toward restrictive laws requiring irrational levels of clear and convincing evidence, most of us would be unable to meet the criteria. Most persons who write living wills cannot accurately foresee which diseases they will encounter and which precise sets of treatments they will want forgone in which medical circumstances. We can write general directives, but these might not meet the requirements of clear and convincing evidence.

Second, the poor and uneducated among us, and possibly the young and the old as well, could be disenfranchised from the right guaranteed to the rest of us. Poor people will not hire lawyers to help them through the potential maze. Medicare and Medicaid do not reimburse physicians for counseling patients on this question. On this issue, the five justices of the majority have been remote from real people in real situations. Clinical experience demonstrates that most people do not have living wills and durable powers of attorney. Loving relatives make the decisions for them. If states were to insist on clear and convincing evidence, many Americans would be forced to endure useless and costly medical treatment. And although Justice Rehnquist is right when he says that decisions to forgo treatment are not reversible, state requirements of evidentiary hurdles are not reversible either. Patients such as Nancy Cruzan would be forced irreversibly into useless death-prolonging treatments, becoming pawns of technology.

We have noted the disadvantages of having decisions such as these made by the judicial system. Research by Steven Miles and Allison August lends further support to the position that these decisions are best made by patient, family, and health care team in the clinical setting. Miles and August present evidence of sexist bias in judges' decisions concerning patient choices to forgo treatment (Miles and August 1990). Courts are more likely to accept such choices when men make them than when women do. In twelve of fourteen cases involving women, courts decided there was insufficient evidence of their choice, whereas only two out of eight men failed similar evidentiary requirements. Requirements of clear and convincing evidence would exacerbate this sexism, since they would necessitate constant involvement of state legislatures and courts to determine whether the precise requirements have been met.

The majority on the Supreme Court feared that relatives might not always act in the patient's best interests. And there is some justification for this fear. But this fear should not be the basis for insisting that all surrogate decisions to forgo life-sustaining treatment require clear and convincing evidence of the patient's wishes. It is this part of the decision and of the Missouri law that is seriously flawed. The solution is not to require a largely unachievable level of evidence for all cases. Rather, the answer is to insist that the decisions reached by surrogates take account of the objective best interests of the patient. This is not as dangerous as some might claim. Doctors and other medical professionals make these kinds of decisions all the time. When they decide that a treatment will be humanly beneficial to a patient, that decision and the knowledge on which it is based has to count. If the surrogate is convinced that these particular doctors are wrong, the surrogate can always get a second or third opinion. But if there is a general agreement among physicians that treatment has a clear chance of being beneficial to the patient, this has to be considered. Surrogates may not (ordinarily) forgo treatment when that treatment is in the objective interests of the patient. Thus, if a treatment is to be forgone, it must be clear that the treatment is morally extraordinary; that is, it must be of little benefit or must impose a significant burden that outweighs its benefit. These restrictions, coupled with civil and criminal laws that can be brought to bear in cases where surrogates decide to forgo treatment out of malice or greed, are already sufficient to prevent an outbreak of the criminal behavior that the justices fear.

Nor is there any evidence that this kind of crime occurs with any regularity. As we see in chapter 20, conflicts today arise more often when physicians want to stop treatment and family members want to continue than the other way around. There is simply no reason to require the kind of evidence of the patient's own wishes that the Supreme Court has allowed states to require. To this extent, the Court's decision is a bad one.

The harm that might result is only potential, however. Indeed, the decision to allow states to require clear and convincing evidence of a patient's wishes before surrogates can forgo treatment need have no effect at all on the consensus we have been describing.

At present, only a few states—New York features prominently among them (Meisel 1989, 255; 1995, 1:43–44, 271–76)—have developed laws or legal precedents that seem to require this kind of evidence when the decision is made, as it should be, at the bedside. The evidentiary standard is more likely to be applied only in judicial review (Meisel 1989, 254). Although the legal variations among states and even within states are complex, hospital experience suggests that in most states and in most cases there is no need for "clear and convincing evidence" of a patient's wish before a surrogate can ask that unreasonable or morally extraordinary treatment be forgone. And there appears to be movement, even in those few states that do have such requirements, to come more in line with the general American agreement not to require such hurdles (Meisel 1995, 1:43–44, 239–46).

In *Cruzan*, the Supreme Court merely upheld an existing Missouri law. It did not require such a law on the federal level or insist that other states pass similar laws. With proper understanding on the part of state legislatures, unnecessary and harmful laws requiring clear and convincing evidence of prior patient wishes to forgo burdensome or nonbeneficial treatment will not be enacted.

One final note on *Cruzan*. The case continues to be misunderstood. While the Court said that states *may* require clear and convincing evidence of a previously competent patient's wishes, it is often said that the decision *requires* this standard. For example, in an article published in 2002 in *Ethics and Medics*, the director of the Linacre Institute at the Catholic Medical Association states concerning *Cruzan* that the decision "established precedents for the states in their determination of who can refuse treatment for incompetent individuals. The court held that there should be clear and convincing evidence of the patient's wishes" (Diamond 2002, 4). This is simply false.

What happened to Nancy Cruzan? It is interesting to note that even though the Supreme Court upheld Missouri's law, the state of Missouri decided shortly thereafter not to insist on feeding her. When her parents again asked the local court for permission to withdraw the feeding tube, the state announced that it would have no objection. Theoretically, the reason the state's attorney general's office gave for this turnabout was that further evidence had been found about Nancy Cruzan's own wishes. A few friends came forward to say that she had mentioned how she would not want this kind of useless treatment. This was enough, said the state, to meet the "clear and convincing evidence" requirement. But the same kind of testimony had been offered from the start, though not from these new sources. The real reason for the state's change of tactic seems to have been that the people of Missouri were angry at the state's position, and there was an election coming up. In the absence of state opposition, the judge agreed with the family. Feeding was stopped and Nancy Cruzan died on December 26, 1990 (Meisel 1995, 1:44–45).

Catholic Controversy over Cruzan

During the course of the *Cruzan* appeal, Catholic pastoral leaders and theologians took widely divergent positions. An exploration of these positions may be helpful in furthering our understanding of the issues and will serve as a review of the relationship between Catholic moral theology and American law, and thus as a study of the relationship among the three pillars supporting the present American consensus on forgoing treatment.

The Problem

The authors of this book have argued—and argue in greater detail in chapter 18—that Catholic tradition judges the forgoing of nutrition in cases such as that of Nancy Cruzan to be morally right. Despite this fact, there has been considerable controversy in the American Catholic Church over this case. The reason for this controversy is best understood by looking once again at the three pillars on which the currently emerging American consensus concerning forgoing treatment has been based. The disagreement is based on the fact, as we have often noted, that there is theoretical controversy concerning the relationship between the first two pillars, the "moral" ones, and the third, the "legal" one, that is, between the two pillars that come from Catholic moral theology (the ordinary/extraordinary distinction and the killing/allowing to die distinction) and the pillar that comes from Anglo-Saxon common law or from American constitutional law (the concepts of liberty, privacy, and autonomy).

This theoretical controversy has not been resolved, despite the fact that courts have been moving toward a practical resolution of this relationship in such cases. In addition, there is debate among legal scholars over whether a legal right to privacy exists in the Constitution, and debate over how far it or similar legal rights and freedoms ought to extend. These debates are basic to the Catholic controversy over *Cruzan*.

Two Catholic Briefs in Cruzan

Among the amicus curiae, or "friend of the court," briefs submitted to the Supreme Court in the *Cruzan* case were two by official Catholic organizations. One position is presented in the brief submitted by the United States Catholic Conference (USCC) (USCC 1989), the educational and research wing of the National Conference of Catholic Bishops, which argues against the request to withdraw the gastrostomy tube.

In the brief, the bishops cannot and do not appeal to their own tradition to argue that it is morally wrong for Cruzan's treatment to be stopped. They cannot and do not claim that their own tradition rejects the right to refuse morally extraordinary treatment, treatment that is of little benefit or that, while of benefit, is of considerable burden. Nor do they claim that the continued treatment of Nancy Cruzan offers her sufficient benefit to make it an ordinary means and therefore obligatory. Nor do they claim that there is no burden involved, certainly to the family or to society, or—in terms of useless affliction and thus of degradation, though not of actual suffering—to Nancy Cruzan herself. Nor do they claim that their own tradition holds that the forgoing of morally extraordinary treatment is euthanasia, that is, is killing. Rather, the Catholic tradition says it is allowing to die, and is morally right in cases like Cruzan's. Nor do they claim that they would want the law to make it illegal for surrogates to choose to forgo other morally extraordinary means, such as ventilation; yet they make no coherent attempt to distinguish medical nutrition from medical ventilation. Thus, they seem to be aware that their own tradition would not allow them to say that the withdrawal of Cruzan's feeding tube is immoral, although they never explicitly state what they think the morality of withdrawal in this case would be.

Nonetheless, they argue that it ought to be illegal. They do so mostly because they oppose the understanding of the right to privacy and autonomy on which the legal submission by Cruzan's family was based. This is at least partly because the bishops fear that the support of such a right to privacy will sustain the so-called right to abortion, which the Church officially opposes. This is clear in the brief itself, where reference is made to abortion on demand as a result of such a right to privacy.

The bishops rightly fear that an absolute stress on the right to privacy and autonomy to the detriment of the state's interest in support of life would create an imbalance not intended in the Constitution, which would support an unrestricted right to abortion and would also open the door to euthanasia. They fear that the right to privacy might support a legal right to assistance in suicide. Therefore, they opposed the Cruzans' petition to remove the feeding tube.

But this means that they argue it ought to be illegal to do what their own tradition says it is morally right to do. This is incoherent. It is also dangerous. If the decision in *Cruzan* had rejected patients' and surrogates' rights to refuse useless treatment, a likely result would have been a backlash, both on the basis of economic impossibility and on the basis of human cruelty to patient and family. That backlash might very well have led to what the bishops fear, legislative action to permit euthanasia. Indeed, there is already some evidence that the *Cruzan* decision has furthered the euthanasia movement.

But a second Roman Catholic brief was submitted in the *Cruzan* case, this one by SSM Health Care System, a St. Louis–based corporation of the Franciscan Sisters of Mary, representing 130 Catholic health care facilities nationwide (SSM Health Care System 1989). This brief makes all the proper distinctions and comes up with the right answer, true to Catholic tradition. Like the USCC's, the SSM brief argues against the absolutizing of the right to privacy such that euthanasia might become a legal right. For the SSM, as for the USCC, sanctity of life is essential. The Constitution does not propose an absolute right to privacy or autonomy. Citizens pay taxes; we have no absolute right to keep all our earnings and do with them what we want. The common good requires sharing, even a sharing legally enacted by the government. Humanly, as well as legally, there is no perfect privacy or perfect autonomy. Privacy and autonomy are unhelpful terms if they are taken to imply a reductionist isolated individualism. Informed consent, a medical ethical process based on the notion of patient autonomy, does not presuppose that the patient makes decisions free from all sources of social influence. This notion of privacy and autonomy is neither possible nor desirable. In arguing against absolutist interpretations of the right to privacy and autonomy, the USCC and the SSM briefs are in agreement.

But, unlike the USCC brief, the SSM brief properly points out that in the *Cruzan* case the withdrawal of treatment is the withdrawal of extraordinary means and is not euthanasia. It insists that beneficial (or morally ordinary) treatment may not legally or morally be withheld by surrogate decision makers, a position with which the courts have generally agreed. It insists on the importance of the benefit–burden analysis. It argues against the two extremes mentioned in chapter 13, the extreme of insisting that everything be done to preserve biological life and the extreme of disregarding the importance of physical life altogether. It is, in sum, well written, properly reflective of the Catholic tradition, and the basis for good law.

The question remains of what to do about persons who are capable of making decisions and who reject morally ordinary treatment. Should this decision on their part be made illegal? Should they be forced to have the treatment? As already noted, it seems that the present agreement of the courts—that persons capable of making these decisions be allowed to refuse any and all medical treatment (that adult Jehovah's Witnesses, for example, be allowed to refuse blood transfusions)—is morally correct. But this is an area where Catholic tradition and American law may be seen, in some interpretations, to disagree. In the *Cruzan* case, however, there should be no such point of contention. Despite recent controversy and some recent Church documents that are reviewed in detail in chapter 18, Catholic tradition is clear that Cruzan's treatment may rightly be forgone since it is the forgoing of morally extraordinary means, which is ethically right, and since it is allowing to die and not euthanasia.

Conclusion to the *Cruzan Decision*

The *Cruzan* case concerns the petition of a surrogate to withdraw morally extraordinary treatment. In this kind of case, the laws of most states permit that decision to be made at the bedside by surrogates in communication with the medical team. But what are the courts doing about cases where surrogates decide to withhold or withdraw treatment that the medical team or someone else claims to be truly beneficial? What role does the best-interests standard play? Fortunately, the correct position on this issue, that the patient's best interests should be considered, is gaining legal support. We turn now to a brief look at two cases of this kind.

Martin and *Wendland* and the Emerging Consensus

State laws differ on the quality of evidence needed before surrogates are allowed to forgo treatment for a patient. But there is a growing convergence of court judgments about what to do when it seems that the treatment may be of benefit to the patient, and surrogates claim that they know the patient would not have wanted it. Cases such as these are difficult because the degree of benefit from the treatment and the kind of life the patient is leading vary from case to case and are interpreted differently by different people. Still, it seems that courts are beginning to recognize that the substituted judgment standard does not trump the best-interests standard after all. Even in states where clear and convincing evidence of a patient's wishes is, quite rightly, not required when surrogates decide to forgo morally extraordinary (not really beneficial) treatment, courts are not allowing them to forgo beneficial treatment unless it is truly clear that the patient said that he or she did not want it.

Martin v. Martin

The *Martin* case was heard in Michigan in 1995. The patient's brain was damaged in a car accident. The Michigan court refused to allow the patient's wife to withdraw the feeding tube even though she claimed her husband had told her he would not want to be kept on machines. The court almost certainly did this because Martin was still able to interact with his surroundings to some extent. Interpreted one way, it might seem that Michigan has joined New York and Missouri as states requiring clear and convincing evidence when surrogates want to forgo treatment (Meisel 2003, 13–15). If so, this would be unfortunate. But, as Alan Meisel points out, "It is essential to note that the court intimated that the holding . . . might not apply to patients more seriously injured than Martin, specifically, patients in a P.V.S. [persistent vegetative state]" (ibid., 15). Whether the court's specific decision in this case was right is not clear; much would depend on details about Martin's condition. And clearly the forgoing of treatment without clear and convincing evidence must not be limited to PVS patients. But it does seem that the general direction of the decision is right in that it supports the legal importance of the objective best-interests standard. Substituted judgment does not automatically supersede best interests.

Wendland v. Wendland

The situation in the 2001 California *Wendland v. Wendland* case was similar to the situation in *Martin v. Martin* (Dresser 2002). Robert Wendland was severely brain-damaged in a car accident. He was incontinent, paralyzed, and on a feeding tube. But he was able to interact and to respond to simple commands. Three family members told the court he had told them that he would not want to be kept alive in this kind of circumstance. They claimed that he had said this often and strongly. When they asked the hospital to remove the feeding tube, an ethics consult was called and the ethics committee agreed. But two other family members opposed this and obtained a restraining order. Two California courts decided in effect that the patient's best interests required that nutrition not be withdrawn. The California Supreme Court determined that a lower standard of evidence than "clear and convincing evidence" of a patient's wishes is enough to allow the forgoing of treatment when the patient is terminally ill or permanently unconscious, but that in cases such as *Wendland*, there has to be clear and convincing evidence that this patient would not want this treatment in this circumstance. The best-interest standard counts.

Again, as with the *Martin* case, the point is not to defend actual decision—that would depend on Robert Wendland's actual condition.[1] But such cases in which patients have suffered from strokes or other brain injuries leading to severe mental impairment are frequent. One of the authors of this book, Dr. Kelly, recalls two cases that were somewhat like *Martin* and *Wendland*. In one of these, the consult team decided that the patient's condition—there was no interaction with the environment at all, although she was not technically in PVS—warranted the family's request to forgo continued nutrition and hydration. In the other case, the patient was still able to interact in a happy if significantly restricted way. The consult team decided that the feeding should not be forgone. Neither decision was without its critics. Some claimed that the correct decision should have been to maintain feeding for both—the team did not sufficiently value life. Others suggested that nutrition should have been withdrawn from both—the team was too vitalistic and did not pay sufficient attention to what the families wanted or to what they said they knew about the patients' wishes. And still others agree with what was done. This kind of judgment is not always easy. But it is clear that the substituted judgment standard and the best-interests standard cannot be seen in isolation from one another. In almost all cases, both the prior wishes of the patient (substituted judgment/subjective standard) and the patient's present condition and the possible outcome of treatments (best interests/objective standard) have to be considered. Substituted judgment does not deserve the automatic hierarchy over best interests that some court decisions have given it.

But this does not mean that the wishes of previously competent persons are insignificant. One of the ways patients can help in ensuring that these wishes will be carried out is by advance directives. We discuss these in the next chapter.

The *Schiavo* Case

The case of Theresa Marie (Terri) Schiavo offers a further look at the issue we are discussing, how to decide whether a surrogate's wishes to forgo treatment ought to be honored. The case became well known—even notorious—with political, legal, and ethical implications. This section introduces the case and briefly suggests its legal implications for honoring surrogate decisions. In chapter 18, we return to it in the context of recent debates in Catholic bioethics.

On February 25, 1990, Theresa Marie Schiavo suffered a cardiac arrest that resulted in a loss of oxygen to her brain. All tests taken then and thereafter showed that she was in a persistent (permanent) vegetative state (Quill 2005, 1630). I return to a fuller description of this condition in chapter 18 and for the moment note only that PVS means a total lack of capacity for inner or outer awareness. PVS patients cannot dream, pray, suffer, or experience thoughts, emotions, or feelings of any kind. They do exhibit movement and their eyes do open and close and wander about, which is often misunderstood, especially by family members, as attempts to communicate (Ms. Schiavo was often shown on television this way). But these movements are completely involuntary and not in response to the environment.

After eight years of caring for his wife in this condition, Michael Schiavo decided to ask that the feeding tube be removed. Members of his wife's family objected. Two Florida courts found clear and convincing evidence that she was in PVS and that she would not want continued treatment were she able to decide (note the importance here of the objective, best-interests standard; there was no advance directive, and evidence of her wishes was not entirely clear). The Florida Supreme Court declined to review that decision (Annas 2005, 1711).

But because of objections from family members who claimed they had new evidence of her condition and new treatment options, another court hearing took place in 2003 (*In re Guardianship of Schiavo*). Again the court agreed with her husband, and again the Florida Supreme Court refused to hear an appeal (Annas 2005, 1711–12). Family members, with support from some religious and political groups, then asked the Florida legislature to enact a law requiring that the feeding be continued, which they did in passing "Terri's Law" in October 2003. The law was drawn up in such a way that it applied only to her and to no one else (Annas 2005, 1712). In the fall of 2004 the Florida Supreme Court ruled this law to be unconstitutional because it was an encroachment by the legislative branch onto the judicial branch of government (*Bush v. Schiavo*). The US Supreme Court refused to hear the case. The feeding tube was removed on March 18, 2005.

In a final attempt to maintain the feeding tube, the US Congress reconvened from Easter recess for the express purpose of enacting a law concerning Theresa Schiavo.

Annas correctly notes the "uninformed and frenzied rhetoric" that was part of the debate in Congress (Annas 2005, 1713). A number of Republican physician-members of Congress claimed to be sure that she was not in PVS, a claim that would be refuted when an autopsy after her death showed clear evidence that that indeed had been her condition. The law Congress passed, which was signed by President George W. Bush on March 21, in effect required a federal court to hear the case. On the next day the federal court ruled. US District Court judge James D. Whittemore refused to order the feeding tube to be reinserted (*Schiavo ex rel. Schindler v. Schiavo*) (Annas 2005, 1713–14). Theresa Marie Schiavo died, still unconscious, on March 31, 2005, more than fifteen years after her last conscious experience.

In the aftermath of this case, with all its attendant publicity, one conclusion commonly drawn was the need to make one's wishes clear in written advance directives (Dombi 2005). Had Terri Schiavo done this, it was said, the strife and the drawn-out court battles would not have occurred. But our discussion of treatment directives in the next chapter uncovers significant reasons why they often do not in fact provide the resolution that is sought. Thus the principal legal conclusion to be drawn from this unfortunate case is, as Rebecca Dresser claims, that there is a need for some sort of objective standard in the law. Dresser points to *Martin*, *Wendland*, and *Schiavo* as three cases underlying this need (Dresser 2005, 21). And this is precisely what we argue for in this chapter. The pure subjective standard (the pure substituted judgment standard), to which courts have all too often given preference, is insufficient. Regarding the *Schiavo* case, Dresser writes: "Much of the opposition to the Florida court rulings was based on weaknesses in the substituted judgment standard. The testimony about Ms. Schiavo's previous statements was general enough to raise doubts about whether she would indeed have refused nutrition and hydration. And years after her brain injury, with her family so divided, could anyone really know what she would decide if she were, in the language of the *Quinlan* court, 'miraculously lucid for an interval . . . and perceptive of her irreversible condition'?" (Dresser 2005, 20).

In *Schiavo*, it is clear that objective evidence *was* considered by the courts and that they properly judged the decision of her husband, Michael, to remove the feeding tube to be the right one. We return to this case later, when we examine some recent developments in the Catholic debate about feeding tubes.

Deciding for the Never-Competent

The issues we have been looking at apply to patients who once were able to make decisions and now no longer can. In these cases, surrogates need to look at the patients' previously expressed wishes as well as at their best interests. In cases of young children or others who, perhaps because of a lifelong mental deficiency, have never been able to make or express autonomous wishes about treatment, the situation is in many ways easier. Now it is clear that only the best-interests standard (pure objective standard) ought to apply. It is sometimes argued that parents and other family members may rightly include their own interests in this decision, but this is not generally accepted and has never been sanctioned by courts. While it is perfectly normal for family members to do this to some extent, health care providers would never be justified in acting contrary to the clear best interests of a child or other never-competent person.

The paradigmatic case here is that of the young child whose Jehovah's Witness parents ask that a lifesaving blood transfusion not be given. In these cases, courts have consistently overruled the parents, and in emergency situations it is clear that physicians must transfuse (Meisel 1989, 417–21; 1995, 2:283–89). In emergency cases it may be possible to get a court order over the telephone, but even if this is not done, emergency transfusion is required. The clear best interests of the child prevail legally and ethically. When the benefit and the necessity of the treatment are less clear, courts are not as quick to override parental refusal (Meisel 1989, 417–21; 1995, 2:283–89).

However, we need to be especially aware that the best interests of the child or other incompetent patient are not limited to the physical or medical. The child will return to his or her family and will have to live with them. If they now reject the child, even unconsciously, because he or she has in their minds been tainted, this is contrary to the child's best interests, not just to those of the parents. If there is an alternative treatment that is likely to be successful, it should be considered.

Illustrative Case: A Hip for a Jehovah's Witness

Dr. Kelly was asked to consult on a case where a child of Jehovah's Witness parents needed a new hip. He was chronologically an adult but suffered from moderately severe retardation. The orthopedic surgeon said that it was likely he would need to be transfused as part of the surgery and said he would not do the surgery unless permission were given for transfusion. The ethics consult team quickly reached the "right" conclusion that the best interests of the child meant the need to override the parents' objection. But a sensitive and very "streetwise" social worker was not so quick. He pointed out that the child might indeed be harmed by the transfusion, not medically but socially and psychologically. Family cohesion is important. So he called neighboring hospitals and found a surgeon who said he knew that in this case he could do the work without the need for blood. He informed the parents of this, and they gladly had him do the surgery. Sometimes the book answers are not the right ones. It is also sometimes the case that Jehovah's Witnesses will refuse the transfusion of whole blood but will accept certain blood products or even autologous transfusion of stored blood. Imagination and sensitivity are required attributes for ethics committees.

Note

1. Indeed, if the facts in the case are properly interpreted by Lawrence Nelson, the attorney who represented Robert Wendland's wife, Rose, who wanted the treatment stopped, then it does seem that continued feeding may not have been in Robert's best interests (L. Nelson 2003). Although Wendland was not technically in PVS, Nelson claims that he was very close to that condition because his interaction was minimal at best. And though the court found he was not terminally ill, he did indeed die (of pneumonia) despite ongoing treatment three weeks before the court issued its decision. Nelson argues that the court's requirement of clear and convincing evidence, despite the exception the court made for PVS and for terminal illness (Dresser 2002, 10), may well be too stringent. Surrogates ought to be able to forgo treatment that is not in the patient's best interests even when there is no clear and convincing evidence of what the patient would have wanted, and this should not be limited to permanent unconsciousness or terminal

illness in the legal sense. This is the very argument made in this chapter in the context of the *Cruzan* case. So the actual decision in the *Wendland* case may have been wrong. Courts are not the best venue for this kind of complex decision. But it is good that courts are beginning to recognize that the best-interests standard does count even when surrogates claim they know what the patient would have wanted, although in this case the court may well have misunderstood what that standard means.

In line with this, scholars are beginning to criticize the all-too-often automatic preference given to autonomy over beneficence. Carl E. Schneider (2004) issues what he calls a cri de coeur (heartfelt cry) about this in a brief piece on a court decision to allow autonomy to override the best interests of a schizophrenic patient who refused medication. He laments that "from the start . . . 'individual rights' and 'autonomy' exude the odor of sanctity, while 'state interests' and 'beneficence' trail the stench of paternalism, even tyranny" (10). Alexia Torke, G. Caleb Alexander, and John Lantos likewise note the inadequacies of the substituted judgment standard and propose that a community standard be used to support the best interests of patients (Torke, Alexander, and Lantos 2008). Legal scholar Rebecca Dresser argues that we must "question not only the absolute priority of substituted judgment over best interests, but also the absolute priority of advance directives over best interests" (Dresser 2009, 3). Bioethics is best served when it serves its patients, which requires considering beneficence (the best-interests standard) along with autonomy (the substituted judgment standard) rather than giving automatic precedence to autonomy.

CHAPTER 17

FORGOING TREATMENT, PILLAR THREE

Advance Directives

Two Kinds of Advance Directives

AN ADVANCE DIRECTIVE (not "advanced") is just that; it is an instruction made in advance by a competent person that lays down what that person wants if he or she should become ill and unable to make treatment decisions.

There are two kinds of advance directives: proxy directives and treatment directives. Proxy directives appoint someone to make decisions if a person no longer can do so. Treatment directives (often called living wills) are instructions, usually in writing, about what kind of care a person would want. Because proxy directives are often more helpful than treatment directives, we will begin with them.

Proxy Directives (Durable Powers of Attorney for Health Care)

A proxy directive, sometimes called a durable power of attorney (DPA) for health care, is a document by which a person appoints a surrogate decision maker. States have different laws concerning these. States may require that they are written according to some approved formula, or law may suggest a form but not impose it. A durable power of attorney refers to a legal device by which one person transfers certain authority to another. Some powers of attorney are not durable. That is, they cease once the person authorizing them loses the capacity to decide and thus to revoke them. Powers of attorney are often granted to authorize others to take care of financial matters, deal with investments, and so on. In some cases of this sort, the person wants to be able to oversee the decisions of the one authorized to act on his or her behalf, and so makes it clear that when he or she cannot do so, the power stops. In the case of health care, however, the entire idea is to appoint someone to make decisions when the person no longer can, so when these are called "powers of attorney," they are durable; they are still in effect after the person loses the capacity to revoke them. Indeed, they do not go into effect or become operative until the person loses decision-making capacity because otherwise the person makes decisions for himself or herself. The name used—"health care proxy" or "durable power of attorney for health care"—does not really matter; it will depend on how the law of an individual state is crafted. All the states now have some kind of law authorizing advance directives of this kind.

This approach is simpler than treatment directives and has a number of advantages. One ethicist has called it the "Committee of the Person" (Maguire 1974, 169–71). I appoint another person or possibly, but not usually, a group of persons to make decisions concerning the treatment to be given in case I am unable to make such decisions for myself. The advantages of this approach are its flexibility and its stress on human friendship and love. I express a trust in another person to do the best possible. No one can ever predict completely the circumstances of a particular process of dying. This approach simply says to a family member or friend: "I trust you. Do what you think is right, what you feel I would want. I trust your motives. If you make a mistake, so be it. It is better for me to put this trust in you than in my physicians, or the courts, or even (possibly) my family."

This approach is admittedly not perfect. There are some aspects of it that might be called disadvantages. What of possible conflict of interest? The person I appoint might turn out later on to hate me, or want my money. What of the burden this might impose on the surrogate? In this approach—indeed, in aspects of this whole question generally—what I think I will want when I am healthy and watching people dying on TV can be quite different from what I actually feel and want when dying. Despite these difficulties, there is much that is humanly attractive in this idea. And there is little or no opposition to it among Catholic ethicists. Assuming the actions taken by the surrogate do not include active euthanasia or physician-assisted suicide, which are illegal in most states, there is no reason for the tradition of Catholic moral theology to reject proxy directives.

The *Cruzan* decision may have increased the importance of proxy directives. In her concurring opinion, Justice Sandra Day O'Connor suggested the possibility of a future Court ruling that surrogates appointed by power of attorney have exactly the same right to decide as the patient would have if capable to do so. If the Supreme Court were to issue such a ruling, this would go beyond the general consensus by allowing legally appointed surrogates to withhold humanly beneficial treatment based on substituted judgment, and would not require that such decisions be in the best interests of the patient. To date this has not happened. As we saw in the previous chapter, state court decisions appear to be insisting that best interests be considered. Still, the *Cruzan* decision does underline the authority of the surrogate and the importance of choosing wisely. It is quite clear that the Court explicitly intended to suggest the durable power of attorney as one of the ways in which states might acknowledge that patients have given clear and convincing evidence of their wishes. So, in the wake of *Cruzan* and of *Schiavo*, especially in those states with strict evidence requirements, durable powers of attorney may be the citizens' best bet.

Treatment Directives (Living Wills)

The second kind of advance directive is an instruction or treatment directive, made through a document often called a living will. This is a document drawn up or a form filled out by a competent person to give instructions concerning the kind of treatment the person wishes if he or she is seriously ill and not able to make treatment decisions. Most treatment directives ask for a limitation of treatment, but that is not required; directives can also request aggressive treatment. There is a standard form of the type of living will that limits treatment, although there are a number of variations of it. The operative paragraph in the form suggested by Concern for Dying, an organization formed to help people prepare for death, is this: "If at such a time the situation should arise in which there is no expectation of my recovery from extreme physical or mental disability, I direct that I be allowed to die and not be kept alive by medications, artificial means, or 'heroic measures.' I do, however, ask that medication be mercifully administered to me to alleviate suffering even though this may shorten my remaining life."

It is clear that in this document there is no question of active euthanasia. Although the document is vague, it enables us to express our general desires concerning treatment. It gives the physician at least a general sense of our wishes. It says, in effect: "Don't do stupid stuff to me!" The living will is morally acceptable for those who find comfort in signing one, and it is in keeping with the Catholic tradition.

Three points about treatment directives are very important and are sometimes overlooked. First, the absence of such a directive is not an indication that a patient wants heroic measures or morally extraordinary means of treatment. Indeed, most people do not have treatment directives. Physicians ought to discuss these matters with patients and get a sense of their wishes. This type of discussion can be initiated in a nonthreatening way while the person is still healthy. Patients may begin these discussions themselves. And family members often, though not always, discuss issues of this kind among themselves. Physicians and nurses should ask their sick relatives if they have talked about this. The lack of documents should never be construed as an indication that a patient would have insisted on aggressive treatment.

Second, living wills do not always mean that patients want treatment forgone. We have presented them that way here because this is usually the reason they are used and is the context envisioned by those who support them and by the state legislation about them. Historically, they were developed to return the authority to forgo treatment to patients from doctors who tended to insist on it. But persons who make living wills are not required to say in them that they want to forgo extraordinary means or aggressive treatment. They can write them to say they *do* want such treatment. In Pennsylvania, for example, the law requires that persons specify in any statutorily enforceable treatment directive whether they do or do not want tube feeding if they are permanently unconscious. It cannot be presumed that they say no. Advance directives have to be read. It is not enough just to chart them.

Third, the fact that a person has signed a treatment directive does not mean that the patient is refusing CPR in the event of cardiac arrest! Unfortunately, it seems that when a patient is asked on admittance to a hospital about a living will and says that there is one, there is some tendency to assign an automatic DNR—do not resuscitate! And this happens even for patients admitted in good health for minor and curable illnesses. Somehow the terms "advance directive" and "living will" are translated in the busy hospital setting to "DNR." Although not common, it happens that some persons with treatment directives deny having one when admitted for minor illnesses, from fear of just this danger.

State Laws

The issue becomes more complex when the question of statutory change in state laws is introduced. These "natural death acts" or "advance directive for health care acts" generally make legally binding (or at least legally recognized) documents similar to, but often more specific than, the living will. There are reasons to worry about some of this legislation, although it is now so widespread that perhaps the risks of these laws are not as serious as some ethicists initially feared. Still, there are problems.

First, natural death acts may suggest the legalization of active euthanasia (a bill introduced into the Idaho legislature, but not passed, fell into this category; a number of initiatives have been introduced to make active euthanasia or assisted suicide legal; in Oregon and Washington, and possibly Montana, as we see in chapter 19, physician-assisted suicide is legal). Moralists who oppose active euthanasia also oppose those statutes that allow active euthanasia or are potentially open to that possibility.

Second, paradoxically, some natural death acts are so specific that they imply that only in this particular case or under these special circumstances can treatment be withheld or withdrawn. These bills tend to reduce, at least implicitly, the flexibility given to the families of dying incompetent patients. In some states, for example, laws specifically ruled out the inclusion of nutrition and hydration as treatments that a person may request be forgone (and such a ruling may now be illegal in light of *Cruzan*). In Pennsylvania, persons who make advance directives must say whether they want tube feeding if they are terminally ill or permanently unconscious; if they fail to fill in this part of the document, they must be given this treatment if it is medically indicated. Persons who do not make an advance directive may be able to escape tube feeding if their families agree. With this kind of legislation, living wills may paradoxically increase the likelihood that treatment will be continued, either because the law forbids including the permission to forgo a certain treatment, or because the document that the person signs does not explicitly include a specific treatment or a particular circumstance in the general permission granted to withhold or withdraw treatment.

Third, there is the similar danger that those who have not signed such a document will find that invasive and useless medical measures are taken to prolong life simply because they have failed to do so. Physicians, and possibly courts, may assume that because a given patient never signed such a document, the patient did not want treatment withheld under any circumstances. The passing of a statute to enact a right that people already have can reduce that right by implying that the state grants it, whereas in fact it is a "natural" right, recognized as such by common law and by the courts in many states. This problem is increased in those bills that require that the document be periodically renewed. What if the person fails to renew it? Does this imply that this individual wants no cessation of heroic treatment even when such treatment would ordinarily be easily forgone with the family's agreement? Does this imply that there is no evidence of the patient's wishes on which to base substituted judgment?

One way in which some state laws try to alleviate these problems is by saying explicitly, as does the Advance Directive for Health Care Act in Pennsylvania, that the law is cumulative legislation. That is, this new law is only an addition to the rights people already had to tell their doctors and families what treatment they would want. If people wish to take advantage of the new law, they write their directive according to its legal requirements. This "statutory" advance directive then has the advantages the law gives it, usually some degree of legal force and some degree of immunity from lawsuit to the physicians and hospitals that follow it. And it has disadvantages as well: it may only become effective under certain circumstances (in Pennsylvania, only when a person is terminally ill or in a state of permanent unconsciousness, for example); it may need to be notarized and witnessed by a certain number of persons. But if the state law is clear that the legislation is cumulative, then people can still make their wishes known in other ways as well, by telling their families or by writing their wishes down in another document. In Pennsylvania, a perfectly adequate treatment directive was written on a single yellow sheet of paper by a woman who signed and dated it and gave it to her children. This was not an "operative" advance directive under Pennsylvania law, but courts, including Pennsylvania courts (*In re Fiori*, 1996), do not usually insist on statutory written documents as the only valid sources for knowledge of a patient's wishes. Yet even when it is clear that the legislation is cumulative, there is a natural tendency to think that since the state law has placed certain limitations on its statutory advance directives, it wants these same limitations placed on other, nonstatutory directives as well. Experience teaches that this is true. Medical personnel become aware of the restrictions in the law—they have to know these—and then are less sure what to do with other, nonstatutory directives that they may be ethically and legally required to consider.

Fourth, one final caution applies to any statute whose purpose is to enable the legal allowing of death. Laws must ensure that such policies are not carried out in order to rid society of individuals it considers burdensome or expensive to maintain. The wealthy have better access to medical care facilities and scarce resources. This results in earlier deaths for the poor and powerless. There is always a temptation to eliminate the poor as a way of eliminating poverty. Whatever laws are enacted, controls are essential to make sure this does not happen.

These risks, inherent in state legislation, may not be reason enough to lead to the conclusion that such legislation is on the whole harmful. Whether statutorily authorized or not, treatment directives make it easier for health care professionals to know that the patient had considered these issues and made some decisions. They relieve the minds and consciences of family members who worry what to do, and they help resolve disputes between family members who disagree about the patient's wishes. For all these reasons, living wills are probably a good idea, even if specific legislation about them may be problematic.

The proxy directive allows greater flexibility than is possible with a living will. Now a trusted friend will decide rather than a physician or the court. And this approach offers something theologically essential: an enhancement of human trust and of trust in God. When the "committee of the person" is made legal by a statutorily enforceable proxy directive or durable power of attorney, the person has ensured as much as is possible that flexible and humanly meaningful decisions about treatment will be carried out. Signing a general living will document is also helpful because it adds another indication of what the person wants.

Most people do not have advance directives. But someone still needs to make decisions for them if they cannot do so themselves. Usually the family acts as surrogate decision maker for the patient. In most states (but these differ, so it is necessary to check in one's own state), when there is no proxy directive and when the family members are in agreement about what should be done, there is no need for court involvement. When there is disagreement, it usually helps to wait for a time so that the family can come to agreement. Sometimes, although this is rare (cases such as *Schiavo*, despite their notoriety, are exceptions to the general process), the only answer is recourse to the court.

Interpreting Treatment Directives

When a person cannot make treatment decisions, the law tries to get us back to the "ace of trump," or as close to it as possible. The law would like to have decisions of this sort be clear and precise. Courts usually do not want to have to make these judgments. They want the patient or the surrogate to make them. As we saw in the last chapter, when the patient is not now able to make decisions, it is seldom possible to achieve this "gold standard." The subjective substituted judgment standard almost always needs to be corrected by the objective best-interests standard despite the theoretical priority the law gives to the former (Dresser 2009). That is because people are seldom able to anticipate exactly their future situation. Thus, the treatment directives they leave for their surrogates to follow always need "objective" interpretation. They are rarely enough in themselves to allow a clear decision about treatment to be made. This interpretation is helped by prior communication. Although it is often difficult to do, the earlier the communication occurs, the better. But communication by the person for whom decisions are going to be made should take place—first, with the surrogate who is likely to help do the interpretation, whether that surrogate is chosen by DPA or proxy directive or simply by family relationship; and, second, with the primary care physician.

The *Conroy, Cruzan, Martin, Wendland,* and *Schiavo* cases that we discuss in the last chapter all concerned the need to interpret a patient's wishes. This applies whether a patient has a treatment directive or not. In the real world of the hospital, this task is usually done by physicians and surrogates. They should take into consideration both what they know of the patient's general wishes and what they know of the medical prognosis and diagnosis. Interpretation thus always involves the objective best-interests standard, whether pure or limited. There are very few cases where a general treatment directive (the kind we make when we are basically healthy) could be sufficiently precise to authorize a surrogate to withhold or withdraw a treatment when that treatment is in the objective best interests of the patient (a directive specifying refusal for a religious reason might be an exception). So the presence of a living will does not change the claim made throughout these last two chapters that the gold standard of legal decision making applies *almost only* to currently competent, alert patients and *almost never* to patients who have lost the capacity to decide, even if they wrote down their wishes in a treatment directive.

Exceptions to the Need for Interpretation

There are three areas of exceptions to the need for interpretation, where treatment directives may give precise orders that can be followed. First, since the area of permanent unconsciousness has been analyzed and dealt with in numerous court cases, persons should be urged, when writing treatment directives, to say whether they want to be kept alive should such a diagnosis be made. They should include whether they want ventilation, dialysis, antibiotics, CPR, and—most important—tube feeding.

Second, there are cases in which there is a well-established religious tradition for refusing treatment. The obvious case is that of a Jehovah's Witness who refuses blood. We consider an example shortly where one of the authors expresses his hesitation to withhold transfusion when the Witness is unable to make a contemporaneous decision. But a well-drafted and clear refusal in a living will might be sufficient evidence of the patient's intentions.

Third, once a person is diagnosed with a certain disease, then it becomes more possible for that person to clarify with the physician what exactly is likely to happen and what the options are, and to write down choices about those options. What do we want to call this document? We might call it a treatment directive (it is one) or even a living will. But it is really not an *advance* directive at all. It is, rather, the contemporaneous decision of a competent patient faced with treatment choices about this illness with these characteristics. For example, a patient is told that such and such will likely happen as a cancer progresses (there is seldom absolute certainty in medicine, but in many cases we can be virtually sure of a disease's progress). At some point, decision-making capacity will be lost. We already know that the cancer has metastasized; we have tried chemotherapy. The last attempt failed. The patient is asked: "Do you want another attempt?" "No." "When you lose your ability to breathe unassisted, do you want a ventilator (knowing that once you are on it, you will not be able to get off)?" "No." In a sense, that is an "advance" directive, but in another sense it is the contemporaneous decision of a competent patient. *This* living will is precise enough to follow exactly.

Check-Box Living Wills

What about the living will forms that try to anticipate different scenarios? In response to the criticism that treatment directives are too vague to be really helpful, it would seem possible to design treatment directives that include a number of illness scenarios with treatment options. Some forms are better than others, but all of them take an enormous amount of intelligent perusal and explanation before the subtle distinctions among the scenarios and treatment options are understood. Experience shows that many people fill out treatment directives like these in contradictory ways. If even doctors sometimes order contradictory treatments or tests, surely we must expect laypeople to do it. At the very least, a person who considers using one of these directives should set up a long appointment with his or her physician to go over the options in detail. Physicians are unlikely to spend hours with each of their patients talking about multiple possible future scenarios. But in the absence of such conversation, the check-box living wills are likely to fail at describing the person's wishes, and are even likely to be dangerous if they are followed (Fagerlin and Schneider 2004, 34–35).

Thus, treatment directives almost always need interpretation. The better a health care institution is at this, the better-trained its ethicists, the better its pastoral care department, and the better it is at understanding cultural diversity among patients and surrogate decision makers, the better that hospital or nursing home will be at understanding and carrying out patients' wishes.

Two Examples

Two cases in which it might seem that a patient's wishes have been precisely expressed but in which perhaps there is still room for hesitation serve to illustrate this. We place both cases in Pennsylvania, which allows us to fill in some actual legal details to make the cases more accurate and more interesting.

First Case: Curable Pneumonia

The first case is a fictionalized version of an event said to have occurred in eastern Pennsylvania. A man writes in his treatment directive that he never wants to be intubated or put on a mechanical ventilator. He checks "no" to every single box where a ventilator is mentioned. He signs it, has it notarized, and carries it in his briefcase. He tells his wife, his children, his doctor, and his malpractice lawyer that he never wants a ventilator. He gets pneumococcal pneumonia. The paramedics who come to his house with the ambulance find him gasping for breath and take him to the ER. His wife and his children go with him. The physicians say they can cure him almost certainly with antibiotics. He will be home and well in a week or ten days. But because the bacteria are now suppressing his respiration, they will need to put him on a ventilator for only a few days while the antibiotics work their medical miracle. But his wife and children point to the treatment directive. The physicians agree not to intubate. And the man dies.

Most who have heard of this case agree that he died because no one had the sense to realize that what he meant was "no ventilator when it means that I will lie in bed terminally ill for months on that machine like my mother did." This man died because procedural justice took precedence over substantive good.

In most states where there are laws about treatment directives, the law says that a treatment directive does not become operative until the person is *both* unable to make decisions *and* terminally ill. In Pennsylvania, one must be either terminally ill or permanently unconscious. Terminally ill in the legal sense means an illness from which one is unlikely to recover regardless of any possible treatment. So in this case, according to state law, the surrogates and the hospital personnel should have intubated. The treatment directive was not legally operative because this man was not terminally ill. They made a serious mistake. But it is understandable that they did so. He wrote it down very clearly. What was not grasped was the need to interpret living wills not simply from the perspective of what the person has written (the pure subjective standard, although in this case one could rightly argue that this is not what he really meant), but from the perspective of the person's best interests as well.

But we need to look again at the idea that they should not have followed his treatment directive because the law says it was not operative. Do we want to make an absolute rule out of that? It would mean that we would aggressively treat everyone not permanently unconscious or terminally ill. What if someone writes in her treatment directive that once her Alzheimer's disease progresses to the point where she is no longer able to interact with her environment, she does not want to be hospitalized and intubated if she contracts pneumonia? She finds herself in the situation where she is aphasic (unable to speak), confined to bed, not only unable to recognize people but also unable to react with joy or with sadness to anything around her. She gets pneumonia. They say it can be cured. The Alzheimer's is not yet to the point where it is terminal in any immediate sense. Does this mean that since the state law says the treatment directive is not operative, she must be treated? No. As we have already seen, the Pennsylvania law (and this applies to many other state laws as well) is quite clear that this is all cumulative legislation. This may not be a statutorily enforceable operative treatment directive, but surrogates and physicians still may and ought to take it into consideration. They look at her wishes; they look at her best interests. They interpret. There is not any perfection in this; there is not any total control. There is seldom any way to be absolutely certain that our wishes will be followed unless we are able, here and now, to say what we want.

If we change this last case a bit, we can again see this need for interpretation and to balance substituted judgment with best interests. A person writes that she wishes to refuse even the simplest life-sustaining treatments such as antibiotics if she is ever in a seriously reduced mental state. Later, with early to moderate Alzheimer's, she is living a significantly reduced yet obviously happy life, content to watch television, root for whatever team is winning, sing along with the other patients, and enjoy eating. The position we propose here is that her present best interests must counterbalance her earlier wishes, especially since she was clearly unable, in her earlier state, to experience what she does now. This is not the "contemporaneous decision of a competent person" and is therefore not the "ace of trump." Simple curative treatments such as antibiotics for curable pneumonia should be provided. This case is sufficiently different from the previous one that proper interpretation and balance leads to a different conclusion.[1]

Second Case: Emergency Blood

This second case was created by one of the book's authors, Dr. Kelly, and, as is clear, represents his own judgments. Hence it is presented in the first person.

There is another case I often use to show this need for interpretation, though I am less sure about my conclusion than in the cases we have just seen. A thirty-year-old man comes to the ER after a traffic accident that has caused a serious internal hemorrhage. He cannot communicate. If he does not get blood *now*, he will die. If he is transfused, the ER physicians think that with uncomplicated surgery he has a very good chance of complete recovery. He has a card in his wallet that says "I am a Jehovah's Witness; do not transfuse." His wife confirms his membership in the Witnesses and refuses to consent to a transfusion. The doctor has only a minute or two to decide. What ought to be done?

Note again that in Pennsylvania, and in other states with similar provisions, this is not an operative treatment directive. Even if the card in his pocket is properly signed and witnessed, which would make it a statutorily enforceable directive in this state, it is not operative because he is not terminally ill in the sense in which the law defines that term. Treatment will probably cure him. But we have seen that nonoperative living wills still ought to be and legally may be taken into consideration. Surely this is enough evidence of his wishes. What is the doctor to do?

Although I am hesitant to say this, I would probably support transfusion. My reasoning would not be the kind of vitalism that overrides patient wishes, though some might judge that in this case I am too close to the "vitalism" side of the spectrum discussed in chapter 13. Here it seems that there is a reasonable possibility (though perhaps a slight one) that the man would not choose *now* to reject the transfusion if he could state his wishes. That is, there is a chance that rejection would not be his contemporaneous decision were he able to make one. There are documented examples of similar cases where Jehovah's Witnesses, when actually faced with this decision, chose to ignore their previously stated wishes and asked for transfusion. And this has happened in my own clinical experience. Impending death focuses the mind in new ways. And it is even possible, though unlikely, that the patient was never truly a believing Witness in the first place. The card may have been for him a way to fit into a family with strong beliefs. This is not a criticism of the faith or the moral courage of Witnesses. Catholics have abortions and use birth control. Circumstances change, and people change their minds accordingly.

It should be clear that if the Jehovah's Witness in this case were able *now* to state his preferences and if he chose to refuse transfusion, knowing that death would (almost certainly) follow, it would then be morally outrageous and criminal assault and battery to transfuse him. For me, however, there is not enough evidence to be sure this would be his wish were he to know his present circumstances. I would need more evidence. For example, if he had previously been in a similar circumstance and had said clearly that even though he might well die, he would not accept blood, then there would be enough evidence to be virtually certain of what he would choose now. Or if the physician had been his longtime internist and if they had spoken together about this over a long period of time so the doctor really did know that he meant it, then that would be enough evidence. But as it stands, in this emergency, I think I would support the transfusion. The same would apply if the man were, in a later reduced mental state, now obviously happy with his life and oblivious of his previous beliefs, to need curative emergent blood. I am aware that this is a controversial conclusion that contradicts the position usually held (Edwards 2011, 368–69).

What about the possibility here of a criminal charge being laid? I very much doubt this would happen (district attorneys do not often bring charges against physicians who save lives) and, if it did, given the flexibility always granted to physicians in emergency situations, the charge would almost certainly be dismissed or the physician acquitted. This is even more likely given the absence of an operative treatment directive. A civil suit is more likely. But if a transfusion were withheld, the physician might also be sued by the man's children who claim that their now dead father had told them that he really was not a Witness but carried the card to keep peace with his wife. Which jury is easier to face, one hearing the grieving children of a man whom you let die and who, they say, did not want to die, or one hearing a perfectly healthy man charge you with saving his life? Theoretically, neither lawsuit should prevail.

Doctors' Orders and Charted Order Forms

Decisions made by the patient or the surrogate must be translated into doctors' orders. The treatment directive is not an order form. The mere fact that an advance directive is on the chart means nothing about what will actually be done until the patient's wishes, properly interpreted by surrogates in communication with physicians, become actual orders on the chart.

The easiest way to make this clear is to use the example of healthy people with living wills who are admitted to hospitals for the treatment of easily fixed medical problems. They should be resuscitated if something goes wrong and they arrest; they are not to be made DNR simply because they have a living will. This is another example of missing the needed interpretation. We have already noted that some people deliberately deny that they have an advance directive if they are hospitalized for a simple illness. If they should arrest during an appendectomy, for example, as a result of an anesthesia reaction, they *do* want CPR. It should not be necessary to hide advance directives. As long as hospital procedures make it clear that hospital staff follow the orders on the chart, and as long as there is proper discussion with the surrogate about how to interpret the living will (or with the competent patient about how to do so should she lose her ability to make decisions) and the resulting treatment decisions are entered into the orders section of the chart, advance directives will not be misused or misinterpreted.

Hospitals should design something similar to the Palliative Care Orders Form that was used in Pittsburgh's St. Francis Hospital. This is an *orders form*. Doctors fill it out and sign it. They are supposed to do so after conversation with the patient (or the surrogate). The Palliative Care Orders Form is more sophisticated than simple code status because often the kinds of treatment chosen are more complex than what could be included in a code status, which is usually something simple, such as "do not resuscitate," "comfort measures only," or "no aggressive treatment." If something goes wrong at two in the morning, the nurses and residents look to the Palliative Care Orders Form and follow it.

But there are sometimes problems even here. If the nurse discovers that the Palliative Care Orders Form is filled out in a way that contradicts the living will, this should be brought to the attention of the attending physician. If this does not resolve the issue, an ethics consult is warranted. People write advance directives because they want their wishes to be honored. Interpreting them is not the same as ignoring them; indeed, it is the very opposite of ignoring them. And in order to give them effect, instructions must be entered in the chart and signed by the ordering physician (usually the attending physician).

Persons without Surrogates

The law also wants to protect the rights of persons who cannot make decisions about treatment, who have left no advance directives, and who have no one (no family, no close friends) who can serve as their surrogate. The way the law has tended to do this is to appoint a guardian and then expect that person to make decisions in accordance with the pure objective standard (the best-interests standard) if there is no knowledge of the patient's wishes, or in accordance with other standards if, as is seldom the case, there is some knowledge of his or her wishes. But hospitals rightly hesitate to do this for a number of reasons. The most important is the problem of conflict of interest. An example might be a case where paramedics bring a man to the ER. He is homeless and has no known family. The doctors decide there is no hope for a meaningful recovery, but there is no one who can decide for the patient. If a guardian is to be proposed to the court, who should it be? Often hospitals propose their own social workers, but these people work for the hospital and are being asked to decide in the best interests of the patient, which may not coincide with what the hospital wants to do. Outside guardians are seldom available, and professional groups who offer this service naturally charge a fee—who will pay it?

For these reasons some hospitals have added to their official policies on forgoing treatment a procedure to follow in some of these cases. At the University of Pittsburgh Medical Center, for example, a policy has been developed that some other Pittsburgh hospitals have adopted. In such a case, if all the physicians agree that treatment cannot be of any benefit to the patient (it is clearly morally extraordinary), then a meeting of the ethics committee is called. For this purpose, the committee must be more than just the usual consult team (see chapter 22). It must include a specified number of members as well as representation from pastoral care, from the legal department, from social work, and so on. If all unanimously agree with the doctors, then treatment is forgone. This seems to be a valid approach, despite the fact that conflict of interest could still be a problem. We surely do not want to go to court for trials on each of these cases. And in the present legal circumstances, as we have noted, guardianship is not likely to be a better solution. This approach has also been proposed by the New York State Task Force on Life and the Law (1993, 21–23).

The Patient Self-Determination Act

In 1990 the federal government passed a law known as the Patient Self-Determination Act (PSDA). The law went into effect on December 1, 1991. It is a rather simple law, although some law firms and some hospital associations seem to have embellished it and suggested added requirements to it that the law itself does not contain.

The federal law obliges all health care institutions that admit patients and accept federal funds (which means virtually all hospitals and nursing homes) to do the following: First, all admitted patients must be informed upon admission about state laws regarding patients' rights concerning choosing and rejecting treatment options. This should be done in writing, in easily read brochures handed to patients upon admission. Some states have a required or a suggested way to do this. It may be in legal jargon. If it is, it is probably best to use it and then to add an explanation written for readers with less advanced reading skills. Second, all admitted patients must be asked if they have an advance directive. The answers go onto the chart. If patients say yes, then they must be asked if they have a written copy with them. If yes, the copy goes into the patient's chart. If no, some attempt should be made to get a copy. Third, the PSDA requires that all admitted patients be told about hospital policy concerning these issues. These policies should be available for patients to take and read. Although the PSDA does not mandate this, if a hospital's policy on these issues is not in line with the usual policies in the region, the hospital should inform admitted patients of what the unusual policy says and how it affects their rights to choose treatment. This might apply especially in any hospitals with so-called medical futility policies (see chapter 20) or in hospitals with unusually restrictive policies on feeding tubes (see chapter 18).

Helping Patients Fill Out Advance Directives

All of this will lead patients to ask questions. They will want to know what a living will is and what a durable power of attorney or health care proxy is, and some may want to make one or both for themselves. Should the hospital help in this? There was some hesitation when the PSDA was originally passed, based on worry about conflict of interest, and some ethicists and hospital attorneys still recommend that hospital personnel not be involved in this process for their patients. This concern is probably overly cautious. Surely at the very least hospitals might suggest that patients choose surrogates to make decisions if they are unable to do so, thus aiding them in making a proxy directive. And many hospitals provide forms and offer some basic help to patients in designing simple treatment directives. More complicated directives, especially those requiring specific knowledge of the patient's present diagnosis and prognosis, should be made by the patient in dialogue with the physician. In any case, hospital personnel should not try to persuade patients in this. And it is better that it be done beforehand. It is also probably helpful if patients are given this information about advance directives again at discharge, although the law does not require this. Then they could look at it away from the traumatic context of the hospital, and they might be better prepared for the next admission.[2]

Conclusion

We have devoted three chapters to the complicated question of who decides to forgo treatment. In general, capable patients may legally refuse virtually any treatment. Legally this is the gold standard or ace of trump. But it does not apply to surrogate decision making. Surrogates may refuse only those treatments that are of little benefit or of great burden (best-interests standard), or that the patient, while capable of choosing, decided against (substituted judgment standard). The substituted judgment (subjective) standard should always be used along with the best-interests (objective) standard. Surrogates may (almost) never forgo treatment that is in the objective best interests of the patient. Advance treatment directives almost always require interpretation.

Notes

1. For an argument toward a similar conclusion, and for references to other scholars on this issue, see Edwards 2011. We agree with Edwards that "the moral authority of an advance directive ought to be constrained by an obligation to respect the independent moral worth of the patient in her severely mentally impaired state" (366). Philosophers debate whether the past and present selves are continuous and thus whether the previous advance directive even applies to the "new" person. Some suggest, as Edwards does, that the present reduced self is not a person but is rather a "post-personhood human" (360–61), a position we do not accept, as is clear from chapter 25.

2. Everything we have seen in the last three chapters points to the importance of communication between patient and physician while the patient is still competent to make decisions about forgoing treatment. Unfortunately, in the United States, political factors have intruded to

make this more difficult. An early draft of the 2010 Patient Protection and Affordable Care Act (PPACA), often derisively called "Obamacare" by its opponents, included a provision to pay physicians for their time in speaking with patients about these matters. But Republican opponents of the plan, led by Sarah Palin, began to call these conversations "death panels," stirring up fears that the Democrats wanted to let people die rather than treat them (Callahan 2011, 25). Although this charge was totally false—there was nothing in the bill that would have included any rationing of treatment—the charge forced the Democrats to eliminate the provision from the bill (DeCamp, Walter, and Goold 2011, 12). Thus, Medicare does not reimburse doctors for this, and too often they and their patients do not have the necessary conversations to ensure that the patient's decisions are known and carried out, as a recent study indicates (Burke 2011, 564).

CHAPTER 18

HYDRATION AND NUTRITION

THE ETHICAL ISSUE OF withholding and withdrawing nutrition and hydration involves a specific application of the general principles developed in the previous chapters. There has been considerable controversy over whether nourishment and hydration can ever be omitted or discontinued for a dying or comatose patient, or for one who is in a persistent vegetative state.

The general agreement reached in the United States is that nutrition and hydration may properly be forgone in some cases. The *Cruzan* decision of the Supreme Court upheld this opinion (*Cruzan v. Director*, 1990). But there was much debate along the way, and some ethicists and some courts have disagreed with the emerging consensus. In addition, over the past decade or so, renewed debate has occurred within Catholic bioethics on this issue, given impetus by the case of Theresa Marie Schiavo (introduced in chapter 4); by an allocution delivered in March 2004 by Pope John Paul II, which, at least at face value, appears to require medical feeding for PVS patients; by recent pronouncements by the Vatican; and by changes in the latest *Ethical and Religious Directives*.

A look at this issue, particularly at some of the related court cases and at the renewed Catholic debate, will allow us to further study the interplay of the three pillars that form the basis of the current American consensus on forgoing treatment. In this chapter, we argue that the Catholic tradition does not require hydration and nutrition for permanently unconscious and similar patients, despite the claims of some that it does.

There are ethical questions as to when hydration and nutrition are morally ordinary and when they are morally extraordinary, and there are legal questions as to which means are always required in the law, which may be omitted and when, and who makes the decision. This issue is one that many hospitals and chronic care facilities face often, and it is a good test case for the meaning of "ordinary" and "extraordinary" and for our care of the dying.

It is important to stress that the issue as it is usually framed is medically assisted nutrition and hydration (MANH), which involves the use of tubes inserted through the nose or directly into the abdomen, not ordinary food and water. Eating and drinking, food and water, have important symbolic meanings for humans (Carson 1989). They connote dining, human relationship, and, for Christians, the Eucharist. They must always be offered to patients who accept them. But this language is not appropriate in the context we are examining. For these reasons, it is better to use the proper words, nutrition and hydration, than the words used for ordinary nourishment.

This does not mean, however, that health care providers are morally required to force food and water on those patients who, while physically capable of taking them by mouth, choose not to do so. Eating and drinking may indeed be morally extraordinary for some patients even if the means are the usual ones and not those of medically assisted hydration and nutrition. In some cases, patients rightly determine that eating and drinking are not of any real benefit to them; they prolong the dying process and add to the patients' discomfort. The patients simply do not have the strength or the will to continue. In the words of the Vatican's 1980 Declaration on Euthanasia, "a correct judgment can be made regarding means, if the type of treatment, its degree of difficulty and danger, its expense, and the possibility of applying it are weighed against the results that can be expected, all this in the light of the sick person's condition and resources of body and spirit" (CDF [1980] 1998, 653). The means may well be simple, but in some cases the patient's "resources of body and spirit" are such that even eating and drinking are morally extraordinary.

Thus, while food and water must always be offered, they need not always be forced. There are cases, of course, when a person refuses to eat or drink as a result of some psychological illness or for some other purpose, as in a hunger strike. These cases present difficulties that cannot be judged a priori. In general, competent persons can legally refuse all medical treatment, even life-sustaining treatment that is clearly morally ordinary from an objective perspective. Usually patients who refuse to eat even when their prognoses are good—they will probably recover from their condition—do so because of some psychological problem, often clinical depression. In these cases, it is better to try to find the cause of the problem than to automatically begin tube feeding. In one case, it was simply a matter of turning on the television set in the patient's room and getting the right flavor of ice cream, a far better solution than a nasogastric tube! Nonetheless, there may be times when tube feeding is required against the wishes of an incompetent patient suffering from severe clinical depression. These cases will almost always concern patients with significant chances for meaningful recovery, however, and not dying patients or those in terminal (irreversible) comas or persistent vegetative states.

Persistent Vegetative State

The issue of forgoing nutrition and hydration often arises in the context of persistent vegetative state (PVS). One of the earliest cases to be decided by the courts involved a PVS patient, Karen Ann Quinlan (*In re Quinlan*). Paul Brophy and Theresa Marie (Terri) Schiavo, whose cases are discussed in this chapter, were both in PVS. And the papal allocution, the Vatican "responses," and the *Ethical and Religious Directives*, to which we return later in this chapter, speak of PVS patients. Thus it is helpful to introduce PVS before continuing. This is not to say, however, that the ethical and legal issues of hydration and nutrition are limited to persons in PVS. But since PVS patients can live for many years with feeding tubes, this condition has given rise to much of the debate.

There are a number of disorders of consciousness, to use the term of Dr. Joseph Fins (Fins 2005). Medicine is learning to better distinguish them. "Vegetative state" is a condition in which a person has lost the use of the cerebral cortex while the brain stem continues to function. Other terms are preferable here because of the pejorative connotations of "vegetable," but this is the medical term used, and we will use it. The lower brain, or brain stem, controls certain bodily activities such as breathing, while the "higher brain," or cerebral cortex, controls the functions we usually think of when we think of human activity, such as thinking, emotion, and awareness of self and others.

A vegetative state is similar to but technically different from a coma. Both comatose persons and persons in PVS are completely unconscious and totally unaware of anything in the environment. But the coma victim is "asleep," that is, the eyes are closed, whereas the person in a PVS has sleep-wake cycles and is therefore at times biologically "awake," with eyes open. Comas do not last as long as vegetative states can; comatose persons die, or become vegetative, or recover.

Because the brain stem continues to function, most PVS patients breathe without any medical support. Their eyes open and close and wander about. There are facial movements that can seem to be facial expressions. Their bodies move and there can be sounds like groans and sighs or other noises. None of these are in response to anything that goes on around them. These unconscious movements occur whether anyone is there or not. It is understandable that loving family will interpret these movements and sounds as attempts at communication—as proof that their loved one is still aware of their presence—but unfortunately such a patient has lost the ability to do this. (The heavily edited tapes of Terri Schiavo that we saw so often on TV, the purpose of which was to convince others that she was conscious, gave an appearance of awareness where there was none. Unfortunately, some who should have known better misdiagnosed her condition based on these tapes and other similar reports. The autopsy done after her death proved beyond doubt that her brain was incapable of any conscious responses to her environment.)

This kind of state is diagnosed as "persistent" or "permanent" after a period of time has passed. The term "persistent vegetative state" is generally used to mean one from which there is no reasonable hope of recovery to a state of even minimal awareness. But this is not always the meaning of "persistent." Sometimes a distinction is made between "persistent vegetative state" and "permanent vegetative state" (Mappes 2003). When this distinction is made, "persistent vegetative state" refers to the original diagnosis that a person is indeed in such a state and that it has persisted for a time, but this diagnosis does not imply that the patient can never emerge from it. Then "permanent vegetative state" becomes a prognosis that no recovery is likely (Mappes 2003, 124). This prognosis requires further observation and further tests, or both.

An important 1994 article in the *New England Journal of Medicine* describes recovery from "persistent vegetative state" to at least a minimal level of consciousness, though not necessarily to functional capacity, as high as 52 percent (Multi-Society Task Force on PVS 1994, 1572). Obviously this is not a permanent state of unconsciousness. In this article "persistent vegetative state" designates the condition after one month, with no implication of permanence (ibid., 1499). Permanence is a prognosis made after further observation—three months postanoxia and six months posttrauma, according to Fins—depending on the cause of the cerebral injury (Fins 2005, 22). This is based on the likelihood of recovery after this length of time. When such a distinction is made, it is possible that a patient can recover some awareness, even significant awareness and function after being in a "persistent vegetative state," but this is not likely after this state has become "permanent." However, the acronym "PVS" is applied indiscriminately to both, and the original term "persistent vegetative state" implied permanence and required waiting until that was reasonably certain. The two different usages result in confusion.

It is better to continue to use the term "persistent" and to wait before making the diagnosis until it is reasonably sure that this indeed means permanence. In hospitals, the distinction between persistent and permanent is generally not observed—"PVS" means "persistent vegetative state," and it implies both the diagnosis of the condition and the prognosis of its permanence. This is the usual medical and bioethical usage. Beauchamp and Childress (2001), for example, use the term this way throughout their standard textbook, and we will use it that way here.

Proper diagnosis of "persistent-permanent vegetative state" is possible when based on laboratory studies and clinical observation, especially when this is supported by positron emission tomography (PET) and possibly by functional magnetic resonance imaging (fMRI). Recovery can be virtually ruled out. A statement to this effect was made by the American Academy of Neurology (American Academy of Neurology 1989; Munsat, Stuart, and Cranford 1989). MRI (magnetic resonance imaging) and CT (computed tomography) scanning can also help by showing structural damage.

The result of PVS, assuming it is truly permanent and has been properly diagnosed, is that such persons cannot think. They are not aware of anything or anyone around them. They are not aware of themselves. They cannot dream. They cannot pray. They cannot recognize music or color or taste or touch. And they cannot experience pain or discomfort. This means that they cannot experience hunger or thirst even if their bodies lack food and water. This is a hard concept to grasp. If we are hungry or thirsty, we experience it; we want food and water. But PVS patients do not. They are entirely unaware of what is happening to them. In this life they are permanently beyond suffering, just as they are permanently beyond joy.

The American Academy of Neurology statement gives clear support to the withdrawal of nutrition and hydration from PVS patients. The academy also insists that PVS patients, despite their ability to breathe and open and move their eyes, are totally unconscious and cannot experience pain or suffering in any way. The withdrawal of nutrition and hydration does not, therefore, cause any sensation of dehydration or starvation.

One must be careful, however, to avoid being too quick to diagnose PVS and permanent coma. These terms are sometimes used inaccurately. Good neurologists will want to be sure of the cause of the problem before deciding that a patient cannot recover from a coma. But the possibility of misdiagnosis cannot mean that we ought to ignore all diagnoses! The only way to be absolutely sure to avoid all undertreatment, in the hope that a diagnosis is wrong and that the patient will recover, is to treat all illnesses aggressively regardless of diagnosis and prognosis, to do everything possible to preserve physical life. And this is not required by the American ethical consensus or by the Catholic tradition.

Legally, PVS and other forms of permanent coma do not fit the usual definitions of terminal illness. State laws usually define terminal conditions as those from which a person is likely to die in a short time (often six months is used) regardless of what treatments are applied. But PVS patients can live on for years, even for decades, with tube feedings and usually with periodic antibiotics to treat infections. In another sense, however, permanent comas are terminal. The patient will die of this condition unless treatment is given. It is a "lethal" condition if not legally a "terminal" one.[1]

The position presented here about the mental status of PVS patients is the one most generally supported; it is, as we have noted, the position taken by the American Academy of Neurology. Yet this position has been criticized by some who claim that PVS patients may have some internal and even external awareness. A 2008 white paper report of the President's Council on Bioethics shows some hesitation to make the claim that PVS patients lack all awareness (Shewmon 2009, 19). And a recent study shows that perhaps some persons diagnosed as being in PVS are capable of some mental response to their environment (Billings, Churchill, and Payne 2010; Fins and Schiff 2010). In a study published in the *New England Journal of Medicine*, researchers at the universities of Cambridge and Liege used fMRI to examine a number of patients with severe brain dysfunction. Some of these had been diagnosed as PVS, others as MCS (minimally conscious state). Some showed fMRI changes that seemed to vary consistently according to different verbal suggestions. When told to "imagine playing tennis," for example, certain local brain changes would occur (Billings, Churchill, and Payne 2010, 18). Some have suggested that this means PVS persons are conscious after all and that we might be able to communicate with them. Deciding this issue requires clinical and scientific expertise beyond our capacity here. But there is reason to be hesitant before accepting the idea that PVS and similar patients may have significant awareness. First, there may be methodological problems with the study, and there have been harsh criticisms of its accuracy (ibid., 17). Second, it is at least possible that misdiagnoses occurred. Third, there is no evidence that the responses showed any significant awareness of what was being spoken to the patients; there is only evidence that a localized blood flow change occurred in the brain (ibid., 18). In another earlier case, a woman diagnosed as in the vegetative state was said to have shown in an fMRI study evidence of a "rich mental life." But the evidence was not clear, and it is likely that her state was not permanent but transitional (sufficient time had not lapsed for the prognosis of permanence to be certain) and that she was in fact in a minimally conscious and not a truly vegetative state (Fins 2006). In any case, "The potential for what most would call a meaningful or even marginal recovery for patients with PVS remains incredibly slim" (Billings, Churchill, and Payne 2010, 20).

But what ethical implications would result even if it were discovered that a few persons diagnosed, or perhaps misdiagnosed, as PVS had indeed the capacity for some minimal awareness? Even if this were the case, it would not be a reason to conclude that they must be kept indefinitely alive by medical means. As long as the condition of permanence is certain, there is no hope of meaningful recovery. In such cases it is indeed likely that most of us would far more dread an existence where we are aware of being unable to communicate in any human way with our environment, to leave our beds, to move our bodies voluntarily, and to escape the technology that was keeping us "alive" than we would dread an existence where we were aware of nothing at all.

The *Brophy* Case

A court case that is particularly helpful in analyzing these issues is that of Paul Brophy, a Massachusetts firefighter (*Brophy v. New Eng. Sinai Hosp., Inc.*, 1986). Both Karen Ann

Quinlan and Paul Brophy were diagnosed, correctly as far as anyone can tell, as being in a persistent vegetative state.[2] The difference between Quinlan and Brophy was that Quinlan received ventilation along with nutrition whereas Brophy received only nutrition, which was provided by a gastrostomy tube (many patients with PVS can breathe without mechanical assistance, since breathing is controlled by the brain stem, which is still functioning). In the *Quinlan* case, the New Jersey court held that the ventilator might be removed, and also that this should not usually be a court decision. Rather, a family member was appointed guardian and was given authority, in conjunction with any ethics committee the hospital might have, to turn off the ventilator (*In re Quinlan* 1982, 170). Most ethicists have applauded the *Quinlan* decision for its conclusion. This kind of decision should seldom be a court decision, and the New Jersey Supreme Court made this clear when it overturned the Superior Court decision that had refused to allow Quinlan's father Joseph to discontinue ventilation. The New Jersey Supreme Court relied on her right of privacy as a basis for her freedom from this kind of procedure (Meisel 1989, 98; 1995, 1:503–4). Quinlan actually lived for years afterward because nutrition and hydration were continued. She never came out of her persistent vegetative state. The argument in this chapter is that nutrition might also have been removed, but this was not requested for Quinlan.

But what about Brophy? Here Judge David Kopelman of the Norfolk County Probate Court in Massachusetts refused to allow Brophy's wife, Patricia, to stop nourishment by the gastrostomy tube. The court made a number of judgments that many ethicists have criticized, though some have supported one or another of them.[3]

First, the court stated that even though Brophy had said over and over again that he would never want this kind of treatment, he had to have it anyway. Brophy had actually thrown away a commendation he received for saving a man from a burning car since the man had later died, and Brophy had judged this kind of treatment to be useless. He had commented to his wife that he never wanted to be like Karen Ann Quinlan.

Second, the court ruled that it would have been right not to insert the gastrostomy tube in the first place (in ethical terms, this meant the judge felt that this was "extraordinary" since it was clearly invasive), but that once the stoma had been created and the tube inserted, the nourishment was a procedure of maintenance only (in ethical terms, the judge might have used the term "ordinary") and must be continued. That is, the judge insisted on a moral and legal difference between withholding and withdrawing treatment.

Finally, the judge stated that removing feeding is different from removing ventilation, since removing ventilation does not include necessarily the intent to terminate life, whereas removing nourishment does. In the ethical terminology we have already seen, he might have said that removing a ventilator is "allowing to die," whereas removing a gastrostomy tube is active euthanasia or "direct" killing.

Four Questions

But was the judge correct in his opinions? In our judgment and in that of most ethicists and jurists, the answer is no. There are four questions involved. Is stopping treatment different from not starting it? Is a gastrostomy tube ethically different from a venti-lator? Is withdrawing nutrition euthanasia, that is, is it "killing" as opposed to "allowing to die"? Who should make the decision to forgo or not to forgo treatment?

First, is there a difference between not doing a procedure in the first place (not creating a stoma and inserting the tube) and withdrawing a procedure that has been started (removing the tube and stopping nourishment)? The judge clearly thought so. With few exceptions, ethicists do not recognize that distinction as morally or legally relevant.[4] It is easy to see what would happen if we insisted on the difference. A person is brought to the emergency room, and the health care team cannot determine easily whether the patient can recover if resuscitation procedures are begun. So they begin them. The result is later found to be merely a prolongation of the dying process, not a treatment that will result in recovery to meaningful human living. If it is now wrong to stop what was started, medical professionals would be caught in an impossible eth-ical bind. Either they do not start treatment and fail to cure some patients, or they start and then are required to continue useless measures for some patients. The Catholic tradition, with the distinctions we have discussed, has been able to avoid this bind. As we saw earlier, there is no moral difference between stopping and not starting. If the treatment is extraordinary, it is right to decide not to start it; it is also right to stop it once started. The American ethical and legal consensus has come to agree with this. As we have already noted, the *Cruzan* decision of the Supreme Court has affirmed this judgment legally. So the judge in *Brophy* was wrong.

Second, is a gastrostomy tube morally different from a ventilator? That is, in PVS and similar patients, is a gastrostomy tube an "ordinary means" of supplying nutrition and hydration while a ventilator is an "extraordinary means" of supplying air? There is some controversy about this among Catholic moralists, but it is clear that the main line of the Catholic tradition has argued that this kind of nourishment, along with intravenous feeding and other methods of nutrition and hydration, are indeed extraor-dinary in cases like this one. This distinction is not as such medical or technical, but moral. Medical procedures that would be quite ordinary in some situations where they might be reasonably expected to help are clearly extraordinary—even unreasonable—in other cases, and the example of Paul Brophy is such a case. Medical feeding and hydra-tion in this kind of situation are extraordinary. They are not the same as offering food and water to a starving or dehydrated person. Indeed, in those cases where nutrition or hydration, or both, are needed for patient comfort, they must always be given. Jesuit moralist Gerald Kelly, the foremost medical ethicist of the 1940s and 1950s, and accepted by all Catholic moralists as being consistent with official church teaching, clearly stated that artificial feeding may be discontinued (Kelly 1950).[5] This is clearly permitted by Catholic medical ethics.

This answer to the second question gives us the answer to the third as well: whether the judge was right in arguing that the intentionality of stopping feeding had to be "to kill," that is, in ethical terms, whether he was right in implying that this was active euthanasia. In the judgment of most ethicists, including—at least until very recently and probably even today—a strong majority of Catholic moral theologians, this was not active euthanasia but was instead the stopping of an extraordinary and unreasonable means of preserving life. In cases like this, it is the disease that kills the patient, not the forgoing of treatment. Thus, the withdrawal of nutrition and hydration in cases like this one is permissible (indeed, since Brophy had clearly stated he did not want this type of treatment, its withdrawal is morally required). But there is still controversy about this question, and it is likely that some of it results from confusion about the complex issue of intentionality that we consider in chapter 14. Families who withhold or withdraw feeding from permanently comatose loved ones do not intend their death in the sense of an end to be sought, even though they may well be relieved that death will mean a way to peace and an end to a life where no human action or experience is possible. And there is no reason to hold that the family's intention when forgoing feeding differs in any way from their intention in forgoing ventilation or other life-sustaining treatments. The Catholic tradition maintains that in cases like Brophy's medically induced nutrition and hydration may be forgone.[6] And this proposal has become, with some disagreement still remaining, part of the American consensus about this issue.

It is interesting to note what finally happened to Paul Brophy. The Massachusetts Supreme Court overturned the decision of the probate court and ruled that the gastrostomy tube might legally be removed, although it refused to compel doctors to remove it. The tube was removed on October 15, 1986, and Brophy died on October 23, three and a half years after he had first lapsed into unconsciousness, and some two years after his wife had first asked that the gastrostomy nourishment be stopped ("Latest Word: In the Courts," 1986; "Latest Word: Brophy Dies," 1986). Most cases of this type have been similarly resolved, some more quickly, some not—for example, New Jersey's Nancy Jobes case (*In re Jobes*, 1987), Danbury, Connecticut's Carol McConnell case (*McConnell v. Beverly Enters.-Conn., Inc.*, 1989), Pennsylvania's Jane Doe and Daniel Fiori cases (*In re Doe*, 1987; *In re Fiori*, 1996), Florida's Terri Schiavo case (*In re Guardianship of Schiavo*, 2003; *Bush v. Schiavo*, 2004; *Schiavo ex rel. Schindler v. Schiavo*, 2005), and a number of others.

The fourth question is who is best able to make the decision? Morally and legally, if the patient is competent, the patient decides. The Supreme Court's decision in *Cruzan* has upheld this. The question in cases such as *Quinlan* and *Brophy* has to do with patients who are not able to decide. Now who makes the decision?

We deal with this question in chapters 16 and 17 and need only make a few points here. In the *Quinlan* case, the court said that Quinlan's father, together with an ethics committee if such existed at the hospital, should decide. This is the best approach. In the *Brophy* case, the probate court rejected the idea that his wife could decide. The Supreme Court of Massachusetts overruled the substance of the decision, deciding that the feeding tube might be removed but did not rule, as in *Quinlan*, that the family should be the ones to decide. And in *Saikewicz*, a similar Massachusetts case, the court agreed that treatment could be stopped but explicitly rejected the New Jersey decision in *Quinlan* and insisted that the court was the only proper place to decide such issues (*Superintendent of Belchertown State Sch. v. Saikewicz*, 1977; Meisel 1989, 238–39; 1995, 1:237–38). The same conclusion was reached by a New York court in the so-called Brother Fox case (*In re Eichner*, 1979) but was later reversed (Meisel 1989, 244; 1995, 1:242). And in some New Jersey cases where nursing home patients have been affected, involvement of the state ombudsman has been mandated (Meisel 1989, 252–54; 1995, 1:269–71).

Legally, therefore, the "Who decides?" question is controverted. There does seem to be a general movement in Massachusetts, New York, New Jersey, and other states away from this unfortunate insistence on court or government action (Meisel 1989, 238–48; 1995, 1:239–46). Most ethicists, along with very many jurists, would like to see a general acceptance of the *Quinlan* decision: in most cases, the decision ought to be left at the level of the family and the health care team, with the hospital's ethics committee as a possible resource. And in most jurisdictions, this is indeed the case.

Consensus and Controversy

Over the past several decades American courts have developed a general agreement that hydration and nutrition may be withheld and withdrawn from PVS and other similar patients. The growing consensus accepts the arguments from the Catholic tradition that medically induced nutrition and hydration may well be extraordinary means and that they may rightly be withheld or withdrawn. This consensus, as we have described it, is the approach taken by the 1983 report of the President's Commission for the Study of Ethical Problems in Medicine and Biomedical and Behavioral Research (1983, 90, 159–60, 196), by the New York State Task Force on Life and the Law (1992, 211–21), and by the Hastings Center in its 1987 *Guidelines* (1987, 59–62). The American Medical Association (1986, 2) advises doctors that artificial nutrition and hydration may be removed from patients who are imminently dying and from those who are irreversibly comatose, provided that the family or other surrogate concurs. Similar positions have been taken by the American Academy of Neurology (1989) and the American College of Physicians (1990).

But there has been and still is some significant debate among Catholic bishops and theologians (May 1998, 1999; O'Rourke 1999a, 1999b). Much of this preceded the *Schiavo* case and the papal allocution. For example, in New Jersey, the state conference of Catholic bishops argued in the Jobes case that artificial nutrition must be maintained (*In re Jobes*, 1987). Yet in a similar case in Rhode Island, Bishop Louis Gelineau agreed that artificial nutrition could be stopped for a patient, Marsha Gray, in a persistent vegetative state. Oregon and Washington bishops issued a statement that supported the possibility of forgoing nutrition for permanently unconscious patients (Oregon and Washington Bishops 1991, 350). So did the Texas bishops (Texas Bishops 1990). Bishop John Liebrecht's statement on *Cruzan* also allows this (Liebrecht 1990). The Catholic Health Association of Wisconsin (1989) issued similar guidelines. But the US Bishops' Pro-Life Committee (1992) issued a statement that makes a strong presumption in favor of continued feeding of permanently comatose persons, a statement that was criticized by Kevin O'Rourke, a strong defender of the received Catholic tradition (O'Rourke and deBlois 1992).

In 1991 the Pennsylvania Catholic bishops issued a statement that seems to require hydration and nutrition of all or almost all PVS patients. Since the PVS patient is not terminally ill, they say, and since feeding tubes are providing a benefit by sustaining life with no burden to the patient, "the feeding . . . remains an ordinary means of sustaining life and should be continued" (Pennsylvania Bishops 1992, 548). These claims are just the ones we have argued the Catholic tradition rejects. Feeding tubes for PVS patients can be said to provide a benefit only by using that term as the Catholic tradition on "ordinary means" and "extraordinary means" does not use it—as a medical term, not a moral one. There is no human benefit to these patients in keeping their bodies alive. Richard McCormick, one of the most influential Catholic moral theologians of the second half of the twentieth century, ends his article on the Pennsylvania bishops' statement this way: "Let me conclude with a fanciful scenario. Imagine a 300-bed Catholic hospital with all beds supporting P.V.S. patients maintained for months, even years by gastrostomy tubes. Fanciful? Not if the guidelines of the Pennsylvania bishops are followed. Appalling? In my judgment, yes—not least of all because an observer of the scenario would eventually be led to ask: 'Is it true that those who operate this facility actually believe in life after death?'" (McCormick 1992, 214).

An unpublished document distributed to American dioceses in 1988 by the Pope John XXIII Medical-Moral Research and Education Center and titled "Feeding and Hydrating the Permanently Unconscious and Other Vulnerable Persons: A Report to the Congregation for the Doctrine of the Faith" requires hydration and nutrition for these patients.[7] But it includes criticisms, some of them rather scathing, by a number of Catholic moral theologians. Among these are rejections of the main conclusions by two "conservative" Catholic moral theologians. On theological grounds, Benedict Ashley correctly rejects the document's central argument that physical life can never be a burden, and argues that the fight against euthanasia is better waged by staying with the Catholic tradition that permits the cessation of unwarranted treatment than by rejecting that tradition. Albert S. Moraczewski, of the Pope John XXIII Center, whose illness prevented him from chairing the drafting group, makes a series of interventions that, on the basis of traditional Catholic moral theology, convincingly refute the main arguments of the document.

The fourth edition of the *Ethical and Religious Directives for Catholic Health Care Services* (2001) included a directive concerning medical nutrition and hydration that was helpful in resolving the controversy. Directive 58 and the introductory narrative to part V, both unchanged from the earlier 1995 *Directives*, made it clear that hydration and nutrition for permanently unconscious patients cannot be said to be always obligatory on the basis of official Catholic teaching. The directive stood in clear contrast to those episcopal conferences that claimed or at least implied that it is obligatory. Directive 58 of the 1995 and 2001 Directives states: "There should be a presumption in favor of providing nutrition and hydration to all patients, including patients who require medically assisted nutrition and hydration, as long as this is of sufficient benefit to outweigh the burdens involved to the patient" (National Conference of Catholic Bishops 1995; USCCB 2001). Unfortunately, the American Catholic bishops have now changed this directive in a more vitalist direction, as we see later in this chapter.

For patients in a persistent vegetative state, there is no benefit in nutrition and hydration that can even remotely be considered a human benefit. In their commentary on the Directives, deBlois and O'Rourke state: "In theological terms, prolonging the life of persons in PVS does not seem to enhance their ability to strive for the purpose and goods of life" (deBlois and O'Rourke 1995, 27). It is interesting to note that the 1995 and 2001 Directives do not require that the forgone nutrition be artificial. If seriously ill patients do not want to eat, and if eating is not of sufficient benefit to outweigh the burdens, this may be forgone. Patients with swallowing reflexes need not be force-fed any more than patients without them need be provided with medical nutrition and hydration.

Recent Catholic Controversy

Disagreement about hydration and nutrition for PVS patients has seen renewed vigor as a result of *Schiavo* and due to a talk given (partially given is more accurate, as we will note) by Pope John Paul II on March 20, 2004 (John Paul II 2004). Following on this papal allocution, the Vatican has issued pronouncements and the American bishops have changed directive 58 in the *Ethical and Religious Directives*.

Schiavo

There is no need to go into detail about the reaction that came from various Catholic bishops, priests, and theologians to the *Schiavo* case as it worked its way through the courts from 2003 to 2005. Some of it was in the context of the papal allocution, and we consider the authority of that speech and some of the different interpretations given to it later in this section. Catholics who commented on the case were just as likely to be misled by the media as were others who, like a number of politicians, insisted that Terri Schiavo was not in PVS. One Catholic bishop, for example, wrote a statement that points explicitly to the media as his source for claiming that "since she is still aware," without hydration and nutrition she would suffer "an excruciatingly painful death" (Wuerl 2005). The statement of the Florida bishops asks for continued feeding until her condition is clarified. They rightly state: "If Mrs. Schiavo's feeding tube were to be removed because the nutrition she receives is of no use to her, or because she is near death, or because it is unreasonably burdensome for her, her family, or caregivers, it could be seen as permissible." This is quite correct according to Catholic teaching. Unfortunately, the Florida Bishops also say that the feeding may be withdrawn "where that treatment itself is causing harm to the patient or is useless because the patient's death is imminent" (Florida Catholic Conference 2005). These two statements, while not flatly contradicting one another, stand in some tension. Treatments are morally extraordinary when their burdens outweigh their benefits, and this does not necessarily require that the treatment itself cause actual harm or that the patient be imminently dying.

This same claim, put even more strongly, that tube feeding is required unless a person is imminently dying, appears in other episcopal statements on *Schiavo* (Burke 2005; Morlino 2005) and in statements of other Catholic commentators (Mulligan 2005). As Thomas Shannon and James Walter (Shannon and Walter 2005a, 656–57) and Kevin O'Rourke (O'Rourke 2005, 549) point out, this requirement of imminent dying is simply not part of the Catholic tradition. To claim that treatment can be morally extraordinary only when a person is imminently dying regardless of whether the treatment is given is to give biological life itself an absolute value that supersedes all other values. This undercuts—indeed, in large measure it eliminates—the entire centuries-old Catholic distinction between ordinary and extraordinary means. It moves Catholic medical ethics toward a vitalism that it has until now correctly resisted.

The Papal Allocution

Pope John Paul II gave a talk on March 20, 2004, to "400 participants in an international congress promoted by the World Federation of Catholic Medical Associations (FIAMC) and by the Pontifical Academy for Life" (Vatican Information Service 2004). In this allocution, the pope seems to have clearly stated that hydration and nutrition are morally ordinary treatment for PVS patients and that forgoing this treatment is "euthanasia by omission" (John Paul II 2004, 740). As should be clear from this chapter, this claim is not consistent with the received tradition of Catholic medical ethics. Since much attention has been paid to this talk, it is important to discuss its authority and how to understand it.

We start with the question of the authority and importance of the talk. Catholic teaching distinguishes internal and external authority. Internal authority comes from the integrity of the arguments and their consistency with the rest of the Catholic tradition on this and similar issues. From what has already been said, as well as from our discussion later in this section of proposed interpretations of the talk, it would appear that its internal authority is not very high. It is not consistent with the rest of Catholic teaching on forgoing treatment and it does not introduce any convincing new arguments as to why that teaching should be changed concerning MANH for PVS patients.

External authority comes from the authority of the author of the document as well as from the way in which it is proclaimed. Papal documents are more authoritative in this sense than documents of individual bishops. Formal encyclical letters are more authoritative than more simple papal statements. Decrees from an ecumenical council, like Trent or Vatican II, which have been approved by the pope and by all the bishops gathered together, are generally seen as more authoritative than encyclicals, and so on. Thus the external authority of this talk is not very high. This is not an encyclical letter or a formal declaration. It is simply a talk Pope John Paul was asked to give to a meeting in Rome. In addition, there is significant doubt about the degree of papal involvement. Unfortunately, when the Holy Father was asked to give the talk, he was suffering from serious effects of Parkinson's disease. It is of course difficult to know exactly how much attention he was able to give—the Vatican is understandably reluctant to speak publicly about a pope's health—but it is known that John Paul II was unable to finish giving the speech. It had to be finished by another, who read it for him. It is quite possible that the Holy Father was unable to give any attention to the talk at all; if this is true, it was simply something he was given to deliver at a meeting of physicians. In any case, the external authority of this talk is not high.

Nonetheless, because it was a papal address, a good deal of attention has been paid to it, and there have been a number of interpretations. Some are careful and explicit, some less careful and implicit. Four will suffice. We will apply these same four later to the Vatican "responses" and to the new *Ethical and Religious Directives*.

The first interpretation is that the talk does indeed mean what it seems to mean, and that it marks a major and dangerous change in the tradition. This is the interpretation of Thomas Shannon and James Walter (Shannon and Walter 2004, 2005a), and their arguments for it are strong. Shannon and Walter claim that the speech "seems to represent a significant departure from the Roman Catholic bioethical tradition" (2004, 18). They worry that this has implications not only for PVS and feeding tubes but for the wider tradition as well. And they point out a number of theoretical and practical problems, some of which we return to later at the conclusion of this section.

The second interpretation, which seems the basis for a number of defenses of this new teaching, is that the allocution applies only to PVS (and, possibly, though not certainly, to other similar states), and that it applies only to feeding tubes and not to other procedures. Thus it does not imperil the tradition as a whole; it is a very limited application issue. This interpretation is not carefully developed. There is no defended basis for making a moral distinction between feeding tubes, which are mandated, and ventilators or other similar procedures, which are not. This seems to ignore the centuries-long requirement that Catholic moral theology has to be reasonable and coherent. Claiming that only feeding tubes are mandated, and that they are mandated only in PVS, introduces incoherence into the tradition. If indeed it is morally mandatory to feed PVS persons for year after year with no human benefit—if this is an ordinary means of preserving their lives—then it is hard to see what could be called extraordinary! Perhaps some treatments that would be enormously painful or overwhelmingly expensive might still fit. But surely we could not continue to say that ventilators and dialysis are extraordinary while feeding tubes are ordinary. And we could not say that the fourth round of chemotherapy for a person with metastatic cancer is optional if that treatment had a small but nonetheless real chance of preserving life for a time. After all, the cancer patient could pray, could love, could think, could suffer—all humanly meaningful purposes of life. The PVS patient can do none of these things. If continuing biological life for the PVS patient is now said to be a human moral benefit that outweighs the costs and other burdens of the treatment, then surely any treatment that, without overwhelming cost or burden, prolongs the life of a conscious person would have to be mandated as well. Thus this second interpretation, that this is a limited change that applies only to feeding tubes for PVS persons, does not stand.

The third interpretation claims that the allocution does not change the tradition because, while it applies "in principal," it still leaves room for individuals to decide that in their own situations feeding tubes for PVS patients are extraordinary and, hence, optional. This interpretation is proposed by Mark Repenshek and John Paul Slosar in response to one of the Shannon and Walter articles noted earlier (Repenshek and Slosar 2004). The authors agree that the tradition proposes a weighing of burdens and benefits. They note, quite correctly, that the tradition has applied not just to medical treatment but to other means of preserving life (ibid., 14), so that simply calling tube feeding "care" and not "treatment" does not make it mandatory. They claim that, "given the origins of the principles . . . the address does not imply that medically assisted nutrition and hydration is obligatory for all patients in a PVS. As noted in the address itself, such care is only 'in principle ordinary and proportionate, and as such morally obligatory.'" They go on to state that "the address does not state that an individual could not judge for themselves that medically assisted nutrition and hydration in the case of PVS would be disproportionate" (ibid., 15). If this interpretation is correct, it seems to mean that the allocution has no required application. It applies to few if any patients. At least it can be said not to apply to people who think it does not apply to them or to their unconscious loved ones. It is rather an "in-principle" exhortation to respect life. If this interpretation can be considered the right one, then it would seem the allocution has little actual clinical impact. We should respectfully receive the exhortation but not think it changes what Catholic hospitals have been doing. As we note in the following, the latest changed directive 58 also includes the words "in principle" and thus is open to this same interpretation.

The fourth interpretation is similar to the third. It claims that the allocution applies only to those in PVS for whom nonfeeding would cause suffering. The important section here from the allocution is this: "the administration of water and food . . . should be considered in principle ordinary and proportionate, and as such morally obligatory insofar as and until it is seen to have attained its proper finality, which in the present case consists in providing nourishment to the patient and alleviation of his suffering" (John Paul II 2004, 739). Norman Ford, after quoting this passage from the allocution, states: "Hence it would no longer be morally necessary to provide MANH if the patient is unable to assimilate it, or if it fails to alleviate suffering, or if it causes suffering" (Ford 2005, 3). Although Ford does not explicitly draw this conclusion, it would seem that, since PVS patients cannot suffer, feeding them never attains the finality of alleviating suffering, so the allocution applies to absolutely no one. Again, here, as for the previous interpretation, the allocution is really an exhortation to respect life rather than a decree that would change Catholic teaching and hospital policy.

Debate over the meaning of the allocution has not arrived at consensus. Some argue that the Pope's speech means that the issue is settled and that Catholics (and, presumably, all persons) are obliged to demand and to provide feeding tubes for all PVS patients (Latkovic 2005, 512; Furton 2005). Others remain faithful to the tradition and insist that hydration and nutrition for PVS patients is morally extraordinary and hence optional (O'Rourke 2005; Eberl 2005; Shannon and Walter 2004, 2005a, 2005b, 2005c). The Catholic Health Association of the United States issued a brief statement on the March 20, 2004, papal allocution, noting that the "ethical, legal, clinical, and pastoral implications" of the allocution require careful consideration, and that "the guidance contained in the current [2001] *Ethical and Religious Directives for Catholic Health Care Services*, as interpreted by the diocesan bishop, remains in effect" (Catholic Health Association 2004). But those Directives have now been changed and the Vatican has issued new statements.

Vatican Responses

In August 2007 the Vatican Congregation for the Doctrine of the Faith (CDF) issued two "responses" to questions posed two years earlier by the American Catholic bishops in the wake of the papal allocution. The first question asks whether nutrition and hydration are morally obligatory for PVS patients excepting only when a patient cannot assimilate it or when it causes "significant physical discomfort." The answer is, "Yes. The administration of food and water even by artificial means is, in principle, an ordinary and proportionate means of preserving life. It is therefore obligatory to the extent to which, and for as long as, it is shown to accomplish its proper finality, which is the hydration and nourishment of the patient. In this way suffering and death by starvation and dehydration are prevented" (CDF 2007).

The second question asks whether this procedure can be stopped when it is morally certain that the patient will never regain consciousness. The answer is, "No. A patient in a 'permanent vegetative state' is a person with fundamental human dignity and must, therefore, receive ordinary and proportionate care which includes, in principle, the administration of water and food even by artificial means" (CDF 2007).

The external authority of this document is presumably somewhat stronger than that of the papal allocution. The CDF had two years to ponder the answer, and the document explicitly states that Pope Benedict XVI approved both responses. This does not mean, of course, that it reaches the higher levels of external authority such as that of encyclicals, conciliar documents, and similar pronouncements. There is certainly no question of infallibility. And the internal authority is still quite weak because it contradicts the received tradition on this issue.

The same four interpretations we have just now applied to the papal allocution might be applied to the "responses." The first would take it at face value and see it as requiring what the tradition has not required and thus as reinforcing a serious and dangerously contradictory change in Catholic medical ethics. This interpretation is certainly possible.[8] The second interpretation would emphasize once again that the requirement is limited only to PVS patients and to nutrition and hydration, and thus does not imperil the tradition as a whole. But, as we noted earlier, this fails to understand that the tradition is supposed to be reasonable and consistent. Changes made to one part of it affect the rest unless convincing reasons are given for the limitation. No convincing reasons are given as to why only PVS patients are included and only feeding tubes are required.

The third interpretation would point out that both responses include the same phrase "in principle" that is in the papal allocution. Thus the same interpretation given to the allocution can be given here. If so, there remains considerable flexibility. Patients can still decide for themselves that feeding tubes are morally extraordinary and thus rightly refuse them. This seems even more possible given the fact that the official French translation uses the phrase "en règle générale," "as a general rule," which suggests more flexibility than might be implied in the English phrase "in principle." On the other hand, perhaps the phrase means to allow only for the one exception that is explicitly stated. If this is the case, then as long as feeding tubes continue to nourish and hydrate the patient, they are absolutely obligatory in fact and not just in principle. As we will see, the same question arises when interpreting the latest change in the *Ethical and Religious Directives*.

The fourth interpretation of the allocution, that nutrition is mandatory only when it alleviates patient suffering (which never happens for PVS patients), would seem not to apply to the responses. The text of the first response limits the finality of the treatment to "hydration and nourishment of the patient" and no longer includes alleviation of suffering.

The 2009 Ethical and Religious Directives

In light of the allocution and the responses, the American Catholic bishops issued a new, fifth edition of the *Ethical and Religious Directives for Catholic Health Care Services*, dated November 17, 2009. The directive at issue is directive 58. It reads as follows:

> In principle, there is an obligation to provide patients with food and water, including medically assisted nutrition and hydration for those who cannot take food orally. This

obligation extends to patients in chronic and presumably irreversible conditions (e.g., the "persistent vegetative state") who can reasonably be expected to live indefinitely if given such care. Medically assisted nutrition and hydration become morally optional when they cannot reasonably be expected to prolong life or when they would be "excessively burdensome for the patient or [would] cause significant physical discomfort, for example resulting from complications in the use of the means employed." For instance, as a patient draws close to inevitable death from an underlying progressive and fatal condition, certain measures to provide nutrition and hydration may become excessively burdensome and therefore not obligatory in light of their very limited ability to prolong life or provide comfort (USCCB 2009a).

This directive, like the allocation and responses, requires feeding tubes for the permanently unconscious. In addition, it states that other patients must receive MANH if this treatment can prolong their lives. The question is whether this is a universal requirement or whether there are exceptions. The directive clearly offers exceptions for patients who are close to death even with tube feeding (there have been debates as to how close they have to be, two weeks or longer, but the directive does not say), and offers exceptions for those for whom the tube feeding would be burdensome for the patient or would add discomfort, presumably to a conscious patient.[9]

But the previous directive 58 is gone. That directive stated simply: "There should be a presumption in favor of providing nutrition and hydration to all patients, including patients who require medically assisted nutrition and hydration, as long as this is of sufficient benefit to outweigh the burdens involved to the patient" (USCCB 2001). That directive was in keeping with centuries-old Catholic teaching that allows for the withholding and withdrawal of morally extraordinary treatment, basing the distinction on a balancing of human burdens and benefits. Most Catholic hospitals and nursing homes interpreted this to mean that for PVS patients, because there was no human benefit to being kept physically alive while permanently unconscious, the burdens of the treatment, the cost, the harm to the families, and so on made the treatment morally extraordinary and hence optional. Now it seems there has been a significant, perhaps radical, change. But is that really the case?

Again we turn to interpretation. As for the allocation and the responses, the first interpretation would take the directive at face value and note with alarm the radical change it makes in the entire tradition. The directive continues the trajectory of the allocation and the responses toward the kind of vitalism traditionally rejected by Catholic ethics. Despite the fact that permanently unconscious patients are unable to carry on the basic purposes of life, life itself is now seen to have absolute or near absolute value. It is important to understand that this is not the same as stressing the undoubted intrinsic value of human life. Throughout this book the intrinsic, immeasurable value of human life has been emphasized. But this does not mean that life itself is of absolute value or that extending it is always of significant human benefit to the patient. "To say that the value of something is immeasurable . . . does not mean that its value is infinite" (Sulmasy 2011, 188). If it did mean this, the entire notion of ordinary and extraordinary life-sustaining treatments, where some are mandatory but others are optional, would be rejected. And this, the first interpretation claims, is what the new teaching does.[10]

The second interpretation would note that only feeding tubes are involved, and only PVS and similar patients are explicitly stressed; it would claim that this does not affect the tradition as a whole. But, as we have pointed out many times, this neglects to recognize the importance in Catholic ethics of reason and consistency. Feeding tubes are required, and other treatments such as antibiotics or simple surgeries are not. No reason is given as to why not. This interpretation fails.

Again the third interpretation would emphasize the phrase "in principle" that begins directive 58 and would claim that this leaves individual patients and their surrogates free rightly to decide that MANH is for them morally extraordinary and hence not obligatory (an earlier draft had "As a general rule" and was probably changed to bring the directive in line with the English translation of the Vatican responses). Whether the phrase "in principle" allows for the possibility of an exception even for some PVS or similar patients depends on whether it applies only to the first sentence or to the whole directive. It is possible that the phrase "in principle" applies only to the first, general sentence and not to the specifics that follow: "In principle, there is an obligation to provide patients with food and water." Under this interpretation, which seems reasonable, the directive then goes on to give examples of when feeding is mandatory and when it is not. It is mandatory in PVS and similar cases; it is not when the patient is close to death. But it is also possible to apply the words to the entire directive. "In principle" we should feed people, including those in PVS, but there may be exceptions, even for PVS patients.

This latter interpretation is made more possible by the inclusion in the directive of an exception that makes feeding treatments optional "when they would be 'excessively burdensome for the patient.'" If this clause is allowed to carry the full weight of the traditional balancing of burdens and benefits, then perhaps nothing serious has been changed in the directive. Treatments that are "excessively burdensome" are optional. This seems to be the interpretation given by Ron Hamel and Thomas Nairn of the Catholic Health Association in an article claiming to reflect the views of the staff ethicists of that organization but not to be an official interpretation of the directive (Hamel and Nairn 2010, 70). Hamel and Nairn include PVS patients among those for whom feeding tubes might be excessively burdensome (71–72). These authors are quite aware that patients properly diagnosed as permanently unconscious cannot themselves experience a burden. The burden must be something else, and it can be excessive only when weighed against a treatment's expected benefits. Indeed, the authors state that "the language of Directive 58 continues to allow for this burden/benefit assessment with regard to medically assisted nutrition and hydration" (72). Whether that is what the directive is intended to mean is not clear. But if the directive is open to that interpretation, then less has been changed in practice than would appear at first reading. Indeed, Hamel and Nairn state that the judgment about excessive burden is to be made by the patient or surrogate and the physician. This approach, if it is accepted as being in accordance with the new directive, will allow Catholic hospitals to continue to honor patients' wishes.

Directive 58 has been changed. Tube feeding is now required for PVS and similar patients, perhaps absolutely, perhaps with exceptions. If the more absolute interpretation is correct and exceptions are limited to cases where patients will die soon even with feeding, and to cases where patients are conscious and thus may experience the burden of suffering, then the directive and the responses and allocation that preceded it require feeding all, or almost all, PVS patients. No patient properly diagnosed as PVS can experience suffering and almost all of them will live on with MANH. But if exceptions are extended to other kinds of burdens, then the change, if there is one, is far less radical.

Reasons against Requiring Feeding Permanently Unconscious Persons

There are a number of reasons why traditional Catholic teaching permitting the nonuse of feeding tubes for PVS and other similar patients ought not to be changed. Here are seven.

1. To do so threatens the whole Catholic tradition of medical ethics. Why this is so should be clear by now.

2. It hurts real people. It keeps unconscious people unconscious, prevents their families from finding closure and moving on, and causes friction and hurt to health care professionals. And, paradoxically, it threatens in a bizarre way to lead Catholic families to refuse treatment for patients who might recover, rather than take the chance that they might lapse into a PVS. This is the possible result of interpretation two of the papal allocation described earlier. The new rule is often said to apply only to PVS and to feeding tubes. There is still flexibility in other cases. Perhaps a loved one has a serious stroke. While still in a coma but not yet in technical PVS, she requires a ventilator. The doctors say there is a small chance that she may recover awareness and even get better and go home. But it is far more likely she will enter a PVS. The family has been told that the allocation and the new directive apply only to PVS and only to feeding tubes, so they believe that they can morally refuse the ventilator now. But if she goes into PVS, they may be faced with twenty years of feeding tubes. So they refuse the vent. This may seem far-fetched, but Dr. Joseph Fins has this exact worry. He states: "If an observant Catholic family were to follow Church teachings, they might be able to discontinue 'extraordinary' measures early in the patient's course when the prognosis was still unknown, but they might not be able to discontinue artificial nutrition and hydration later on, once it was clear that the patient would not make any progress from the vegetative state. The paradox is startling: A Papal statement intended to promote life might have the unintended consequence of limiting the chance of recovery for some" (Fins 2005, 23). There has been rumor of such cases having actually occurred.

3. It threatens Catholic hospitals. Stories are already circulating that some Catholic hospitals are refusing to honor advance directives, and this may indeed be the case. People are starting to warn each other not to go to them. If Catholic hospitals were to be told not to honor advance directives about feeding tubes, as some writers insist they are (Furton 2005), they would be required by federal law (the Patient Self-Determination Act that we note in chapter 17) to tell all admitted patients this, which would severely threaten the hospitals. They and their doctors might even be open to criminal assault charges if they put tubes

into patients whose directives refused them. Hamel and Nairn are quite clear that Catholic hospitals must never do this (Hamel and Nairn 2010, 71).

4. It suggests no belief in an afterlife: keep them here as long as possible. Richard McCormick's statement about this was quoted earlier in this chapter.

5. Surely it is a violation of justice to spend so much on those who cannot benefit and who do not want the treatment in the first place.

6. It lends support to the euthanasia movement. This is despite the fact that many who would change the tradition and insist on MANH are motivated, at least in part, by a desire to stem the movement toward the legalization of euthanasia and physician-assisted suicide (PAS). In this they quite correctly interpret and apply the received tradition of Catholic medical ethics. But the identification of refusing MANH with suicide, implied in some of the bishops' documents and in other writings, is more likely to lead to the acceptance of PAS than to its rejection. If we allow suicide when we allow patients to forgo treatment, then why not make assisted suicide legal, too? In the next chapter, we note that this very claim, made by Justice Scalia in the *Cruzan* decision, was used by the Second Circuit Court to support its decision that laws against PAS are unconstitutional (Annas 1996, 684). Ironically, requiring PVS patients to submit to years of continued nonconscious life further motivates the very movement the bishops and others who would require MANH seek to oppose. It is clear that one of the major reasons for the current support of proposals to legalize PAS and euthanasia is the fear of loss of control. To require decades of unconscious existence in nursing home beds with virtually no chance of any conscious or even subconscious neurological activity is to give ammunition to those who claim that the only way to avoid this is to have the right to kill oneself or to be killed by another. The next chapter develops and defends arguments against the legalization and practice of physician-assisted suicide and euthanasia. These practices are largely unnecessary and potentially dangerous. But if people are forced to choose between being killed quickly and being stuck unconscious in a bed for twenty years with their families constantly in agony about it, many—even those opposed to it in theory—will ask for euthanasia.

7. It lends support to ethical relativism, that is, to the belief that there is no real basis for discovering right and wrong, and that it is all a matter of personal, baseless opinion. When internal incoherence is introduced into Catholic medical ethics, it and the Church it comes from are relegated to the realm of the "quaint." "Isn't it interesting," people think, "the Jehovah's Witnesses won't take blood and the Amish drive buggies and the Catholics feed the permanently unconscious. Who knows what's right? It's all a matter of opinion." This danger is increased when Catholic moral theology moves in the direction of a decreed or posited (we used to say one thing, but now the Vatican has spoken so we say another instead) rather than a discovered body of knowledge (we know what is right and wrong because we can discover it using reason and experience to examine the nature and purpose of the human person as creature of God). Thus, one of the last traditions of ethics (perhaps *the* last one) actually claiming to be reasonable and coherent and based in human purpose becomes but one more

example of an interesting contribution to contemporary ethical chaos, reduced to an arcane subject for study in graduate school.

Debate concerning the meaning of the documents we have discussed continues. And while some Catholic ethicists continue to hold to the earlier teaching that MANH is optional for PVS and similar patients, others claim that it is now mandatory.[11]

Practical Advice

The following practical suggestions for Catholic hospitals may be of some help. If a Catholic hospital decides to initiate tube feeding on a capable patient who rejects it, or on an incapable patient whose surrogate refuses it, having properly followed the legal standards of surrogate decision making that we saw in chapter 16 (substituted judgment and best interests), that hospital and its personnel are liable for criminal prosecution for assault and battery, although the local district attorney might well opt not to prosecute. There would also be liability for civil action for malpractice, and the likelihood of that would depend on the patient or the family and the outcome would depend on a jury. Catholic health care institutions should not break the law in this way. Some claim that the usual conscience clause exempting religious institutions from violating their beliefs would allow this, as Catholic hospitals must follow Church teaching. But conscience clauses usually apply to a hospital's refusal to do a procedure, such as an abortion or a sterilization. Hospitals can refuse to do certain things. But this is different because here presumably the hospital would be doing something to the patient that the patient does not want. The only solution—and it is not a good one—would be to transfer the patient to another institution that would agree to follow the patient's wishes.

In a case where a feeding tube has been legally and properly inserted and feeding begun, but *now* the patient or surrogate refuses to continue, a Catholic hospital might try to transfer the patient to a facility that agrees to remove the device. Remember that there is no legal or moral difference between withholding and withdrawing treatment. If the patient or surrogate has the right to withhold, he or she has the same right to withdraw. It might be hard to find a place that would accept the transfer, of course, but a good residential hospice would be a likely choice. If no one agrees to do this, it seems that continued feeding would itself be subject to the same rules as insertion in the first place, and thus liable to criminal and civic action. Catholic hospitals should not break the law.

The Patient Self-Determination Act that we discuss in chapter 17 requires that all health care institutions accepting federal funds—and that means almost all because almost all accept Medicare patients—must inform patients about their policies upon admission. The policies have to be available to patients to read if they wish. The PSDA does not explicitly require that admitted patients be informed if a policy is not in line with the usual policies. However, it does seem that if a Catholic hospital has a policy that it will insert feeding tubes in all patients who need them to survive and who are not immediately terminally ill, and that it will not honor treatment directives or patient or surrogate decisions in this area, then it needs to make this very clear upon admission despite the likely financial harm this will bring to the hospital. Even with such a statement, however, it does not seem that criminal and civil liability would be eliminated, although the statement might mitigate civil damages. Patients cannot legally immunize hospitals from assaulting them any more than one person can give permission to another to beat, enslave, or kill him and expect that this permission will immunize the perpetrator. Even if a hospital were to require of every admitted patient an explicit statement that he or she agrees to feeding tubes whenever the hospital deems it necessary, patients would still have the right to change their minds and refuse, and if the hospital treated against the patient's wishes, the hospital would violate criminal law.

Similarly, a Catholic hospital might include in its admissions documents a statement to the effect that patients have the right to refuse treatment and to create an advance directive "to the extent permitted by law and the Ethical and Religious Directives for Catholic Health Care Services," a clause taken from one Catholic hospital's admissions packet. This is an excellent idea, but, for reasons just given, such a statement would not allow the legal treatment of patients against their wishes or against the proper and legal wishes of their surrogates.

The new directive 58 includes the words "in principle" and allows for an exception when the treatment is excessively burdensome to the patient. It does seem reasonable to interpret these phrases as meaning at a minimum that Catholic hospitals are not required to impose MANH on patients who refuse or whose surrogates properly and legally refuse. In any case, there has been no official statement that would reject this interpretation.

The final point does not concern hospital policy but speaks to the moral obligation of individual Catholics to follow the presumed new change in Catholic teaching. As we have noted, there is no question here of infallible teaching. This is not a *de fide* teaching, a matter of faith. Catholic are certainly free to form their own consciences and may follow the teaching as it has been for decades, even centuries, rather than adopt the latest restrictions. Catholic moral teaching is supposed to be coherent and reasonable. Insisting on tube feeding for the permanently unconscious and similar patients is not consistent with Catholic principles. Catholics may rightly disagree with this policy and ask that tube feeding be withheld or withdrawn when its human burdens outweigh its human benefits.

Medically Futile?

One further related issue is the question of whether artificial nutrition might be removed from a permanently comatose patient against the wishes of the family or other surrogate. Currently, it is unwise and probably illegal to do so. The consensus as it has emerged thus far in the United States considers decisions such as these to be not medical decisions in the strict sense but value decisions or "quality of life" decisions. That is, no medical decision can be made that hydration and nutrition (as well as ventilation and other similar modalities) are medically futile in cases such as *Quinlan*, *Brophy*, and *Schiavo*. Such treatment cannot be called medically futile in the strict sense, such that physicians might unilaterally decide to forgo it. We return to the issue of medical futility in chapter 20.

Starvation and Dehydration?

When a person has irreversibly lost consciousness, there is no possibility that he or she will experience any of the effects of malnutrition or dehydration. But the ethical issue of forgoing hydration and nutrition is not limited to those in this condition. It can be morally extraordinary to use feeding tubes in other patients as well, as long as the principles for determining this are properly applied. Thus, the question arises as to whether hydration (and perhaps nutrition) are always required as a comfort measure for conscious patients. It seems clear that for very sick and dying patients the effects of dehydration are often actually benign (Printz 1989; Miller and Meier 1998). There is less fluid to cause breathing problems. Whatever discomfort there is can probably be alleviated by "maintaining moisture in the mouth with water, ice chips, or various forms of artificial saliva" (Billings 1985, 809). There is even medical evidence to suggest that tube feeding may be contraindicated in patients with advanced dementia who are not imminently dying, as its burdens often outweigh its benefits in such cases (Gillick 2000). According to one study, it does not provide comfort and does not even significantly prolong the patients' lives (Finucane, Christmas, and Travis 1999). Thus, it may be right to forgo it for patients with advanced dementia; the debate on this question is now under way (Burke 2001b; Kahlenborn 2001; Burke 2001a).

Terms such as "starvation" and "dehydration," while in one sense technically accurate, include implications that are almost never valid in the kinds of cases we have been considering. Clearly, if hydration and nutrition are necessary for the patient's comfort, they must always be used. But usually in cases such as these they are not necessary for comfort. Rather, they serve only to prolong the patient's dying process and may in fact add discomforts of their own. Thus, they are morally extraordinary and may rightly be withheld or withdrawn.

Determination of Death

PVS patients and the permanently comatose are not dead by current American legal standards. The Uniform Definition of Death Act (UDDA) makes it clear that death is the irreversible cessation of all cardiopulmonary function, or, in the presence of ventilators that keep that function going, death is the irreversible cessation of all brain function, including that of the brain stem (usually interpreted as all integrating brain function—random electric events are not signals of life) (Meisel 1989, 134; 1995, 1:625). All fifty states have accepted brain death as meaning legally that a person has died (Meisel 1995, 1:625). PVS patients have not lost function of the brain stem, which means that many continue to breathe on their own. Thus, in this chapter we have spoken of living but lethally ill persons, patients who will, unless morally extraordinary means are used to keep them alive, inevitably die of their condition.

Brain Death

Treatment is not "forgone" for the dead. No treatment can be given to the dead body of what once was a human person. Only the respect owed to corpses is proper. But there has been some development since the 1970s regarding how to determine that death has occurred. Prior to the use of mechanical ventilators that can keep the heart beating by providing it oxygen through the lungs, the determination of death was relatively simple, at least in theory. When a person stopped breathing, death was declared. There were in fact a considerable number of cases where persons in comas were thought to be dead and were buried alive. Devices were sometimes used to ensure that such people could signal were they to wake up in such a dire circumstance, but in theory the issue was easy enough. No breathing and no heartbeat meant that death had occurred. But that changed with the use of ventilators, creating the issue of "brain death."

Brain death, according to the UDDA, is not different from any other kind of death. It is death pure and simple. It is arguably unfortunate that the term is used, because many think it means a different kind of death, or an earlier death, or even a preventable death. It is better, for example, when doctors must tell families that this has occurred, for them to say simply that the patient has died rather than to say that the patient is brain-dead. Of course, if the family wants to know the details, or has been involved in the process of the diagnosis, physicians have to be clear about what has happened.

"Brain death" refers to criteria used to determine that a person has indeed died when the usual criteria for determining this event (cessation of breathing and heartbeat) are not available because heart and lung function are being forced by machines. But no one who is declared brain-dead would have been thought to be alive before the criteria and the machines that necessitated them were invented. Total brain death, when properly diagnosed, means virtually instant cessation of cardiac and pulmonary function in the absence of machines, though some cases have been reported of persons diagnosed as brain-dead whose hearts continued to beat for a few days or even as long as two weeks (Shewmon 2009, 19). Both the higher brain, the neocortex, and the lower brain and brain stem are dead. The person is dead. Heart and lungs may be forced to work, but this does not mean that human life of any sort continues. This is now almost universally accepted. Continued treatment of the brain-dead is treatment of a cadaver and is thus contrary to the standard of medical care. It is, in the meaning we give to the term in chapter 20, medically futile.

Recently there has been a good deal of controversy about the theoretical consistency of the definition and of the criteria for brain death (Shewmon 2009; Crowley-Matoka and Arnold 2004, 321; Fost 2004; Miller and Truog 2008, 2009; Chiong 2005). Some claim that brain death is not really death, but should be called "total brain failure" (Shewmon 2009, 19). These issues, which are usually posed in the context of organ retrieval, need not concern us here.[12] Most scholars, including most Catholic ethicists, agree that when the tests are properly applied and a person is found to permanently lack all integrative brain function, including that of the brain stem, the person has indeed died.

There is also some controversy about how to respond to persons who, from religious bases, reject the notion of brain death and insist that the hearts and lungs of such persons be forced to continue to function in the body, arguing that the person is alive. The most common judgment made here is that religion cannot legitimately reject a medical fact, and that this is indeed a medical fact and not a question of faith or of personal philosophy. Death is an ontological state and not, as such, a social construct (though there is much that we socially construct about the process and meaning of dying and death). Persons who are dead cannot properly be claimed to be alive. No medical treatment may be given to the dead. A dissenting opinion is given by those who believe that patient and family autonomy should always prevail in such cases and by those who reject brain-death criteria. The prevailing opinion, that this is a medical determination that cannot be denied on other bases, is held by a majority of ethicists and physicians. At the very least, anyone insisting on ongoing treatment for the brain-dead—that is, for dead persons—should be asked to bear the total cost.

Another controversial issue concerns the determination of the status of persons in irreversible comas and persistent vegetative states, those whose higher or neocortical brain functions have permanently stopped. These patients are not brain-dead since their brain stems continue to function. But they have irreversibly lost all higher brain function. They are "vegetative" and will remain so, but their hearts and lungs will continue to function, usually without mechanical ventilation. In this chapter, we have discussed the ethical and legal issues concerned with forgoing medical nutrition and hydration in such cases. But these issues would be moot if we were to declare these persons dead. Some argue that this is precisely what we should do (Meisel 1989, 134–35; 1995, 1:627–30; Veatch 2004).

There may be a legitimate theological argument for this approach, although thus far it has not been generally accepted.[13] It is clear, however, that society is not willing to claim that breathing bodies may be dead, not willing to bury breathing corpses. In addition, there is a serious danger of backlash against organ transplantation, especially since it is mainly the transplant specialists who are proposing that higher brain death be sufficient for declaring a person to have died (Meisel 1995, 1:627; Campbell 2004, 309–12). The context of harvesting cadaver organs is a bad one for making this kind of decision. This is also true of the proposal to declare anencephalic infants to be brain-absent and therefore dead.

This may change, but for now only total brain death, including death of the brain stem, should be considered to mean that the patient has died. Total brain death simply introduces a new set of criteria for determining the same moment of death. But neocortical criteria, according to which the irreversibly comatose would be declared to have died, would indeed push death earlier: patients who would, decades ago, have been thought to be alive would now be said to have died. Physicians would have to intervene to stop the heart and lungs. Society is not ready for this and probably doesn't need to accept it. With the sensitive forgoing of treatment, persons in irreversible comas can be allowed to die. They need not be declared already dead.

One final argument supports this position. Decisions to forgo medical treatment for the living need not be traumatic, but they should not be automatic either. Declaring a person to have died allows an easy escape from what should be a decision requiring serious thought. Ethics should offer comfort and relief from false guilt and fear, but it should not adopt moral or legal shortcuts to turn important decisions into thoughtless ones. Comatose persons should not be declared dead; brain-dead persons have indeed died.

Notes

1. PVS patients are indeed dying; they are dying from the brain injury that makes it impossible for them to eat and drink, just as patients with end-stage lung disease are dying because

their disease makes it impossible for them to breathe. Medically induced ventilation can keep breathing for them, but they are still said to be dying patients, and if the ventilator is withdrawn, they die from the disease, not from the withdrawing of the ventilator. The same is true for patients in irreversible coma or PVS. They are dying of a disease that will kill them unless these morally extraordinary means are used to keep them alive. As another example, the cause of death in patients with end-stage heart disease is the disease, not the forgoing of a heart transplant. If this analysis were not true, forgoing extraordinary means of treatment would always be the cause of death, and thus would be a direct killing. However, this is not the case, either according to American law or according to Catholic medical ethics.

2. The court in *Quinlan* used the word "comatose" (*In re Quinlan* 1982, 170), and the two terms are often not properly distinguished.

3. On the *Brophy* case, see Annas 1986; Paris 1986; Bresnahan and Drane 1986; Rothenberg 1986. For an opinion given at the trial, insisting that the treatment be maintained, see Derr 1986.

4. No secular ethicist, to our knowledge, insists on the moral relevance of this distinction. Some religious leaders insist on such a distinction, and the Orthodox Jewish tradition has claimed such relevance (Bone et al. 1990). For a different interpretation of the Jewish position, see Feldman 1986, 91–96; Dorff 2000b, 348–54; Mackler 2003, 97–98.

5. For citations in context by contemporary authors who are arguing the issue, see Paris 1986; Flynn 1990, 79; McCormick and Paris 1987, 358. Gerald Kelly says that artificial means such as oxygen and intravenous feeding "not only need not but should not be used, once the coma is reasonably diagnosed as terminal" (Kelly 1950, 220). Some argument might remain about what is meant here by "terminal," but it is most likely, given the rest of Kelly's argument about benefit and burden, that what we now call "irreversible coma" and "persistent vegetative state" would fit. In this article, Kelly argues that these means are "ordinary" but "useless" and therefore optional, thus adding a confusing distinction that is not necessary if "ordinary" and "extraordinary" are considered as moral rather than medical terms, as we have proposed, and as is more in consonance with the development of the distinction in Catholic medical ethics. Kelly's later use of these terms clears up his confusion here (Kelly 1958, 129).

6. A particularly helpful brief review of the issues from the Catholic perspective is O'Rourke 1989. Another source, often cited, is the doctoral dissertation by Daniel A. Cronin, later bishop of Fall River, Massachusetts, who supports the position that nutrition and hydration are not mandatory (Cronin 1958). A list of key citations from Catholic authors recognized as orthodox is given by McCartney 1986. An excellent analysis of the issues is given by Shannon and Walter 1988.

7. See also McHugh 1989; May et al. 1987. This last is a summary of the report sent to the Congregation for the Doctrine of the Faith.

8. The responses include a commentary that tries to show continuity of the required treatment with previous Church documents. But the citations are selective, and no recognition is made of the wider tradition we have described or of the reasons that tradition has given for concluding that MANH is indeed morally extraordinary for PVS patients.

9. This may be the case for some persons with Alzheimer's disease (Gummere 2008). While Peter Gummere insists that Church teaching now requires tube feeding for all PVS patients, he says that MANH imposes suffering on some (conscious) Alzheimer's patients and may not even prolong their lives. Thus it is not mandatory in these cases.

10. One of the reasons often proposed for the claim that MANH is obligatory for PVS and similar patients is their undoubted intrinsic dignity (for example, CDF 2007, Comm. no. 2). But is it indeed true that accepting the intrinsic value of life means that life itself is a benefit? Is life itself a benefit that must be weighed in all its immeasurable value against the burdens of a

treatment that extends it? Specifically in the context of PVS patients, who cannot consciously experience their lives, is extending life a benefit? In an important article, Daniel P. Sulmasy shows how the transcendental value of life itself is of a different order than the burdens and benefits to be weighed in determining whether a treatment is morally ordinary or extraordinary. Life itself is of intrinsic value. It is not weighed as a burden or a benefit. And while length of life is a benefit to be weighed along with other benefits and burdens, it is to be considered "only as one among other possible benefits and burdens of treatment, not as something of a special transcendent order that has automatic primacy. . . . Length of life is not the value of life" (Sulmasy 2011, 195). Sulmasy makes it clear that quality of life judgments must be made:

> It is contradictory to hold that it might be justifiable to forgo life-sustaining treatments but also to hold that one is prohibited from making quality of life judgments. The burdens and benefits of treatment are predicates of the patient, not of the treatment. It is Mrs. Jones, not the ventilator, who is benefitted or burdened by the ventilator. A judgment about the net sum of the burdens and benefits of continuing treatment for Mrs. Jones is a judgment about the quality of her life (ibid., 193).

It is certain that the Catholic tradition allows the forgoing of life-sustaining treatment in some (many) cases. It does this by weighing the burdens and benefits of treatment for the patient. That is, it requires that the patient's quality of life now and after treatment be evaluated. The mere fact that a patient will continue to live with MANH is not of itself reason to require it.

11. One recent suggestion has been made that while enteral nutrition and hydration (the tube is inserted into the stomach or the intestines) may be mandatory under the changed guidelines, parenteral nutrition (nourishment is given by IV directly into the bloodstream, thus bypassing the gastric tract) is not (Becker 2011). The latter is said to be a medical treatment whose burdens are greater than those of enteral MANH, and which can thus be discontinued under the usual criteria (burden and benefit) for distinguish ordinary and extraordinary means. But despite recent documents there is no reason to hold that enteral MANH is anything other than a medical procedure. It, too, should be judged according to burden and benefit. And while its burdens may in some sense be said to be less than those of parenteral MANH, its human benefits for terminally ill or permanently unconscious patients are virtually nil. For these patients, both enteral and parenteral procedures are morally extraordinary and, hence, optional.

In support of the tradition's claim that MANH may be optional for PVS patients, and for an excellent summary of and critique of the move toward vitalism, see O'Rourke 2008. See also Dugdale and Ridenour 2011. For claims that MANH is always mandatory in these cases, see Gummere 2008. For an argument that the new directive 58 is more flexible than the Vatican responses, see Dugdale and Ridenour 2011. These authors also note that some critics of the vitalist trajectory we have been tracing think it is based on "a perverse interest in prolonging suffering in order to save souls." This is certainly not the case. The move is toward an unfortunate and dangerous vitalism, and it may well result in increased suffering, but that is not its purpose. Still, Catholic teaching has often been accused of increasing the suffering of dying people. Concerning the slow death of her grandfather, who was afflicted with advanced Parkinsonism, Alice Dreger writes in a bioethics piece that it was "the Catholic Church that I came to resent, as it seemed to put us in the position of having to endlessly torture a man we could not have loved more by treating what I think came to eighteen rounds of pneumonia" Dreger 2010, 3). That never should have happened, of course; Catholic teaching has never required extraordinary means of this kind. Sadly and tragically, someone must have misunderstood the tradition. Hopefully the vitalist trajectory of recent pronouncements will not be seen as reason to cause such tragedy in the future.

12. Because there is virtually no chance of a person properly diagnosed as brain-dead recovering any level of consciousness or interaction, the debate is usually framed in terms of whether the dead-donor rule—the requirement that donors must be dead before vital organs are taken—should be kept, changed, or discarded. Few argue that organs not be taken in such cases. But there is a kindred controversy concerning the retrieval of organs from those declared dead after cessation of heart function, or "donation after cardiac death" (Marquis 2010; Miller and Truog 2008). Here it seems that the issue is more than theoretical because organs are often retrieved after as few as two minutes of cardiac arrest, a time lapse that would not preclude the possibility of medical resuscitation, even to a conscious and interactive state. Those who consider death an ontological state and not a social construct must consider it likely that some such donors are living persons. For a defense of donation after cardiac death with a five-minute time lapse as compatible with official Catholic medical ethics, see Driscoll 2012. For the claim that donation after cardiac death is forbidden by Catholic teaching, see Sanchez 2012.

13. See Janssens 1983. For an analysis of this argument, see Kelly 1988.

CHAPTER 19

PHYSICIAN-ASSISTED SUICIDE AND EUTHANASIA

Introduction

WE HAVE SEEN that the American consensus on forgoing treatment has as one of its ethical bases the claim that there is a difference between killing terminally ill patients, on the one hand, and allowing them to die of their underlying condition, on the other. The general agreement has been that while it is often right to withhold or withdraw medical treatment that would prolong the lives of dying persons, it is not right to kill them or to help them to kill themselves.

There have always been, of course, those who disagree with this position. But only recently have we seen major turmoil in the United States about the ethics and about the law concerning euthanasia or physician-assisted suicide (PAS). Some states did not have laws forbidding assisting at suicide, and some states did (and still do), but until 1996 no cases had been decided concerning the constitutionality of such laws. Prior to this, there had been no real legal attack on the "second pillar" of the consensus.

Recent Legal Decisions

In 1996 two important court decisions reached conclusions opposed to the general legal consensus about active euthanasia and physician-assisted suicide. And then, in June 1997, the US Supreme Court reversed those decisions, returning the legal status to what it had been but in doing so underlining the possibility that states may indeed proceed to pass laws legalizing physician-assisted suicide and, presumably, even active euthanasia.

The US Court of Appeals for the Ninth Circuit (Washington, Oregon, California, Alaska, and four other western states) and the US Court of Appeals for the Second Circuit (New York, Connecticut, and Vermont) both decided in 1996 that certain state laws (those of Washington and of New York) forbidding physician-assisted suicide were unconstitutional (Meisel 2003, 479–93). Although neither of these decisions affected practices in other jurisdictions—and even in these states the practical effect was minimal as everyone waited for the anticipated Supreme Court appeals—there was for a time a real worry (or hope, depending on one's viewpoint) that all state laws forbidding physician-assisted suicide might be found unconstitutional.

The Ninth Circuit claimed that there is a constitutional right to choose the time and manner of one's own death that extends at least to terminally ill people, so that they may ask physicians to help them commit suicide (*Compassion in Dying v. Washington*, 1996). It appeals to the *Casey* abortion decision (*Planned Parenthood v. Casey*, 1992) and to *Cruzan v. Director* (1990) as supports for a liberty interest that is, or approaches the status of, a fundamental right to choose how and when to die. Thus, laws making this illegal are unconstitutional (Meisel 2003, 479–88).

The Second Circuit argued more narrowly that the equal protection clause of the Fourteenth Amendment does not permit states at the same time to let terminally ill people choose to withdraw life-sustaining treatment, and thus to die when and how they wish, *and* to forbid terminally ill people from asking doctors to help them kill themselves (*Quill v. Vacco*, 1996; Meisel 2003, 488–93). This, said the Second Circuit, illegally discriminates against those unfortunate enough to be dying and not be on forgoable life-support. These persons were not equally protected under the law. Both circuit courts claimed that the long-held distinction between killing and letting-die is a false one. The Second Circuit cited Justice Scalia's minority opinion in *Cruzan* equating refusal of treatment with suicide as one of its bases for this judgment (Annas 1996, 187).

The Ninth Circuit decision includes bad history and bad analysis (Schneider 1997; Kamisar 1996). The court did not even take the time to understand the meaning of some of the ethical terms it was using. For example, it seems to have equated the distinction between withholding and withdrawing treatment with that between commission and omission, or active and passive euthanasia. As we saw in detail in chapter 2, withholding and withdrawing are *both* permitted as "passive euthanasia," a term that is, as we have already noted, confusing and probably ought to be avoided. Withholding and withdrawing are both the nondoing of treatment and may well be right. The Second Circuit decision was better argued but still ultimately flawed. Despite Scalia's opinion, refusal of treatment is *not* the same as suicide. And there are other reasons as well for rejecting the decisions of both circuit courts that we note later in this chapter.

In June 1997 the US Supreme Court reversed the decisions of both of the circuit courts (Meisel 2003, 493–510). It held, against the Ninth Circuit, that there is no constitutional right to choose when and how one dies, and it rejected the argument of the Second Circuit that there is no difference between forgoing life support and suicide, holding that it is not contrary to the equal protection clause of the Fourteenth Amendment to allow withdrawal of life support but to forbid assisting at self-killing and euthanasia.[1] Thus, the Supreme Court stated that the Washington and New York laws forbidding assisting at suicide are constitutional, or, to be more precise, that they are not unconstitutional on the grounds claimed by the circuit courts. We are thus back to where we were. States may pass laws forbidding euthanasia and forbidding assisting at suicide. States need not pass such laws, of course. They may have no laws at all. Or they may specifically permit these practices, as Oregon and Washington have done for PAS.

The 1994 Oregon referendum and subsequent law (The Oregon Death with Dignity Act, 1998) and the 2008 Washington referendum and law (The Washington Death with Dignity Act, which was explicitly based on the Oregon law) permitting physician-assisted suicide were not rejected by the Supreme Court's decision. Another federal court decision rejected the Oregon law as unconstitutional, but the Supreme Court overturned that decision. In November 1997 another referendum in Oregon that would have reversed the first referendum, thus making PAS again illegal in Oregon, failed by a 60–40 vote. Various attempts by federal and local initiatives, including rulings that using drugs for suicide would violate federal laws, also failed (Meisel 2003, 43–45), and the Supreme Court ruled in January 2006 against the attempt by the Bush administration to criminalize this use of drugs (Baron 2006). Thus, PAS is now legal in Oregon and Washington.

In sum, although we are legally back where we were, much has been legally clarified, and the next battleground will be state legislatures. Their decisions are not easy to predict. After the decision in Oregon many thought that other states would soon legalize PAS. To date this has happened only in Washington, and perhaps also in Montana where, on December 31 2009, the state supreme court ruled that physicians may not lawfully be convicted of homicide if they prescribe lethal drugs in accordance with certain state rules (Robinson 2010, 15–16).[2] Some other states have passed laws forbidding PAS or have strengthened their own laws against the practice. As of 1999 thirty-seven states had laws specifically forbidding assisting at suicide, eight forbade it by common law or case precedent, and four were unclear (Doerflinger 1999b).

This chapter is divided into three main sections. First is a brief sketch of the definitions and distinctions necessary for an understanding of the issue. Second is a description of alternatives to physician-assisted suicide. The third section is a brief personal chronology of the changing judgments of Dr. Kelly, one of this book's authors, on the question about whether PAS and euthanasia are morally right and ought to be legal. The chapter argues against active euthanasia and physician-assisted suicide, and develops the bases for the arguments against these practices, suggesting which bases hold and which do not.

Definitions and Distinctions

Physician-assisted suicide is generally understood to mean the action by a licensed physician of providing to a legally competent person some means to use in the committing of suicide. Although it is not formally part of the definition, a context of the person's terminal illness is often assumed and has been part of the prerequisite conditions in all proposed laws thus far as well as in the two decisions by the US circuit courts. But this is not a formal part of the definition of physician-assisted suicide as such, since physicians might be permitted to offer such aid to those who wish to kill themselves for other reasons. In fact, many advocates include conditions that are not terminal in the sense the law commonly gives to that term, that is, a condition that will probably cause death within six months regardless of what treatments are applied. PAS is different from the withholding or withdrawal of life-sustaining treatment, on the one hand, and from the actual killing of the patient by the doctor (physician-administered euthanasia), on the other. The former action (withholding or withdrawal) is legal and is recognized as ethically right by the present American ethical consensus and by official Catholic teaching. The latter (active euthanasia) is forbidden as criminal homicide in all fifty states, and the recent court decisions do not address it directly, though, as we point out later, once we allow PAS, we will almost of necessity have to allow active euthanasia in at least some cases.

A distinction is often made among voluntary, nonvoluntary, and involuntary euthanasia. Voluntary euthanasia is the killing of a person at that person's request. Nonvoluntary euthanasia is a killing in the absence of such a request and is usually proposed and debated in the context of incompetent persons. Involuntary euthanasia is a killing of a person who explicitly rejects the offer. Physician-assisted suicide in the strict sense presupposes a voluntary act because it is the patient who consumes the drug. Pressures that would reduce voluntariness might be brought to convince persons to accept the offer and take the drug. Similarly, less-than-competent persons might be allowed to choose to kill themselves and then might be given lethal drugs. These two reductions in voluntariness are admittedly also possibilities when patients must decide whether to accept or forgo life-sustaining treatment.

Alternatives to Physician-Assisted Suicide

There are two humane and morally proper alternatives to PAS that are supported by the present consensus, along with a number of inhumane ones that unfortunately often occur. The inhumane alternatives to PAS include abandonment of patients to their own devices, refusal to care for them because their insurance is insufficient, inadequate pain management, and paternalistic insistence, against their wishes, on aggressive (morally extraordinary) life-sustaining treatment.

The two humane, legal, and morally proper alternatives are, first, the ethically right and legal forgoing of life-sustaining treatment, and, second, proper pain management. Even such a strong advocate of PAS as Timothy Quill supports these as alternatives when PAS is illegal (Quill 2008, 18–19). It is clear that if we were better at these than we are, we would reduce the perceived need for helping patients kill themselves, though we would not eliminate it altogether. As we saw in chapter 14, the process of dying inevitably brings with it what James Walter calls "agent narrative suffering" as distinguished from the "neurophysiological suffering" that pain relief can eliminate (Walter 2002, 6). Eliminating this existential anxiety that comes to so many of us as we die and eliminating the loss of bodily and mental control that accompanies dying will doubtless remain reasons for requesting euthanasia and PAS. As we have already seen, however, even these can be alleviated with the care and compassion of health care providers, family, and others.

The Ethics of Assisted Suicide and Euthanasia

Even with the proper forgoing of treatment and proper pain control, there remain some reasons for physician-assisted suicide and euthanasia. What, after all, is the difference between giving dying persons enough sedation to keep them unconscious until they die and simply killing them now or helping them to kill themselves while they still can? Why not just get it over with? Why maintain this antiquated notion that killing and allowing to die are ethically different?

We need to return to the reasons supporting the second pillar of the consensus, the claim that there is a moral difference, and that there ought to be a legal difference between killing and allowing to die. To get at these reasons, I will trace my own moral journey on this issue.[3] I hope this will not be totally idiosyncratic and will help in an understanding of the claims made and the justifications given for them. My own moral judgment on this issue has gone through four stages, and I will use this as a framework.

Stage One: Euthanasia Is Intrinsically and Always Wrong and Must Be Illegal

When I was in college and during my early graduate work, I was convinced that the reasons proposed by the received tradition of Catholic ethics for concluding that the direct killing of innocent people is absolutely wrong were valid. There are two basic reasons given. First, it is argued that God keeps to God's self the right to kill the innocent, giving to humans only the right to kill the guilty and the right sometimes to allow the innocent to die. Second, it is argued that such killing of the innocent is an intrinsically evil or intrinsically wrong action apart from intention, circumstances, and consequences. In this first stage I accepted these reasons as valid. Thus, I held that euthanasia (and PAS, which was not really an issue then) was always wrong and ought to be illegal.

Stage Two: Euthanasia Is Often Right and Should Be Legal

When I was working on my doctoral dissertation on the history and method of Catholic medical ethics (Kelly 1979), I became convinced that neither of the reasons worked. Since we have already, in parts I and II of this book, looked at both of these reasons and the bases for rejecting them, it is enough here to say that the first reason, the one about God, turns out to depend on the second, the one about intrinsically evil acts. I did not think, and still do not think, that a person can make valid ethical judgments based solely on acts themselves apart from human circumstances, intentions, and consequences. I had shifted my answer to question 2 of normative ethical theory from deontology to some form of consequentialism or proportionalism and had moved from physicalism to personalism. I accepted the arguments proposed by Daniel Maguire (1974) and concluded that euthanasia was sometimes morally right and that it ought to be legal as well.

Stage Three: Euthanasia and PAS May Be Morally Right but Should Be Kept Illegal

In 1981, when I began teaching at Duquesne University and working on ethics committees in Pittsburgh area hospitals, this experience and the reading I did around the issue began to worry me. I became more aware of what I perceived to be the social consequences of a practice of euthanasia, and more concerned about slippery-slope social results. So, in *Critical Care Ethics* (Kelly 1991), I argued that although euthanasia might be morally right at least some of the time, it should not be legalized. My reasons against the legalization of PAS and euthanasia, which I think are still valid, include the following:

> 1. Any increase in the number of exceptions to the general principle against killing makes other exceptions easier. Our nation has decided that killing is legally permitted

in properly declared wars, in court-ordered capital punishment, in abortion, in self-defense, and in some circumstances in defense of private property attacked criminally. Active euthanasia is not the same kind of killing as these others, but to permit it legally would add one further allowable exception to the law forbidding killing. This first reason is not convincing to everyone because of the difference between euthanasia and PAS and other kinds of legal killing. But I am convinced that there is simply too much violence, and for me this remains a violence.

2. It will be very difficult, if not impossible, to hold the line at physician-assisted suicide and resist moving to voluntary and to nonvoluntary active euthanasia (New York State Task Force on Life and the Law 1994, 144–45). This much is clear to me. If one accepts PAS, one must accept logically, and will have to accept legally, some kinds of euthanasia—certainly voluntary and probably nonvoluntary. I do not mean by this that I think that euthanasia advocates are really Nazis in disguise who want to do away with the old and the infirm. Far from it. Most are caring physicians and ethicists dedicated to helping the dying and to alleviating suffering. But I do not see any valid moral reason for refusing a merciful death simply because a patient is not able, here and now, to ask for such a death and to do it unaided. Although laws might at first limit the practice to physician-assisted suicide, it would be hard to draw the line there, since one might logically insist that those incapable of choosing and of killing themselves should also have the right to be freed of the dying process that presently competent persons might legally escape. Surely, if we cross the line to allow physicians to provide lethal drugs to help in the suicide of a dying patient, we owe similar help to those competent dying persons unable to kill themselves—for example, to a quadriplegic who requires assistance to take the pills. In this case, the action would technically be euthanasia because the physician would have to put the pills in the patient's mouth. And if this is done, there is surely good reason to do it by injection instead, since lethal agents can be better introduced that way.

And what about those who asked for euthanasia in documents they wrote after they were diagnosed with a terminal illness? These people want to live on until they can no longer function humanly. So they ask that the drug be administered to them, not now while they still have reasons for living and can take it themselves, but later, when they are no longer able to interact. Surely these people have greater reason to have their lives ended than do those who wish to take the pills while they still can. And this is clearly a case of euthanasia by previous directive. I think it is still voluntary euthanasia, but it is less immediately clear what the person would want now.

What about those who request euthanasia in an advance directive written before any specific diagnosis? If they suffer a sudden trauma that makes them permanently unconscious, should we refuse to honor that directive simply because they never had the chance to ask for drugs and to take them themselves? This will open up the problems of interpretation we discuss in chapters 16 and 17.

And what about those who have never been able to ask for this help, such as children and those with lifelong severe mental illness? We will certainly have to allow loving families to request that their dying loved ones be killed—or "euthanized"—just as we now allow them to request the forgoing of treatment. It makes no sense not to do that (Jones 2011).

And finally, what about a person who is not terminally ill in the strict sense but who is diagnosed with a long-term chronic illness such as Lou Gehrig's disease (ALS)? What reason do we have to refuse "aid in dying" to such a person? Although perhaps we can hold the line at terminally ill or permanently unconscious persons, why would we want to do that? Medication can eliminate pain in the dying patient, but it will not help the quadriplegic walk again. It does not allow persons with long-term progressive illnesses to escape the limitations those illnesses bring. So in some ways there is greater reason to help nondying persons commit suicide or to kill them when they ask us (active euthanasia) than there is to do this for the imminently dying. Nonterminal patients may be assisted in suicide in the Netherlands, Belgium, and Switzerland (Appel 2007, 21).

It is important to note that there is reason to think that once we legalize PAS, we will be required to legalize euthanasia for at least some of the categories of persons I have described. It is quite probably contrary to the equal protection clause of the Fourteenth Amendment to limit such help to conscious persons and to refuse it to others. The Supreme Court overturned the decision of the Second Circuit Court of Appeals on PAS, but it did not repeal the Fourteenth Amendment. Rather, it said that there is a relevant difference between forgoing treatment and PAS. It does not seem that there is such a relevant difference among the kinds of patients I have been describing. I think it is likely that someone in Oregon and Washington will argue that the state laws there are unconstitutional because they unjustly discriminate in favor of persons currently able to ask for and to consume the lethal drugs and against those who cannot. The Supreme Court may well have to rule that since these states have permitted PAS, they must permit active euthanasia as well.

A great deal of controversy has arisen concerning evidence from the Netherlands on this question. For some time, although euthanasia remained technically illegal, there was an agreement that physicians who practiced it would not be prosecuted as long as they followed certain criteria (euthanasia under these criteria is now technically legal in the Netherlands). One of these criteria is that the person to be killed must ask for it. But there is clear evidence, based on the Dutch government's own 1991 "Remmelink Report," that a significant number of those killed do not ask for it (Marker and Smith 1996, 84–85; Hendin, Rutenfrans, and Zylicz 1997; Keenan 1998, 17). Infants, children, and the unconscious seem to be candidates in some cases. The same is clear from a more recent report, which notes that in 2001 more than 25 percent of cases of euthanasia in Holland were without request on the part of the person killed. And in Switzerland the Swiss high court upheld the right of the mentally ill to assistance at suicide (Appel 2007).

None of this is compelling proof in itself against the legalization of PAS. But it is compelling proof that it is naive to think that one can support the legalization of PAS but not also support the legalization of voluntary and of some kinds of involuntary euthanasia. The same reasons support both.

3. There is the ever-present danger, especially in a time of necessary resource allocation, that PAS and active euthanasia would serve as a socially acceptable form of cost containment (Wolf 1996; Burt 1996, 169–72; New York State Task Force on Life and the Law 1994, 143). The temptation to eliminate poverty by eliminating the poor might be hard to resist. This will be especially tempting to insurance companies, which might offer lower premiums to persons who agree ahead of time to commit suicide if they are diagnosed with a terminal or chronic illness. Minority populations may perceive themselves to be especially vulnerable (King and Wolf 1998). And even if laws were passed forbidding this, there would remain the inevitable subtle and not-so-subtle pressures exerted in families and even among the elderly themselves. If the elderly see their peers agreeing to PAS or euthanasia in order to eliminate a burden on their families, they may feel a responsibility to do the same. Social and cultural pressures might become hard to resist.

Admittedly these same pressures already exist when it comes to refusing life-sustaining treatment. So this argument is not itself totally compelling. That is the problem with "slippery slope" arguments. But there *is* a difference. PAS and euthanasia, once accomplished, are definitive choices. Decisions to forgo treatment can be changed if conditions warrant it. Perhaps of greater importance is the fact that persons simply must have the legal right to be free from unwanted medical intervention; if this right were not granted, we would needlessly increase suffering and attack personal autonomy. We do not want to go back to where we were. And so we grant this right, even though we know there can be cases where unjust pressures are brought to bear on poor persons to forgo treatment they may really want. We try to safeguard against this by insisting on criteria for surrogate decision making and by trying to be sure this is what patients want. But the same is not true of PAS and euthanasia. The right to have help in killing oneself or the right to be killed is not an essential basic human right or human need. This practice would add further risks to the ones we already face in a basically unjust health care system of discriminating against people unable to pay for their own care, an issue we discuss in chapter 28. It is a line we should not cross.

4. The distinction between killing and allowing to die has been one of the pillars on which the present American consensus, which legally permits the forgoing of certain treatments, is based. The absolute legal prohibition of active euthanasia (and, thus far, the legal prohibition in most states of PAS) thus serves as a protective barrier against going too far and serves as a valid argument against those who think that forgoing treatment is itself euthanasia. If we remove that barrier, there may be fear on the part of some that we have gone too far already (Kamisar 1996, 495–96). There may be, in other words, a backlash against the present consensus that forgoing treatment is in many cases legally and morally right. The legalization of active euthanasia may lead politically to a restriction of the present consensus as the pendulum swings back.

There is already, in the court decisions we have examined, the kind of confusion that might lead to a strictly vitalistic legal code insisting on aggressive treatment for all persons regardless of likely outcome. If the Second Circuit Court was right when it said that the equal protection clause required that we make no distinction between persons on life support and those not on it, then perhaps, if we want to avoid euthanasia, we must insist on treating even against patients' wishes. If withholding or withdrawing treatment is itself euthanasia, as the Second Circuit implied, and as Justice Scalia explicitly claimed in *Cruzan*, then to avoid euthanasia we would have to refuse quite proper requests by patients or surrogates to withdraw life-sustaining treatment. Only by maintaining the distinction can we avoid this confusion.

5. The final reason concerns the integrity of the medical profession. Doctors are not now allowed to kill their patients. Permission to do this might possibly lead to mistrust on the part of some patients. The American Medical Association and the American College of Physicians both oppose PAS on this basis (Nelson and Ashby 2011, 35). Admittedly, this reason can be said to beg the question. Those who support PAS argue that physicians would in this way be able to help their patients die, and thus greater trust would result. Thus far in Oregon there is no evidence that trust in doctors has been lost (ibid., 33). But there is still some reason for concern. In Australia a law legalizing euthanasia in one section of the country was revoked, in part because Aboriginal peoples, fearing white doctors, worried that the doctors would kill them. Similar fears are often found in minority populations in the United States (King and Wolf 1998).

Thus, for these reasons, I concluded that although euthanasia and suicide might be morally right, they should not be made legal.

Stage Four: PAS and Euthanasia Are (Usually) Wrong and Should Not Be Legalized

My present judgment is not far removed from stage three. Perhaps the difference is too minor to worry about. But the more aware I become of the possibilities of pain management, the more I think that, when proper pain control is available, it is morally wrong for persons to request PAS or euthanasia. If I am right that legalizing physician-assisted suicide and euthanasia would be bad for our society, then, since even dying persons have social responsibilities, dying persons should not further the move toward legalization by requesting this for themselves. I do not believe this moral obligation holds in some circumstances where pain relief is not available. Thus, in "deserted island" cases, and possibly in similar circumstances in developing nations (but I cannot know without knowing the likely social results of proposing a practice of euthanasia in those societies), euthanasia and assisted suicide may be morally right. It is true that in the United States pain relief is not always properly provided, but the answer in such cases is to insist on getting it, or to fire the doctor, or to change hospitals. There may be other exceptions in addition to the absence of pain relief, although I do not think they are many or common. So I continue to disagree with the judgment that active euthanasia and suicide are absolutely morally wrong. But the exceptions are rarer than I used to think they were, and I now consider the dangers greater that I once did.

I am aware, as I have noted, that there is always a problematic remainder beyond pain, a remainder of "agent narrative suffering," loss of control, and family grief that, at least arguably, only quick killing can eliminate. This remainder calls for care. It should not be dismissed. But I do not think this remainder is enough to lead us to the judgment that active euthanasia and physician-assisted suicide are generally morally right. I am too much worried about the social effects of the widespread practice of euthanasia. So, even though it might be better for *me* to be killed now, or to kill myself now, rather than wait for death to come, it is better for *us* that I wait.

Notes

1. For a claim that this finding was based on the principle of double effect; see Black 2011.

2. The Montana case, *Baxter v. Montana*, overlooked the essential distinction between forgoing treatment (allowing to die) and killing or self-killing (Robinson 2010, 16). Once again we see how the vitalist claim that since both are the same, neither should be permitted, made by Justice Scalia in *Cruzan* and by many of those who insist on MANH for the permanently comatose, is reasonably used by their opponents to defend euthanasia and PAS. If withdrawing treatment is already euthanasia, they say, then both should be legal. In 2012, a ballot initiative in Massachusetts to legalize physician-assisted suicide was defeated by a very narrow margin.

3. This section is written in the first person by David Kelly, one of the book's co-authors. The conclusions expressed here are shared by the other authors of the book, at least in general, but the chronology obviously is not.

CHAPTER 20

MEDICAL FUTILITY

Introduction

MUCH OF THE BIOETHICS LITERATURE of the 1970s and 1980s, and all of the early court cases involving conflict between hospitals and doctors on one side and patients' families on the other concerned situations where the hospitals and doctors insisted on continuing treatment and the families wanted to stop. The medical ethical literature suggested that the paradigmatic case of conflict would set the physicians' medical model against the more humane moral sense of patients and families. Physicians, and possibly other health care providers, would see the main enemy as disease and death, and would try to hold it off at all costs. It would be the families who would ask that their loved ones be allowed to die with dignity, free from disproportionate medication and technology.

By the late 1980s, at least in teaching hospitals in big cities, the exact opposite was more likely to occur. Although conflicts did and still do arise along the lines of the earlier model, there had been a major shift in the type of conflictive case. The most contentious cases now are likely to be those in which the families insist on aggressive treatments while the physicians want to stop, often arguing that the treatment is futile. From this context has arisen the debate about the meaning of and the criteria for "medical futility."

The literature on medical futility began around 1988, but the term "futile" had been used before that, even though its exact meaning had not been specified. It is often found in hospital policies on forgoing treatment. When used in these policies, it refers generally to procedures that doctors are not required to offer because they are contrary to the standard of care; they are medically useless in a generally recognized way. Policies would say simply that physicians are never required to provide futile treatment. Only more recently has there been argument as to what exactly that means. The medical futility debate has arisen because some have attempted to expand the notion of futility to include treatments that were not included earlier in the category of procedures doctors ought not to provide. That is, treatments that physicians might have argued for in an era of physician paternalism, sometimes against the wishes of patients and families, were now to be rejected by physicians, against the wishes of patients and families, on the basis of futility. The question is whether this expansion is ethically justified. The short answer to that question is that it is not justified, but nuances of the debate and of that answer to it are important.

The Importance of the Issue

In chapter 18, the chapter on hydration and nutrition, we discuss and argue against a movement that criticizes and would radically change the "first pillar" of the consensus concerning end-of-life treatment, the distinction between ordinary and extraordinary means of preserving life that we discuss in chapter 13. It would do that, we saw, by claiming that what has generally been seen as extraordinary and thus optional is really ordinary and thus mandatory. This challenge comes from the "right," or "conservative" wing. In chapter 19, the chapter on physician-assisted suicide and euthanasia, we discuss and argue against a movement that criticizes and would radically change the present American consensus by rejecting the legal and ethical notion that there is and ought to be a distinction between killing and allowing to die. Proponents of physician-assisted suicide and euthanasia would thus change (or eliminate) the "second pillar" of the present general American approach to these issues, the pillar we develop in chapter 14. This challenge comes from the "left" or "liberal" wing. The medical futility debate challenges the third pillar of the consensus, the procedural or legal pillar supporting the legal rights of patients or surrogates to decide about treatment options. It involves a proposal to allow physicians to reject on the basis of their medical knowledge certain treatments desired by patients or surrogates. Criteria have been proposed for determining medical futility that would expand the applicability of this concept from its traditional restricted usage.

We have just seen one indication of the importance of this topic: the shift in the kind of conflictive case from the older typical case where the physician insists on aggressive treatment against the family's wishes to one where the patient or family insists on treatment against the advice of the health care team. Why has this shift occurred? The number of articles dealing with the topic, starting in the late 1980s, indicates that it is a general phenomenon. Physicians and ethicists are increasingly interested in what to do when doctors want to stop and families want to treat. Clinical experience and anecdotal evidence suggest that this shift at first occurred more in urban hospitals than in rural ones. That is, in rural hospitals physicians were, and perhaps still are, apt to insist on aggressive treatment for the terminally ill despite family wishes, whereas in urban hospitals conflicts are now more apt to be the other way around. It is probable, however, that changes like this began in the urban teaching centers and are now making their way to the rural institutions.

Why the Shift?

There are three causes for the growing concern about cases of this type and thus about medical futility. First, American health care providers have become more aware of the importance of patient autonomy. There is a greater emphasis on informed consent and other issues of patients' rights. Certain decisions about treatment are made by the patient or the patient's surrogate, not by the physician or the health care team. One reason for this change was the general acceptance of a criticism made against the older paternalistic approach. In 1973 Robert Veatch, one of the strongest critics of medical paternalism, attacked what he called the "generalization of expertise" (Veatch 1973b). By this he meant the tendency of health care professionals, especially physicians, to assume that their considerable expertise in medicine gave them expertise as well in ethics and in determining correct human values for their patients. Physicians are professionally trained to make medical decisions, he said (and, as will become clear, this includes decisions that a treatment is medically futile) but not necessarily to make decisions about what patients ought to do with respect to the values they cherish. To assume they could was a fallacy, the fallacy of generalization of expertise. Medical ethics has generally accepted this criticism of paternalism, as has recent American law. Although it is quite true that patient autonomy cannot stand as an absolute value in automatic preference to all others—a point being made with increasing frequency, especially in the context of allocation of medical resources—the importance of autonomy is well recognized. Physicians have come to understand this. Legally and morally, the patient is to be seen as more than a disease to be treated. The patient is also a person who makes decisions and whose values count.

It may seem puzzling to say that this is a reason for proposals that would reduce patient and surrogate authority by returning to health care professionals some of the decision-making authority that has been transferred since the 1960s to patients (or their surrogates). But this change has brought with it a reduction in the automatic technological imperative that preceded it. Because physicians realize that patients and surrogates must enter into the decision-making process, they are more apt now than they used to be to hesitate before automatically going ahead with treatment. Perhaps ironically, therefore, the emphasis on patient autonomy has led to a situation where physicians, no longer insisting on treatment in all cases, have begun in some cases to reject their patients' desires to continue aggressive treatment. There is also a growing sense that perhaps the American consensus has moved too far in the direction of the autonomy of the individual patient.

A second cause of the shift from cases where providers insist on treating and patients or families refuse treatment to cases where providers want to stop and families or patients insist on continuing is the ongoing increase in medical knowledge and development of outcomes assessment. Health care providers are becoming more aware that certain procedures that initially showed great promise may not be appropriate in many specific clinical situations. This has quite properly contributed to a hesitation in performing procedures that physicians and nurses know will do little or no real good.

The third cause of the shift is more problematic: the developing restrictions of resources available to health care and to health care institutions. In the growing market-based approach to payment and insurance, hospitals often take serious losses by continuing treatment that family members wish but that physicians consider unwarranted. Prospective payment schemes, such as diagnosis-related groups in which hospitals are paid a set fee according to diagnosis, have largely replaced the retrospective fee-for-service approach in which doctors and institutions are paid for whatever they do. This has resulted in major hospital losses in some cases where families insist on treatment that physicians consider inappropriate. Physicians naturally defend the fiscal viability of the hospitals in which they work. And hospitals and health maintenance organizations (HMO) put pressure on physicians not to treat needlessly, since now the hospital or the HMO will take a loss if the cost of treatment exceeds repayment. Capitation schemes and other payment plans that penalize physicians who treat "too much" further increase this disincentive to treat. Clearly this is a different financial incentive system from the one that formerly prevailed, which rewarded physicians for continuing aggres-sive treatment. Physicians find themselves more and more besieged by those who threaten their employment, usually implicitly but sometimes explicitly, if they spend "too much" on their patients. They are urged to decide against some treatments on the basis that they are unnecessary or "futile."

The Wanglie *Case*

A court case heard in Minnesota is typical of the medical futility argument (*In re Wang-lie*, 1991). It has been called "a case of Cruzan-in-reverse" ("Courting the Issues" 1991, 1). Hennepin County Medical Center went to court seeking to turn off Helga Wanglie's respirator and artificial nutrition. Like Nancy Cruzan, Helga Wanglie was in a persistent vegetative state. Her care was paid for by Medicare and an HMO, so the hospital was not losing money. Rather, it claimed that the treatment was medically inappropriate, though its legal claim was explicitly that Helga's husband, Oliver, should not be the decision maker in the case. He was insisting on continuing the treatment, arguing this on the basis of their Lutheran Christian beliefs, and what evidence there is suggests that Helga herself would have wanted it continued as well. District court judge Patricia Belois decided in early July 1991 that Oliver Wanglie was the proper decision maker. The hospital did not appeal and continued life-sustaining treatment. Helga Wanglie died three days later, on July 4, 1991.

The Concept of Medical Futility

With this as background, we turn to the issue of medical futility itself. What precisely is it, and what are the proper criteria for determining that a treatment is medically futile?

What medical futility means (or at least what it ought to mean) as a formal concept is quite simple. Medical futility, however its criteria are chosen, characterizes those treatment modalities that must not be used because they are of no medical benefit to the patient. The treatment is, for this patient in this situation, contrary to the standard of medical care. Once a treatment has been categorized as medically futile, physicians must withhold it or withdraw it, regardless of the wishes of the patient or surrogate. This is a medical decision, not an ethical one, and depends on the proper application of medical expertise. Physicians—not ethicists, patients, or patients' families—will apply the criteria of medical futility in individual cases.

The term is used in policies on forgoing treatment and seems to refer generally to treatments that doctors need not give. Policies might say simply that physicians need not provide "medically futile," or simply "futile," treatment. For example, the Forgoing Treatment Policy at the St. Francis Medical Center in Pittsburgh, written in 1990, said simply: "If the requested treatment is clearly futile or non-beneficial, it need not be provided" (St. Francis Medical Center 1995, 6). What was almost certainly meant, although the lack of clarity makes it hard to prove this, was treatment that provided no benefit at all.[1] The context of such policies supports the claim that it was not intended to mean life-sustaining treatment that did indeed maintain life but that some or even most persons might not want. Those treatments, the policies would say, should be provided to patients who ask for them. Although not spelled out in any detail, whatever "futile" meant, it meant something that physicians were right to refuse.

Besides medically futile treatments, there are treatments that some might call humanly futile treatments: morally extraordinary or optional treatments that some patients consider useless for themselves but that other patients choose—for example, chemotherapy associated with a 10 percent chance of a two-month remission. But this kind of treatment was never considered futile in the sense that the treatment must never be given regardless of who wants it. Nor was, for example, hydration and nutrition for a permanently unconscious person considered futile in this sense, something that doctors must never do, something contrary to the standard of medical care.

It seems preferable, then, that when we use the term "medical futility," we ought to mean that a treatment thus characterized should never be offered regardless of who wants it. It is contrary to the standard of medical care. Doctors who offer it or give it show by this that they are bad doctors. Only this formal definition of medical futility allows us to do anything with this concept that we cannot do with words we already have, like "extraordinary" or "aggressive" or "unreasonable."

Doctors Do Have Expertise and Authority

We have already stated agreement with Veatch's position criticizing the generalization of expertise. But this criticism does not mean that health care professionals have no expertise whatsoever. It does not mean that physicians are reduced to giving their patients a list of options, a bibliography of articles in the *New England Journal* and the *Annals of Internal Medicine*, and telling them to go home, read up on it, and come back with a choice of treatment. Physicians, nurses, physicians' assistants, and other health care professionals are still the experts in medicine and health care, and unilateral decisions can be made, even without consulting the patient or the patient's surrogate.

A silly case makes this clear. If a man goes to a dialysis center with a head cold and demands dialysis as treatment, offers one thousand dollars in cash, insists that he is an autonomous person, quotes from the literature against paternalism and the generalization of expertise, and threatens to sue if the center does not do what he wants, the physician is required ethically and legally to refuse his request. The man does not have any idea what he is talking about. Medical expertise must override the silly request. His demand contradicts the standard of care. There is no need to try to refer him to another physician or nurse who might (illegally and unethically) do what he requests. The dialysis center must simply tell him that dialysis is not treatment for a cold and send him away (unless there is reason to suspect he might be crazy and self-destructive, and then possibly one might try to get him committed for psychiatric observation).

Physicians have no obligation to give medically futile treatment to any patient. Indeed, they must *not* give it. They are not obliged to inform the patient or ask the patient's permission or that of the family. This applies to CPR, antibiotics, and all sorts of treatments that in other circumstances might be warranted if in this case they are medically futile.

Criteria for Medical Futility

We turn now to the criteria for medical futility. Concerning them there are a number of important points to be made.

Who Decides on the Criteria?

The criteria for determining medical futility are crucial. But are these criteria within the purview of medicine, or of ethics, or both?

An analogy, though it is not perfect, will help here. The physician has the expertise needed to determine that a patient has died. In the case where cardiopulmonary function is being maintained by machines after brain dysfunction has occurred, the neurologist has that expertise. The neurologist runs tests to determine whether the criteria for total brain death have been met in any given case, and if those criteria have been met—if total brain death has occurred—then the patient is declared dead. The fact that relatives may say the patient has not yet died because they can see breathing is irrelevant. No further treatment is given. The decision is a medical one.

However, the choice of what "kind" of brain death will mean the determination that the patient has died was not and is not a purely medical decision. As we note in chapter 18, our society has decided that only total brain death means that a person is dead. We have rejected the arguments that irreversibly comatose persons have already died. The cessation of all higher brain function is not enough, we have said, to allow us to declare a person to be dead. We do not want to bury breathing corpses, or to stop them from breathing and then bury them. This decision was an ethical and social one, not merely a medical one, although medical professionals had an important role to play in the discussion that led to the decision.

Now that the criteria are ethically and legally established, doctors are the ones who apply them. Doctors decide on the proper tests to use to determine if a person is or is not "brain-dead." But the establishment of what kind of brain dysfunction counts as death—that is, the establishment of the kinds of criteria used to determine that death has occurred—involves social, legal, and ethical decisions, not purely medical decisions. This becomes clearer when we recall that there is still some discussion, largely in the context of organ procurement, concerning whether our nation ought to add anencephalics and possibly the irreversibly comatose to the ranks of the truly dead. No one suggests that the American Academy of Neurology can, by itself, decree this kind of a change.

The same applies to the issue of medical futility. Once a treatment is determined by the physician to be medically futile, the physician must not offer it or continue it. But the determination of the kinds of treatment that are going to be included in this category, that is, the determination of the kinds of criteria that must be met before medical futility is to be declared, is a societal, ethical, and legal issue, not a purely medical one.

Four Proposed Criteria

What then are the criteria proposed for determining that a treatment is medically futile? Stuart J. Youngner lists four criteria that might be proposed (Youngner 1988). We will argue that the first two are valid but the last two are not.

Physiological Uselessness

First, a treatment is clearly medically futile if it will fail in strictly physiological terms. The dialysis will not clear the blood, the vasopressor will not increase the blood pressure, electric cardioversion will not start the heart, arrhythmia control will not stop the fibrillation. Perhaps these procedures are tried and they fail. Perhaps, as in the silly dialysis example earlier, the treatment is entirely worthless for the patient's condition. No one disagrees with this first criterion. In such circumstances, physicians must refuse to perform the procedure regardless of patient or surrogate requests. The procedure is in this case contrary to the standard of medical care. It is medically futile.

Irrelevance to the Real Condition of a Dying Patient

Second, a treatment is futile if, although it works in the direct or local physiological sense, it does not postpone death in a dying patient for even a very short time. The cardioversion does start the heart, but the heart stops again almost immediately, and this continues each time CPR is done. The dialysis does clear the blood, but because the patient is immediately moribund from another cause, the dialysis is in fact irrelevant to the patient's underlying disease. A family member insists on knee surgery to remove a cartilage spur in a dying patient who will never leave the bed.

What counts as "a very short time"? If a ventilator will keep a dying patient alive for an extra day or two, but not longer, is use of it medically futile? If intubation or other intensive care unit (ICU) procedures will not reverse or even significantly affect the patient's "death spiral," but will probably postpone death for a day or two, can the physician refuse a request to admit to the ICU on the grounds that ICU treatment will not change the patient's "immediate dying" and is thus medically futile and violates the standard of medical care? There is no consensus about the definition of immediate dying. It is likely that dying in two or three days can usually be considered immediate dying; hence, the procedure in this case is usually medically futile. On the other hand, death in two weeks or more is probably not "immediate"; in such a case physicians should not unilaterally refuse a patient's or a surrogate's request for treatment. The intervening time of delay is less certain, and there is no clarity here in ethics or in law, though it seems most unlikely that any legal action would be successful against a physician who refused treatment when medical science clearly indicated that the treatment could not have prolonged the patient's life by as much as two weeks. But note that the word "usually" has been added to the agreement that two or three days is "immediate dying." There may well be cases where patients or families have valid reasons for asking that treatment try to extend life for that short time, such as when family members are traveling to be with their loved one before death. So, although it is quite clear that treatment that does not alter the patient's death spiral *at all*—that is, treatment that does not prolong life for even "a very short time"—is medically futile, this is not as clear about treatment that is likely to postpone dying for a day or two.

However, prescinding from the problem of what counts as "a very short time," there is near universal agreement that if either of these criteria of futility is met, the futility is indeed "medical futility," and the treatment must be forgone by the physician. No consent is needed by the patient. The treatment is useless in the strictly medical sense. The decision about its uselessness is made by the medical expert.

The third and fourth criteria are the ones around which the medical futility debate has centered. Those who propose an extension of the meaning of medical futility argue that they should be included. Those who oppose the extension reject them.

Poor Quality of Life

Third, a treatment is futile if it fails to meet the quality-of-life criterion. What if the treatment does indeed prolong physical life for a few weeks or longer but cannot lead to the patient's recovery? With treatment, the patient will not survive until discharge but is likely to survive for a time in the hospital. Or what if the treatment does result in discharge from the hospital, but the patient's level of living is such that he or she cannot continue to carry out the basic purposes of life? What about the patient in a persistent vegetative state maintained for many years on medical nutrition and hydration?

Low Probability of Success

Fourth, the treatment is futile if it has a low probability of success. What if the physician estimates that a treatment is 75 percent likely not to postpone dying; 20 percent likely to do so, though not until discharge; and only 5 percent likely to lead to discharge? In these cases, who makes the decision? Is this still the kind of futility that can properly be called "medical futility," so that the physician may make a unilateral decision to forgo treatment?

Debate about the Criteria

There has been considerable controversy in the literature about the question of medical futility, although the amount of published research on the topic has decreased in recent years.[2] One early article argued that a very low quality of life after a successful procedure, or a very low probability of success, should mean that the treatment is medically futile (Schneiderman, Jecker, and Jonsen 1990). This is not acceptable. The correct answer is clear, and it has been generally supported.[3] The health care professional, usually the attending physician, may decide unilaterally to withhold treatment when it is medically futile, and medical futility is based on the first two criteria noted earlier and not on the last two. That is, treatment is medically futile if the answer to either of the following two questions is no: First, will the treatment do, in the immediate local physiological sense, what it is intended to do? If the answer is no, it is medically futile and must not be given. Second, if the answer to the first question is yes, and if the patient is imminently dying, will the treatment and its resulting local physiological effect cause a postponement of physical death? If the patient is imminently dying, and the treatment does not postpone physical death, even though it does accomplish in the local physiological sense what it is intended to do (it does purify the blood or balance the electrolytes), the fact that physical death is not postponed by even a very short time means that the treatment is medically futile and should not be given. It is medically futile to treat a secondary and clinically unimportant symptom in a patient imminently dying of another cause.

There is, of course, an obvious exception to this. Treatment that relieves pain or other patient discomfort is not futile just because it does not postpone physical death. With this exception, however, these two questions can serve to define medical futility. Treatment that might be called futile for other reasons is not medically futile in this sense, and the decision to forgo it must be made only after consultation with the patient or surrogate, and only with his or her approval. Perhaps a patient wants to be kept alive to see a Steelers game, even though he knows he will never leave the hospital. This reason may appeal only to someone who roots for the Steelers, but it does appeal to him. Or perhaps a patient wants to live until after the marriage of a son or daughter; this reason would probably appeal to most of us as a valid reason for resuscitation, even if the patient is virtually certain to die before leaving the hospital. Or perhaps a surrogate wants to continue treatment for religious reasons or even out of fear or guilt. Now the reason may not appeal to most of us. But the consensus in our nation is that this cannot be called medically futile treatment, and the decision to forgo cannot be made unilaterally by the physician, the health care team, or the hospital.

The other criteria that have been proposed, criteria three and four on Youngner's list, should be rejected as bases for medical futility, that is, as bases for the conclusion that physicians must unilaterally refuse to perform the procedure. Some argue that in addition to the quite restrictive criteria we have been supporting, medical futility can be determined as well on the basis of small probability of success or on the basis of society's agreement that even a medically successful outcome is not humanly beneficial.[4] This set of criteria would enable physicians to unilaterally forgo a treatment if it had a minimal (perhaps less than 1 percent) chance of success, and/or if the medically successful outcome was one that most of us would not want for ourselves (perhaps continuing life in a persistent vegetative state).

The "and/or" in the last paragraph is important. These two criteria could be conjunctive or disjunctive. That is, both could be required or either one could suffice. There is a major difference. If both are required before a treatment can be said to be medically futile, then, although medical futility is expanded somewhat from the restrictive set of criteria we have suggested, it is not expanded as much as it would be if the proposed criteria were to be disjunctive. For example, if the criteria are conjunctive (if both are required), nutrition and hydration for most patients in persistent vegetative states would not meet the criteria for medical futility. The treatment might be said to yield an outcome that most of us (the "reasonable person" standard) would consider to be humanly undesirable. But the odds of reaching this medically successful outcome are great. With this conjunctive use of the proposed criteria, surrogates would still get to decide, not physicians. But if the criteria are disjunctive, that is, if either would suffice as a basis for determining the medical futility of a proposed treatment, physicians could unilaterally choose to end nutrition for patients such as Wanglie, Cruzan, or Schiavo, since the reasonable person would have decided that the outcome was not truly beneficial. Under this disjunctive use of these criteria, a Steelers fan might not get to see his team play, or a parent might not get to see a child marry.

Criteria for Medical Futility Summary

Criteria based on probability of success and societal determination of benefit should not be used as reasons for declaring a treatment to be medically futile. Despite the literature that recommends this, physicians should not make unilateral decisions to forgo treatment on these bases. Patients and families get to decide whether to forgo a treatment with small probability of success and/or with poor quality of life as a result of success. This means that although we do not agree with those who require hydration and nutrition for PVS patients, we do not think physicians ought to be empowered to reject such requests unilaterally. Such "treatment" may be morally extraordinary, humanly useless, or even silly or demeaning. But it is not medically futile.

Problems with This Restrictive Approach

The approach to medical futility proposed here and generally supported in the literature is very restrictive. Most treatments that providers rightly and humanely want to stop will not fit into this notion of medical futility. As the Consensus Statement of the Ethics Committee of the Society of Critical Care Medicine puts it: "The concept of futility is generally not useful in establishing policies to limit treatment. Futile treatments, as we have defined them, are rare, and are usually not offered or disputed" (Ethics Committee of the Society of Critical Care Medicine 1997, 888). Some families will continue to demand aggressive therapy for very sick patients who would be kept alive by such procedures but who would never truly benefit from them.

Physicians are often disturbed, even angered, by such requests. Why should patients and families think themselves capable of making these decisions? In the American context, part of the answer comes from the fact that for years many physicians and health care institutions supported a technological imperative: if treatment that could prolong a patient's life is available, that treatment ought to be tried, regardless of the quality of the outcome or the probability of success. In the American retrospective-payment (fee-for-service) context, in which the more a doctor or hospital did for the patient, the greater the profit, patients and families often found they were unable to persuade health care providers to stop treatment. In all the early related court decisions in the United States, families asked that treatments be withdrawn, and hospitals or physicians refused to do so.

But the ethical consensus and the law changed to allow patients and surrogates to make these choices. The Patient Self-Determination Act, advance directives, and state laws supporting them added and still add to this shift in decision-making authority from doctors to patients. A social sense concerning which treatments ought to be done and which forgone has not emerged. Unlike many other nations, the United States has fostered this ethos of individual choice. Individuals ought to be able to receive what they want. Today's physicians and health care institutions are right to question the insistence by patients and surrogates that patients receive inappropriate treatments that are often costly and are at best unlikely to benefit them. But it is important to recognize that the social context for this is one that American medicine has supported and still supports. Other social contexts, such as those found in Europe, in which a general societywide vision of proper care prevails, and in which access to health care is guaranteed by and regulated by governments or other public bodies, provide a better basis for decision making at a higher, civic level. In these other contexts, individuals are less apt to feel they have a right to anything they request. Only systemic changes in American medicine will end the medical futility debate.

Reducing Demand for Inappropriate Treatment

There are options that can be tried to reduce patient demand for inappropriate but not medically futile treatments. Some of these would require the kind of systemic change America has thus far rejected. Ten options are listed here.

1. Any system of national health insurance could rightly refuse to pay for such treatments. A good national health system will also specifically tell hospitals and providers that they need not give such treatments to patients who cannot pay for them. Unfortunately, American resistance to governmentally mandated single-payer universal coverage, exacerbated by televised political warnings of the horrors of government interference, makes such an alternative unlikely in the near future. Chapter 28 returns to these issues.

2. In the absence of such a system, states might pass futility policies. All states do have laws about what to do when patients or surrogates disagree with physicians, but these laws, except for one in Texas, simply urge continued dialogue and provide for the transfer of patients to another facility when that is possible (Miller 2007). The 1999 Texas law, which might be called an actual "futility law," sets a ten-day deadline for the end of dialogue, allowing physicians to stop treatment unilaterally with the agreement of the hospital's ethics committee (ibid.). It seems that most cases are resolved without the need to invoke the ten-day provision for unilateral action, as patients die or are transferred, or families agree to stop treatment (Traveline 2007, 796, 801). The ten-day deadline and the power given to the ethics committee have been criticized as coercive, and in at least one case a Texas court granted an injunction extending the time for debate (Miller 2007). And the criteria for determining futility are not clear. Still, the Texas law does provide a legal mechanism for protecting society from the unending costs of caring for persons for whom ongoing aggressive treatment is inappropriate.

3. Private insurance companies, medical care organizations, preferred provider organizations, HMOs, and the like may also rightly refuse to pay for these treatments, although the legal implications of hospitals refusing to treat would be unclear without federal or state statutory indemnification. But because private insurers are ethically and legally required to tell their clients what treatments they will and will not pay for, and because American health insurance is largely private and highly competitive, insurance companies are unlikely to refuse to cover inappropriate treatments. If one insurer told potential clients it would not pay for treatment that another covered, the former might be at a disadvantage in a market in which clients want access to all possible medical care.

4. Hospitals could establish public policies rejecting specific treatments in certain situations. A hospital might say, "We do not treat patients who are in a persistent vegetative state because we believe the resources should go to our well-baby clinic instead." That is not a medical policy in the strict sense; rather, it is a social-ethical decision based on a wide range of factors including, but not limited to, the strictly medical. But hospitals are unlikely to take this approach,

given possible damage to public relations in a competitive environment. Attempts by hospitals to establish "futility policies" are unlikely to be able to define exactly which procedures are to be unilaterally denied in which cases; thus, hospitals are likely to fall back on a policy that asks for better communication with patients (Wear et al. 1995) or a policy that admits of exceptions when, despite all attempts, families insist on continuing treatment (Saint John's Hospital and Health Center 1995).

5. Hospitals or individual physicians can always go to court to try to get a guardian who will agree to forgo the inadvisable treatment. A judge is unlikely to rule in the hospital's or physician's favor, however, unless it can be shown either that the surrogate is unfit because of a conflict of interest or that the treatment is not only unreasonable but hurtful to the patient, which, with proper pain relief, should never be the case.[5]

6. Early review can often be helpful in reducing the number of cases of inappropriate treatment. If primary care physicians take the time to speak with their patients about these issues, many of these patients will opt against inappropriate treatment and will perhaps leave advance directives that can help forestall it later on. In this context, it is important to note that physicians act ethically when they advise patients and surrogates against procedures that offer little benefit. Health care providers are rightly expected by patients to give such advice. They are not supposed to behave as neutral observers and offer a list of options. Unfortunately, as we noted in chapter 17 (note 2), attempts to have Medicare pay physicians for conversations like this were rejected as "death panels" in opposition to the health care reform bill of 2010.

7. Time spent with the family can be of great help. It takes time for families to let go. Hospital personnel should try to keep families well informed of the deteriorating condition of patients. If the ICU attending physician tells a family on Monday that he hopes that a series of diagnostic procedures will suggest a solution, even though he knows that in cases like this a favorable prognosis is highly unlikely, then when the physician who comes in on Tuesday tells them that in this case there is no hope for recovery, it is hardly surprising that they are unable to let their loved one die. They want the Monday doctor back!

8. General education of the public is important. It seems clear that the medical community does significant harm with its competitive advertising. People are continually told only about the miracles that occur in hospitals. They naturally expect that another miracle is possible. And there is the problematic fact that medicine is not and cannot be an exact science. Stories often appear in the popular media about patients whom doctors gave up on but who survived and even thrived. People naturally want that chance for themselves and their loved ones.

9. Living wills and durable powers of attorney may help families follow the expressed wishes of dying patients to forgo unreasonable life-sustaining treatment. These documents are most helpful in assuaging family guilt. Instead of having to decide for the patient, the family can instead agree to do what the patient would want.

10. It is always correct for a physician or other provider to withdraw from a case if the treatment demanded is against his or her conscience, but the provision, as always, is that some other provider will agree to care for the patient, which is unlikely in this kind of situation.

Conclusion

In the light of recent legal decisions and of the present American ethical consensus, physicians and other providers ought not to declare medical futility when a treatment would prolong the patient's life by any humanly significant length. Such treatment may well be inadvisable, too costly, silly, or even degrading. But this kind of quality-of-life decision should be made by the patient or the surrogate, not unilaterally by the physician. It is not strictly a medical decision but a decision that includes ethical and social dimensions. Perhaps in the future, American support for individual decision making in health care will be balanced by a recognition of the needs of society and of the common good. But until systemic change occurs, the decision belongs to the patient and not to the physician.

Notes

1. But the coupling of the term "medically futile" with the less precise term "nonbeneficial" shows a lack of detailed development of the meaning. Indeed, the policy goes on to say that physicians who refuse to give such treatment, such as those who object on ethical or religious grounds, may withdraw treatment but must transfer the patient to the care of another. The meaning of medical futility that we are arguing for here would neither require nor permit such a transfer.

2. In addition to Youngner's work (1988), articles include Blackhall 1987 (Blackhall gives more latitude to physicians' unilateral decisions than we believe is appropriate); Tomlinson and Brody 1988 (these authors make very helpful distinctions between medical futility and quality-of-life futility); Murphy 1988 (Murphy argues that physicians may unilaterally write a DNR order when the future quality of life is low [2100], a position we do not accept); Brennan 1988; Boyle 1988; Lantos et al. 1989; Paris, Crone, and Reardon 1990; Callahan 1991 (whose approach is similar to ours); Solomon 1993; Schneiderman, Faber-Langendoen, and Jecker 1994; Youngner 1994; Laffey 1996; Council on Ethical and Judicial Affairs of the American Medical Association 1999; Halevy 1999; and Helft, Siegler, and Lantos 2000.

3. This approach to medical futility is supported by the statement of the Ethics Committee of the Society of Critical Care Medicine (1997) and by the New York State Task Force on Life and the Law (1992, 195–204). It is also implied in the American Medical Association's statement (Council on Ethical and Judicial Affairs of the American Medical Association 1999). That published statement does not suggest that quality-of-life decisions may be made unilaterally by physicians. See also Helft, Siegler, and Lantos 2000. The authors note that the futility debate has largely ended because the attempt to expand the criteria has been medically, legally, and ethically unsuccessful. The authors also note that attempts at objectifying and quantifying outcomes of treatments have failed, thus making it difficult, if not impossible, to base decisions about quality of life and probability of success on clear and certain medical criteria. Attempts at designing medical futility policies have been process-based and have rejected any unilateral decisions by physicians based on quality of outcome and probability of success, which of course is exactly

what expanded medical futility is supposed to enable. The approach suggested here is also supported in Lantos et al. 1989; these authors argue that patients are best able to make decisions of this kind because their personal values and goals differ. Arthur Caplan rightly argues that the solution is not to use medical futility as a way to reject patient and family wishes but is rather to increase the trust patients have in doctors (Caplan 1996). In her book-length treatment of the topic, Susan Rubin also argues against allowing unilateral decisions by physicians when patient values are at issue, but she seems also to reject even the most basic physiological understanding of medical futility, which seems to go too far in rejecting physicians' competence to make medical decisions (Rubin 1998, 88–114).

4. These criteria are proposed in Schneiderman, Jecker, and Jonsen 1990. These authors argue that either a very small probability of medical success (less than 1 to 3 percent; no successes in the last one hundred cases) or an outcome that does not benefit the patient as a whole (the treatment only prolongs the life of an unconscious patient, or the treatment maintains life but the patient remains dependent on intensive medical care) is a sufficient warrant for declaring a treatment medically futile. They want these criteria to be independent; meeting either one is enough. They propose that nutritional support for a patient in a persistent vegetative state be considered medically futile, and that physicians withhold or withdraw such support regardless of the wishes of the patient or the family (950). If medical care does not offer patients the opportunity to achieve any of life's goals, physicians must refuse to give it, regardless of the wishes of patients or surrogates (949, 952–53). In a later article written to answer critics, the authors admit that more empirical outcomes assessment is needed in order to support their proposed approach, but they otherwise continue to propose it (Schneiderman, Jecker, and Jonsen 1996).

5. The *Wanglie* case is one example. See also Helft, Siegler, and Lantos 2000, 295. These authors quote Daar 1995 as saying that almost every court case of this kind has been resolved in favor of the patient. They list one notable exception (*Gilgunn v. Massachusetts General Hospital*, 1995), but that was a jury decision, not a court ruling. Alexander Morgan Capron analyzes this case and concludes that both judge and jury erred in applying the law; Mrs. Gilgunn's daughter's demand that treatment be maintained for her permanently comatose mother should have prevailed (Capron 1995).

CHAPTER 21

PAIN AND PAIN MANAGEMENT

Introduction

THE TREATMENT OF PAIN is a major component of American health care, costing about $100 billion annually (Kalb 2003, 45). American medicine has not had a very good record of dealing adequately with pain, but in recent years this has improved significantly. Painful ailments such as fibromyalgia that were once thought to be imaginary are now known to have physical causes (Underwood 2003), although some physicians still refuse to accept clear proof of this. Many hospitals now have programs devoted to pain management, and physicians are far more likely now to take seriously patients' complaints about pain. Ethics committees and ethics consults have contributed to that advance, and consulting teams are likely to ask that pain be given attention.

In chapter 14, we discussed the most common ethical question asked about pain management, whether it is ethically right and legal to alleviate pain in a dying patient even though the medication may hasten (co-cause) death. Here we first review some of the Christian approaches to the meaning of pain and suffering. Then we discuss some of the spiritual issues of pain and pain management. Health care professionals may well ask these questions not only relative to their patients but also in the course of their own spiritual journey. Finally, we turn to some of the practical ethical questions of pain management and to the role of the clergy in hospital ethics.

The meaning of the word "patient" is instructive. The word comes from the Latin *patiens*, which means "to undergo." The patient is the undergoer, the sufferer, the one put-upon. A number of sociological and psychological studies have been done about the patient's "role," and these studies have been partially responsible for the insistence over the last two decades on patient autonomy, informed consent, and patient participation in treatment decisions and implementation. Still, the patient is more the done-to than the doer. The patient is poked and prodded, dressed and undressed, looked at and talked about, often by large numbers of strangers who "round" in teaching hospitals. While there are better and worse ways of doing it, that poking and prodding and looking at and talking about is all part of good medical care. But it symbolizes and reminds the *patiens* daily that she or he is the sufferer, the one in pain.

It is helpful here to distinguish between pain and suffering. Pain is largely physical. Suffering is largely spiritual and mental. As was noted in chapter 14, there is a difference between "neurophysiological suffering," or pain, and "agent narrative suffering" (Walter

2002, 6). People often insist that the pain itself is not the worst of it, and good pain management can effectively reduce and often eliminate pain in the strict physical sense. But we need to remember that even in the absence of pain, real human suffering may remain to the *patiens,* to the one who undergoes.

It is important to realize what the hospital environment does to patients. The professional is in control; it is where he or she works. For the patient, the experience is totally different. Every noise is a sign that something is wrong. As a patient in the ICU, I fear that the beeps and the buzzes are *my* beeps and buzzes, that the nurses and the doctors are talking about *me.* In teaching hospitals, usually early in the morning, I am talked about by all sorts of strangers who come in large groups. What is so awful about my illness that all these smart women and men want to talk about it? The doctors must all be lying when they tell me I am getting better. They tell me to relax, but I'm bathed in light and surrounded by noise (Dr. Kelly recalls one patient whose complaint was about the ICU computer printer set next to her bed that never stopped running).

There is clear evidence that the attitude of the patient has a considerable effect on the success of medical treatment. The well-known placebo effect, where patients who are given inactive pills do better than those who get nothing, is proof of this. And patients who actively participate in their own recovery do better than those who do not. Trust is one of the most important aspects of the patient–doctor relationship. Human illnesses are never purely physical, since the human person is always psyche and spirit as well as body. The more a patient is actively and confidently involved in the healing process, the more likely it is to work. Yet often the overwhelming frenzy of the hospital reduces patients to passive recipients and decreases the very participation that helps in their recovery. Doctors and nurses might try to stay for one twenty-four-hour period in an ICU bed, taking on the "role" of patient. Professionals all too seldom have actual experience of what it is to undergo a stay in a hospital.

The Problem of God and Suffering

The principal theological problem with pain and suffering is why God permits it. The question of why God causes or permits evil is known in theology and philosophy as the problem of "theodicy." Theodicy is the "justification of God": how can a God who permits evil be justified in so doing? This is a complex theological question.

In simple terms, the problem can be described as a dilemma arising from three factors. First, God is said to be all-good. God wants us to be happy; God loves us. God's purpose in creation is to extend divine love to us, God's people. Christians claim that God sent Jesus to reveal himself to us and to save us from sin and death. Second, God is said to be all-powerful. God can do anything God wants. God is God, after all. Third, the world we live in includes a significant and sometimes overwhelming presence of evil. If God is a loving God who is omnipotent, then why doesn't God eliminate the suffering, agony, and pain we experience ourselves and see around us in our world?

For many people, the problem of theodicy is a reason for concluding that there is no God. God cannot be justified. Theodicy is impossible. It is easy to see why this answer is appealing. For some atheists, human experience demonstrates clearly that there is no way a real "God" could have created or tolerated a world like this one. But if human life and the universe itself are seen as an accident, a fortunate (or unfortunate, depending on where you stand) mixing of atoms with no plan behind it, then pain and suffering are simply part of that great accident, and there is no need to explain them. Many major thinkers have made this judgment, and it is not wise of those who believe in God to simply dismiss it. This kind of atheism comes from deep insight, from a grappling at some considerable depth with a real human and religious issue. It is sometimes closer to real faith and to real Christianity than what often passes for more normal forms and expressions of Christian living. Probably many of us at one time or another have asked the question. Perhaps now and again we think this answer has some merit. Why, after all, does God cause, or permit, all this agony?

There are three general sets of answers possible. First, we can conclude that God is not really good, or at least not all-good. Perhaps God is really a big computer in the sky. God has control groups who do not get cancer as children, and experimental groups who do. God is simply interested in knowing what happens to the different groups. This answer is not too different from denying God altogether. God started the universe and now sits back and watches the experiment with some interest but with no real desire for one outcome rather than another. God is an "objective" research scientist with various hypotheses, and we are the experimental subjects. Or perhaps God is a sadist. God delights in pain and suffering. The only reason God permits good, pleasure, and happiness is so that people can know what they are missing when they are in pain.

A second answer is that God, while all-good, is not all-powerful. God would eliminate evil if that were possible, but God does not have the power to do so. There are a number of possible ways in which this answer is made. Some have believed that there are two gods, or two sources for creation. One of these is good; the other is evil. The evil god keeps the good god from eliminating pain and suffering. The evil god inflicts it, and the good god reduces it. But since each is as powerful as the other, neither is omnipotent. Religions that have held this belief have generally seen the good god as the god of spirit, and the evil god as the god of matter. Clearly, Christianity has rejected this answer, but remnants of it remain in the notion of a devil: "The devil made me do it; blame him." Still, in Christianity it is clear that the devil, whatever this myth really means, is a creature of the one God. Theoretically, God should be able to control or even eliminate the devil. So the question remains.

Some Christians, among them those who follow "process theology," hold that God is growing along with creation. God as God transcends creation, that is, is above and beyond it, but God is also within creation and in that sense is struggling with the rest of creation to work toward the good, to eliminate pain, suffering, and death. But this answer also questions or at least is in tension with one of the basic doctrines of traditional Christianity, that God is indeed all-powerful, and most Christians have not accepted it. So the theodicy question remains.

Christian Answers

The third set of answers to the theodicy question accepts the idea that God is all-good and all-powerful. There are a number of approaches Christians use within this set of answers, and as we mention these it will become clear how this is important to health care workers and to patients.

The most widespread traditional answer is that God is not really responsible for evil. We are. God's original plan for creation did not include the presence of evil, but humans sinned and thus introduced evil into the world. To some extent, this answer works for the evil caused by sin, but it is at least partially problematic when applied to physical evils such as pain, illness, and death. It is true that the story of Adam and Eve in Eden, if accepted literally as a historical document, can be interpreted as reporting this kind of event. Eden is claimed by some to be a historically existing place where disease, accident, sin, and death were nonexistent. Mosquitoes and lions did not bite; stones did not fall on anyone; there were no storms; no one caught cold. But today we know that this is inaccurate. Pain and disease exist apart from peoples' sins and always have.

Despite the problematic nature of this answer, however, it contains important theological and ethical truth. Many physical evils are indeed the result of human sin and error, ecological mismanagement, greed, violence, and so on, and this attempt at an answer does have the important advantage of urging us to live more virtuous lives and thus reduce the pain our actions cause.

Even the reality of death as we know it is made humanly traumatic by the fears and lack of trust that sin causes and exacerbates. Death can, in some real way, be said to be "caused by original sin." As we experience it, death is not the simple passage from this life to heaven that Christians believe to be envisioned and desired by God but is rather a wrenching and often fearful experience dreaded by most of us. In some cases, a morally wrong act causes it directly (homicide, for example); in other cases, structural moral evils cause death (poverty, injustice, racism, sexism, the lack of a just health care system, etc.). In still other cases, with which nurses and doctors are all too familiar, family conflicts caused by greed, envy, intrafamilial rivalry, and even hatred greatly increase the human suffering that goes along with a patient's death. These even affect treatment decisions. So human sin does indeed inflict pain and suffering. Yet it is not possible to conclude that all physical evils—all pain, disease, and accident—are caused by human sin.

The answer that people's sins cause pain and suffering can even be destructive. It is one thing to think of Adam and Eve and blame pain and suffering on them. It is another to blame it on ourselves. Sometimes, of course, as we have just seen, we are right to do so. But this can be dangerous, and the danger reveals another important problem with this answer to the theodicy question. "Bed 18" may have cancer because she smoked; "bed 12" may have AIDS because he used drugs. Empirically this might be true. But why does God cause this result for this kind of behavior? Did God create the AIDS virus to punish homosexuals and drug users? Did God create cancerous lung cells to punish smokers? And what about the child with leukemia? Such answers return us to God the sadist. Those who propose this explicitly, for example, those who preach that AIDS is God's punishment for sexual sin, are in fact blaspheming against God.

Still, many patients may think that their illness is God's punishment for sins, real or imagined. And this may be an obstacle to recovery or to pain management. If one believes, for example, that a disease is God's punishment for sin, what right do we have to try to change God's righteous punishment? What right do we have to undo what God wants done? The idea that disease is God's punishment for sin can be a major problem for health care.

Another theologically and humanly distorted notion is the idea that God uses pain and suffering to test us. A remarkably large percentage of college students seem to find this answer congenial. Pain and suffering are tests from God. Perhaps college students are so often being tested that this appeals to them. The introduction to the biblical story of Job, where God agrees with Satan to test Job, leans in this direction, though Job's final answer does not.

The tester God seems too much like the sadist God or the experimenter God. Lovers ought not to inflict pain on their loved ones to see if they can remain steadfast. The Christian God is not like this. But if patients believe this about God's relationship to their pain, they may be ambivalent about pain management. They may feel guilty about analgesics because it might seem that they are avoiding the test. In fact, it is much more likely that pain, at least too much of it, will get in the way of spiritual peace and will make it harder for the dying patient to prepare for death.

Persons who see pain as a punishment from God or as a test from God have an answer of sorts to the question we began with, but it is not a sufficient answer. It makes it very hard for those who believe this way to love a God who is constantly punishing and testing them.

Helpful Ideas

What then is left? Not any easy answer. Not any answer that will solve this difficult issue of theodicy. But there are three ideas that may help. First, in creating, God could not create perfection. That is because only God is totally perfect, and God cannot be created or God would be a creature and not God. This means there must be some sort of limitation in creation. And God chose to create a physical universe, where innumerable physical wonders exist. A necessarily limited physical creation means union and separation, growth and decay, death and new life. In some sense, then, if God were to create a wondrous yet necessarily limited physical universe where people are embodied and not just angels, God had no choice but to include the limits of physical reality. In that sense, God can even be said to cause evil.[1] This does not answer the question of why children get leukemia, but it sets it into perspective. A loving God creates a universe that of necessity offers both beauty and rot, life and death, pleasure and pain. God might have created something entirely different, but the wonders of this kind of creation would have been lost had God done so.

A second helpful idea is the notion of human freedom. The Adam and Eve story tells us this. God chose to create people free. This freedom is our glory and our burden. In order to give us the glory, God needed as well to give us the burden. This helps us understand only those evils and sufferings that result from human action, and is dangerous when we think it means that all pain and suffering is God's punishment for human sin. But it correctly reminds us that much human agony does result from our sin, and it urges us to do better.

Third, by suffering we learn better how to relate to others and help carry their burden. This does not mean that we choose suffering for its own sake. Christianity is not supposed to be masochistic. But it is clear that the experience of human hardship and suffering makes it possible for us to understand what others are enduring, to be less judgmental of them and of their behavior, and to join them in empathy and sympathy. This is the principal reason why suffering can truly be an ennobling part of human living. It is central to the theological concept of redemptive suffering. In this sense, suffering helps us to mature. Sensitive persons are better caregivers than those who lack this virtue.

Does this solve the problem of evil? No. The theodicy question remains a mystery. That is the final answer of the book of Job. Only God can really know why there is evil. Yet the Christian God remains a loving God—not a punishing God, not a testing God, but a loving God despite the evil that exists in a physical universe where people are free.

Anger

Thus far, we have arrived at no complete answer to the theodicy question. The punishment and test answers, at least in their crude form, have been rejected. The idea of a physical creation where people are free helps set a context for the right answer, but this context does not solve the question of the presence of pain. Innocent persons suffer, so we often get angry at God. Whom do we blame for the dead baby? The theoretically right answer is that we blame no one. People of faith try to remember that God does not delight in this, that somehow it is part of God's providence. And for some of us, some of the time, the belief that God takes the child to heaven is of help. But often this is not enough, so there is often anger at God. Health care providers need to accept this. It proves we care.

The Ethics of Pain Management

Previous chapters have addressed the question of sedating a dying patient even though sedation may hasten the moment of death. We have seen that this is morally right and legally proper. A few remarks on the ethics of pain management are helpful here in addition to those already discussed.

First, what about the patient who asks not to be sedated? This may be for a good reason (to be alert to talk with visiting relatives) or for a reason we might think is a bad one (to suffer more for past sins and thus escape God's wrath). The ethical answer to this question is that if patients are capable of making treatment decisions, the decision to reject sedation must be followed. Clearly, it would be ethically wrong, and arguably illegal, to sedate them without their knowledge. This applies even when the lack of sedation causes problems to the health care team. Of course, if the lack of sedation makes it impossible to treat, the patient must be informed of this, and there might be very rare cases where doctors and hospitals would be justified in telling such a patient that they could no longer offer care. Surrogates may never reject proper pain management for patients who are not capable of deciding for themselves. This would be against the best interests of the patient.

Second, what about the problem of addiction? This is a complex issue, but it ought to be possible to avoid two extremes. The first extreme is the theory that addictive drugs should never be used in physically addictive amounts. It is clear that physical addiction is not a major problem for a dying patient, but that pain is. Morphine dosages that would be criminal apart from the patient's condition may well be quite proper for the patient with terminal cancer. The second extreme is the theory that addiction is impossible or irrelevant for the elderly. This is the "quick fix" theory and is in use at times in nursing homes and other institutions where the staff wants quiet patients. When addiction to drugs is likely to prove harmful to the patient, which may well be the case when the patient is not dying, the possibility of addiction must be considered and reduced or eliminated if possible.

The Role of the Clergy and the Chaplain

Clergy and chaplains can be of help to patients as they struggle with pain and with their illness generally. What is the role of the clergy or chaplain in health care ethics? The terms "clergy" and "chaplain" are used interchangeably here, even though all churches have clergy who are not trained as chaplains, and many have chaplains who are not ordained.

All clergy and chaplains have a major role to play, regardless of whether they have any specific knowledge about, much less expertise in, health care ethics. First, they need to recognize that they do not have such an expertise if in fact they lack it. Clergy who are unfamiliar with medical ethics are not helpful when they try to make judgments based on their own personal opinions and force these on patients and their families. For Catholics, this sometimes happens when priests who have not kept up with their own tradition insist that the church's teaching is what it is not.

Second, sensitive clergy and chaplains should not impose themselves on patients and families who do not want them. Clergy should not take such rejection personally (except in the rare case in which it is indeed their own fault) and should make it clear that they are available if the patient or family should want to speak with them.

But all sensitive clergy, including those who have little or no knowledge of medical ethics, can be tremendously helpful in three areas. First, patients and families want clergy and chaplains to help them deal with the spiritual aspects of illness and of dying. Different traditions have different ways of doing this, but, whatever the mix of personal praying and sacramental symbol, the presence of this help as part of the process of dealing with illness and of preparing to make treatment decisions can be quite reassuring.

Second, clergy and chaplains can help mitigate false guilt and fear. This does not mean that they should always help do away with guilt and fear. Guilt can be real. Fear can be salutary. But often patients worry that their illness is a punishment from God. They may fear that this same God is preparing them for eternal damnation.

The Christian belief in an afterlife ought to serve as a consolation for the dying patient and his or her family, not as a source of fear. Christians ought to believe that the God of Jesus Christ is a merciful and forgiving God, a God who wants all persons to live eternally with God in Jesus, in this life and after death. Christians ought to believe that the God of Jesus Christ offers them, and all human persons, the grace that makes this happiness possible.

Yet often fear of hell or of purgatory overwhelms the trusting confidence God asks of us and offers to us. Dying patients may fear meeting God. Sensitive clergy can be of great help in talking through these issues with the patient and with the family. This is an important part of the spiritual preparation for death; it is indeed an important part of the spiritual dimension of any illness. Good chaplains can offer important help to patients and their families during this difficult time.

In particular, chaplains might help patients understand that their pain is not caused by a vengeful God. Most Christian theologies approve pain management; few propose the idea that God wants us to suffer when help is at hand. Pain is more likely to interfere with a dying person's spiritual preparation for death than to enhance it. Chaplains can also console patients by reminding them that Jesus did not inflict pain but often removed it with his healing touch. In this way clergy can help in the management of pain.

Another aspect of the problem of guilt and fear arises when families worry needlessly that their decision to continue or to forgo treatment means that they are not doing the loving thing for the dying patient. This is especially true when they decide to forgo life-sustaining treatment. Clergy, even those not familiar in any depth with the tradition of medical ethics, can be helpful in supporting families who obviously love the dying patient and are trying to make the right decision. They can help the family understand the difference between relief at the end of an ordeal and malicious desire for the death of their loved one. They can help them recognize the difference between intending to kill and resigning themselves to the inevitability of death.

Third, chaplains can help facilitate communication among family members. Families need help in coping with illness and death and in making difficult treatment decisions with some degree of equanimity. Clinical experience demonstrates that families with strong religious backgrounds are often those most easily able to make difficult decisions about forgoing treatment. Such families are more apt to have spoken about death and to share common values about which kinds of treatments they feel to be humanly reasonable. They may share a belief in a loving God who will welcome them to heaven. They may share a sense that purely biological life is not of ultimate value, and thus share a degree of resignation when medical treatment can no longer be of real help. Such families will agree that "death was a blessing," even as they mourn their loss. Clergy and chaplains will support this. Indeed, chaplains and other clergy will very often find their own faith enhanced and their fears of death reduced by working with and listening to such families.

But this is not always the case. The anticipated death of a family member can also cause rancor within the family. Some relatives will insist on treating; others will want to stop. This can pose a major problem for physicians and for hospitals and nursing homes. The presence of a chaplain or clergyperson can help in getting the various viewpoints expressed with less acrimony and may help in resolving the crisis.

All of this can be done by clergy and chaplains whether or not they are knowledgeable in health care ethics. Clergy who do know something about medical ethics can do all this and more. The minister may be the only one present who understands the basic consensus that has developed about the moral and legal rightness of forgoing treatment. If he or she does know this (the "if" is important—it cannot be presumed), then he or she can serve to help articulate the issues involved. Physicians and nurses are often unaware of what the difference is between substituted judgment and best interests, or of how to determine the difference between medical futility (where the doctor decides) and other kinds of value decisions (where the patient or family decides), or what the law allows and forbids. Some hospitals may have literally no one on staff who is aware of these issues in any depth. The hospital counsel may be a good contract lawyer, but may not have done any research into the laws and cases about who decides to forgo treatment and on what bases. The hospital may not have a resident or consulting ethicist. Often the rabbi, priest, minister, or hospital chaplain is the only one there who knows what the general consensus is on these questions.

In addition to knowing the general American consensus, knowledgeable clergy know their own religious tradition. This is less easy than it sounds, as any good theologian will testify. Within religions and within denominations, some differences remain as to specific issues. Clergy should not force this tradition on a family but are certainly able to help the family come to an informed decision, based at least in part on the religious tradition family and minister may share.

Roman Catholic clergy and chaplains—if they understand their tradition (experience shows that some do and some do not)—can be of significant support by explaining to families how flexible the Catholic tradition is in this area. Catholic tradition rejects direct euthanasia, but it has been very much aware that not all medical treatment is mandatory even if it will prolong life. Treatments that are of little or no real human benefit to patients, or whose burdens outweigh those benefits, are not mandatory in the Catholic tradition. And the American consensus has come to agree with this long-standing tradition. Similarly, the American consensus has come to agree that there is no moral difference between withholding and withdrawing treatment. Catholic clergy and chaplains who know their tradition can thus give moral support to families faced with this difficult decision.

Note

1. The notion of God actually being in some sense responsible for evil, or causing it, comes from Karl Rahner's notion of transcendent causality (O'Grady 1975, 66–67). God does not cause suffering as its efficient cause. But because God could have prevented evil by not creating a physical universe with free and transcendent human creatures, God can in some sense be said to be the transcendental cause of evil.

CHAPTER 22

ETHICS COMMITTEES

Introduction

THIS CHAPTER EXAMINES the institutional ethics committee (IEC), also called the hospital ethics committee (HEC). As previous chapters have made clear, from the 1960s to the present there has been a significant increase in the importance of medical ethics in the United States. The growth in the literature has been remarkable. Whereas only *Hospital Progress* and *Linacre Quarterly*, two Roman Catholic publications, had been devoted to the study of health care ethics prior to the 1960s, such periodicals now abound, led by *The Hastings Center Report*, which began publication in 1971. Medical ethics think tanks have grown up all over the country; the federal government and state governments have commissions and task forces focused on bioethical issues and policies; law courts hear cases; hospitals and medical schools hire ethicists; and medical journals publish articles on ethics. Hospitals also have ethics committees. Indeed, there are now associations of ethics committees, and there are consultants hired to assist them.

Since the 1976 decision of the New Jersey Supreme Court in *Quinlan* in which the court properly suggested that decisions about forgoing life-sustaining treatment might rightly be made by hospital ethics committees (Veatch 1977b, 22), the number of these committees has risen rapidly (Levine 1984, 9). The influential 553-page report of the President's Commission for the Study of Ethical Problems in Medicine and Biomedical and Behavioral Research, issued in 1983, titled *Deciding to Forego Life-Sustaining Treatment*, gave significant support to the role of ethics committees (President's Commission 1983, 160–70, 443–57). A survey prepared in the early 1980s for that report found that only 1 percent of the nation's hospitals had at that time a functioning ethics committee (ibid., 446). But by 1988, the growth of ethics committees was such that *The Hastings Center Report* added a new section concerning them, and noted that more than 60 percent of hospitals with two hundred beds or more had them (Cohen 1988a). A 1992 estimate set the figure at 60 percent of all hospitals (McCartney 1992a, 222). A 1992 survey by the American Hospital Association set it at 51 percent (Fletcher and Hoffmann 1994, 335), as did a 1989 survey of hospitals in New York State (New York State Task Force on Life and the Law 1992, 287). A 1993 survey of the Catholic Health Association member hospitals received responses from 329 of 600 hospitals, and of those that responded, 92 percent claimed to have an ethics committee, and the remaining 8 percent were all institutions with fewer than 200 beds (Lappetito and

Thompson 1993, 34–35). Nearly two thirds of these committees were established between 1983 and 1989. An earlier 1978 survey of Catholic hospitals received responses indicating that 27 percent had "medical-morals committees," but these are not the same as ethics committees (President's Commission 1983, 161n124).

In 1992 the Joint Commission on Accreditation of Healthcare Organizations added the requirement that institutions must have procedures for dealing with ethical issues. This does not mandate an ethics committee as such, but it does mandate that hospitals provide for the functions that such committees carry out. Although the Patient Self-Determination Act (PSDA) did not mandate ethics committees, the bill originally introduced in Congress had included such a provision ("Ethics Committees" 1990), and the PSDA as it was finally passed in 1990 has stimulated the growth of these committees. Maryland's 1993 comprehensive statute on surrogate decision making includes the provision that hospitals must have "patient care advisory committees" (Medical Ethics Advisor 1993; Hoffmann 1993, 679), thus continuing an earlier 1987 Maryland law that made it the first state to require such committees (Hollinger 1989, 23). In the revised so-called Baby Doe regulations, the federal government issued guidelines about treatment for handicapped infants and suggested that all hospitals have infant care review committees (Meisel 1995, 2:335). These developments have all provided impetus for the establishment of institutional ethics committees. Virtually all hospitals now claim to have some form of ethics committee, though these vary widely in training and in quality.

This rapid growth in ethics committees is due to a variety of factors, among them the increase in medical technology, the prolongation of the dying process, increased costs, insistence on patient autonomy and criticism of physician paternalism, and the consumer movement. On the more practical level, the immediate impetus for institutional ethics committees came from court cases and federal guidelines that referred to them (Meisel 1995, 1:264–65).

It is a perfectly good idea to have ethics committees, but the governmental context needs to be looked at with some hesitation. Hospital ethics committees are internal to hospitals and ought to be voluntary. Were the government to mandate their existence, it might also mandate their role. Especially in the light of the *Cruzan* decision, with the danger that states might impose regulations making it difficult for surrogates to choose to forgo treatment, IECs might become an arm of the state for imposing and administering such restrictions. The context for infant care review committees, under the original Baby Doe regulations, was one of investigation of possible criminal activity, which does not set the proper context for ethics committees. IECs are internal organs within health care institutions that serve as one resource among many for enhancing the hospital's purpose: the health care of its patients.

It is important to note that the hospital ethics committee is not the only or even the most important source of ethical reflection or of ethical decision making within the hospital. It does only a very small part of the ethics that hospitals must do. If the various constituencies in any institution get the idea that they can pass off ethics onto this committee, much as decisions about patient competency are handed over to a consulting psychiatrist, or pulmonary diagnoses to a pulmonary specialist, or follow-up care to a social worker, then the hospital will lose, not gain, by the presence of such a committee. Medicine has become specialized. Health care ethics must not become one more specialization. It is true, of course, that ethics committees ought to develop certain skills that other members of the hospital community may not develop in the same theoretical or even practical way. That is why we have them. But ethics is not a specialization in the same sense that other specializations are. All members of the hospital community need to make ethical decisions, and indeed are faced with these issues all the time. The ethics committee, if it is a good one, will help in this. But it must not be seen as a dumping ground for ethical decisions. The ethics committee is but one community of wisdom and concern within the hospital.

Finally, it is important to note that an ethics committee is, after all, just one more committee, and, like all other committees, it will have no intrinsic value. Ethics committees do not make hospitals ethical. They do not have automatic expertise about ethics just because they have the title. Some of them are excellent, some good, some fair, some worthless, and some meddlesome. That is not specific to ethics committees; it is the way committees are.

Although ethics committees continue to proliferate, disagreement remains about their proper function and about how they ought to exercise that function. Some of these disputes concern ethical method, asking questions about the proper theoretical direction that ethical consultation ought to take (Drane 1990; McCartney 1992b; Murray 1988). These may mirror conversations within applied ethics as to whether principle-based or case-based approaches are better. There is also discussion concerning the problem of inconsistency among the recommendations made by members of different ethics committees (Fox and Stocking 1993). Additionally, even supporters of ethics committees rightly point to the need for continual evaluation and examination (Lo 1987; Fletcher and Hoffmann 1994; Sugarman 1994; Hollinger 1989). Some voice uncertainty about the role of committees, especially in case consultation (Siegler and Singer 1988; LaPuma and Toulmin 1989). And finally, a minority among ethicists and health care providers reject ethics committees altogether as usurpations of physician authority, and argue that only clinically trained professionals, preferably physicians, should carry on the role of case consultation (Siegler 1986).

The Makeup of the Ethics Committee

We begin with what an ethics committee is not. We then speak of how it might be structured within the hospital. Finally we turn to the makeup of the committee itself.

What an Institutional Ethics Committee Is Not

First, an institutional ethics committee is not an institutional review board (IRB). An IRB is required by law to serve as a kind of screening and approval committee for any experimental protocol where research is to be done using human subjects and where federal funds are involved. An IRB has decision-making authority within the institution and serves as a gatekeeper and a regulator of experimental research, and it clearly has functions that are of ethical import. It is wise to have a member of the institution's IRB on the ethics committee, or some other way of maintaining contact. But an IEC is not an IRB.

Second, an IEC is not a "medical morals committee." This is of no importance for most hospitals, but it is in some Catholic hospitals. The medical morals committee was often the body charged with enforcing official Catholic teaching on the hospital. Some of these, I am sure, did function validly as ethics committees. Others were merely watchdogs and censors. An ethics committee is not this.

Third, an IEC is not a quality review board. Nor is it a risk management committee. These serve valid functions in the hospital, and proper risk management and quality review are part of good ethics. Liaison between the IEC and these other entities is essential. But the functions performed by each are quite different.

Fourth, an IEC is not a prognosis confirmation committee. This is legally important as well as logically apparent. At times, courts have tended to confuse the two, asking ethics committees to comment on the patient's prognosis (Meisel 1995, 1:266–67). Even the report of the President's Commission includes prognosis confirmation as one of the tasks of an ethics committee (President's Commission 1983, 160). And hospitals sometimes do the same thing, especially if a court case is anticipated. Prognosis is clearly an essential datum for making the ethically right decision about treatment. But physicians, not ethics committees, make prognoses.

Fifth, an IEC is not an infant care review committee. As we have seen, federal guidelines suggest the establishment of such committees. Actually, "infant care review committee" is a bad name for them, since their proper function is not to review diagnoses and prognoses but to review the ethical and legal rightness and wrongness of treatment decisions for infants. An infant care review committee is really an infant bioethics review committee or a pediatric ethics committee. There is no reason why this should not be a subcommittee of the IEC, but in many hospitals it was established first, and such a subordination, while logical, might be politically difficult.

The Institutional Structure of the Ethics Committee

There are a number of possible ways the hospital ethics committee can fit into the already established hospital structure. First, it can be a medical staff committee. The advantage of this is that physicians may accept it better as one of their own, and this position properly symbolizes the committee's internal relationship to medicine. The disadvantages are that it becomes a physicians' committee so that the input of other members may be reduced, that it may tend to split up into specialized fields in the manner of most medical staff committees, and that the areas it treats may be reduced to those of immediate practical importance to physicians, who constitute an essential part of any hospital but who are not the whole of it.

Second, it can be a committee of the hospital administration. This properly symbolizes the inclusive nature of the committee. But with this positioning, the committee may be perceived by clinicians as one more imposition on the health care side by the money-and-regulation side of the institution.

Third, it can be a committee of the board of trustees. This may be helpful if the health care side of the hospital sees the administration side as more bothersome than supportive, but the disadvantage is that the committee might be seen as even more "outside" than an administrative committee would be.

Fourth, it could be a nursing committee. Although few if any IECs have chosen this structure, there is no theoretical reason to reject it. It is not really any different from making it a medical staff committee. Some have suggested that a second committee be established to deal with ethical issues specific to nurses ("Nursing Ethics Group" 1989), although if this is done, it would seem better to have this be a subcommittee of the IEC. If the IEC itself were to be a nursing committee, this would carry with it the disadvantage that it would be seen as representing a part of the hospital rather than the whole. Physicians might be unlikely to participate.

Fifth, and finally, the IEC could be a committee of some other area of the institution. For example, it could be a pastoral care committee. But ethics is not the same as pastoral care, although the pastoral care division must surely be represented. Similar objections can be made against making it a committee within social work, psychiatry, and so on.

Where then should it fit? It should fit wherever it will work best within the individual hospital. Idiosyncratic features of each institution will be more important here than wider theoretical considerations. Theoretically, the most logical structure is probably an administration committee. But some hospitals may find a medical staff or a board committee politically advantageous. The 1993 survey of Catholic hospitals found that 31 percent of those ethics committees were board committees, 19 percent administration committees, 17 percent "hospital or system" committees, 15 percent medical staff committees, 8 percent interdisciplinary committees, and 10 percent were some other type of committee (Lappetito and Thompson 1993, 38).

Ethics Committee Membership

It is generally accepted that a hospital ethics committee should be more or less evenly divided among physicians, nurses, and others. The size of the committee should vary according to the size of the hospital, but it should probably have ten to twenty-five members (McCartney 1992a, 223), though some are smaller and some larger (Lappetito and Thompson 1993, 37). Since a portion of its work will be done by subcommittees, a too-small committee will find itself handicapped. The membership should be balanced as to gender and race, if possible; committees should try to avoid having all the physicians male and all the nurses female.

Nonphysician, Nonnurse Others

If possible, IEC membership should include an ethicist with some theoretical background about the state of the art of ethics. A 1993 survey of Catholic hospitals found that 58 percent of ethics committees claimed to have one (Lappetito and Thompson 1993, 38). She or he should be acquainted with the general consensus and debates about many of the major ethical issues in the health care community, and about the theoretical and methodological questions that underlie them. This expertise, despite its theoretical nature, will help the IEC in its deliberations. Some hospitals will wish to find ethicists with clinical experience, or to hire full-time or part-time ethicists whose work goes beyond their presence at IEC meetings. These must know, or be willing to learn quickly, the clinical and structural aspects of the hospital, so they are able to apply theoretical knowledge to the clinical environment and to modify theory when clinical reality requires this. Ethicists can be very helpful in pointing out the issues to be considered and in presenting the majority and minority opinions. But they are also likely to have made their own judgments, sometimes strongly, about certain issues, and they should be able to distinguish these from the general consensus when there is a difference. The IEC at St. Francis Medical Center in Pittsburgh, on which Dr. Kelly served, had no fewer than four ethicists with doctorates, who represented Catholic, Protestant, and Jewish perspectives.

There has been some sporadic controversy as to whether the hospital lawyer should be on the committee (Mitchell and Swartz 1990). Some who argue that the lawyer must be a member worry that otherwise the IEC might unwittingly enter into illegal or legally unwise decisions. Those opposed to a lawyer's presence worry that the committee will stop doing ethics once a lawyer cites the relevant law. They also rightly note that many hospital lawyers lack knowledge of patient care law, emphasizing instead contract and litigation law. The Catholic hospital survey found that 52 percent of those ethics committees had an attorney as a member (Lappetito and Thompson 1993, 38).

Lawyers who know patient law and are interested in ethics are invaluable to the committee's work. But the committee has to watch out lest the meetings become two-way conversations between the lawyer and the ethicist. If a hospital decides not to have its lawyer on the committee, then the committee should take care to consult with her or him often. Some IECs have resolved this issue by inviting a lawyer who is not the hospital counsel. The intent here is to avoid possible conflict of interest. But most IEC members are hospital employees or staff, and it is not clear that the hospital counsel would suffer more from such conflict than other members.

IEC membership is enhanced by including administrators, social workers, and board members. Administration attendance and support is essential. Clergy representation is also important. Depending on the committee's size and the religious diversity of the community, the committee might think of inviting members of the clergy from various religious perspectives. The College of Chaplains, in its 1992 *Guidelines for the Chaplain's Role in Bioethics*, emphasizes the role of chaplains in the work of IECs (Phillips 1993).

There is some controversy over whether the committee should have a "patient advocate." This might be a member of the lay public or a representative from some patient advocate group or patient rights group. The argument in favor of this is that otherwise the committee can become too elitist. The arguments against it are that having only one person from the public on the committee would be simply tokenism, that the patient advocate would be overshadowed by other members of the committee, and that a patient advocate group would see its mission as pushing strongly for one position. If a lay member is chosen, she or he should probably be a person of some importance within the community, should be acquainted with how committees work, and should be unafraid to speak up. Though it is not exactly the same thing, perhaps a member chosen from the hospital board of trustees could help provide a lay perspective.

Physician Members

Physician members should represent various departments and divisions within the hospital. It is important that the physician members include some of the hospital's "biggest wigs," some of its most important doctors. A top surgeon should serve. The head of medicine, or of the intensive care unit, or of the emergency room might be invited. It is virtually essential that one member be on the medical executive committee, especially if the IEC is not a medical staff committee. The IEC simply will not work unless the medical staff consider it part of medical care in the hospital, just as informed consent, for example, does not work when physicians see it as a legal and bureaucratic imposition rather than as an essential and intrinsic part of good medical care. If the IEC of a teaching hospital consists mostly or only of residents with maybe a fellow or two, it will not work. However, membership ought to include some newer members of the staff, perhaps including one or more fellows or residents.

It should be obvious that physician members who have an interest in ethics, and perhaps even some background in the area, will be of greater value than those who do not. If none of the "big wigs" are concerned about ethics, or if most of the department heads think ethics is one more invasion of outside expertise intended to plague the doctor, then the hospital is in a muddle anyway, and the ethics committee will have a hard time of it. This should not be the case in any hospital; good hospitals are not like this.

Nurse Members

Nurses are essential to the IEC (Murphy 1989; "Nurses Bring Holistic View" 1993). The same criteria that are true for physician members are true for nurses. Some of the nursing members should have authority and influence. A nurse-administrator should be on the committee. Nurses are often the group most sensitive to ethical questions, and nurses are always involved in patient care and in treatment decisions. Nurses from different specialties should be members. Some nurse members should be floor nurses who can speak from day-to-day clinical experience. There should be enough nurse members (this is why the one-third rule is important) to give them a true voice. Like the physician members, all should have an interest in ethical health care and have, or be willing to gain, knowledge in the field.

Chairing the Committee

Who should chair the IEC? Probably not the ethicist, since ethicists are not usually long-term hospital staff personnel. If the ethicist has been a long-term hospital employee, accepted as an essential member of the health care professionals of the hospital, this might be acceptable. The chaplain is usually not a good candidate, for similar reasons. The best idea may be to have a physician as chair, though this is more a politically practical than a theoretical decision. After the committee is established, it may be possible to rotate the chair, but this carries with it the danger that continuity and interest will flag. It is most important that the chair be intrigued by ethics and recognize the importance of the work of the committee. No one else is going to call the meetings and set up the work agenda.

Changing Membership

A final issue is how to handle changing membership. Inevitably, some members will quit expressly, and others will simply stop coming. The committee needs to have some way of asking those whose attendance falls to leave the committee to make way for others who are more interested. One of us (Kelly) worked with a committee that sent out a report card of attendance at the end of each year, telling each member his or her percentage of unexcused absences. Members were asked to call the chair's office if they could not attend. Surprisingly, there was little resentment of this, and the technique helped. Committees might require that members with unexplained absences of more than a certain percentage leave the committee.

The Function of the Ethics Committee

The IEC has three generally recognized roles, although some ethicists subdivide one or other of them (McCartney 1992a, 223-24; Lappetito and Thompson 1993, 35; Bell 1993; Gibson and Kushner 1986, 10; Van Allen, Moldow, and Cranford 1989, 23). The IEC educates hospital staff, creates policy, and provides consultation.

Ethical Education

Self-Education

Education is the sine qua non of any IEC (Slomka 1994). Without this, the committee has no function. No IEC ought to attempt any other function until it has made a considerable start at this for itself, and has at least begun to do it for the hospital. This takes more time than is usually anticipated. It is reasonable to postpone policy development and case review for perhaps two years after the IEC is established. There may be exceptions to this in cases of emergency. But hospitals have always had emergency need for case decisions and policy development, and the new IEC simply cannot consider itself able to develop policy and review cases until after it has gone through a period of self-education. If it attempts to do so, this will rightly be rejected, and its ongoing mission will be seriously jeopardized.

Techniques for self-education are many. The hospital might provide stipends for the committee to bring in outside experts to give lectures on various aspects of health care ethics. Members might be reimbursed for travel to seminars or for courses and even graduate programs. Some process whereby the committee members meet on a consistent basis to read and discuss issues is indispensable. An ethics journal club session at each meeting, where a book chapter or an article or two are assigned to the committee, is a good way to do this. One member is assigned to report. Inevitably, focused and meaningful discussion ensues. The presence of an ethicist at these sessions is helpful, but even without one, the members of the committee, if required to work through the material, will educate themselves. Beginning with the practical issue of forgoing treatment is a good idea. Members might be urged to subscribe to a health care ethics journal. The self-education process can also proceed by using cases from the several case books now available, or by having physicians and nurses present cases for discussion (Veatch 1977a; Cohen 1988c; Ackerman and Strong 1989; Perlin 1992; Crigger 1998; Gervais et al. 1999; Pence 2000; Freeman and McDonnell 2001). If the purpose of the case presentation is the education of the committee, however, and not case review as such, care should be taken to make sure that the committee does not know who the patient is, and that there is no feedback to the actual people involved. Educational cases are better when some changes are made in them so that they are theoretical rather than actual cases, since the purpose is the education of the committee and not consultation as a help in resolving the case.

The self-education of the committee never ends. After the committee has completed its self-imposed period of education and has begun other functions, those very functions will require ongoing education. And IECs will have changes in membership. While it is impossible to repeat the entire process of education for each new member, the ongoing tasks of the committee are themselves educating, and new members will become aware of the issues, approaches, terminology, and so on. New members might be asked to read a certain number of books and articles. In any case, the presence of new members is itself an educational resource for the committee because they help the committee avoid shortcuts that assume what should not be assumed.

Education of the Hospital Community

In addition to self-education, the IEC will involve itself in the education of the hospital community. This task need not await completion of the committee's self-education. Ways of implementing this role include grand rounds, special lectures, seminars, journal clubs, in-service workshops, and weekend symposia. If the hospital is a teaching hospital, ethics grand rounds should be part of the residency curriculum, and other hospital personnel may be invited to attend. Consistent case review also contributes to this process (Glaser and Miller 1993).

Policy Development

The second task usually taken on by IECs is policy development. Although some argue that IECs are not the proper way to make policy (Murray 1988), a majority disagree and consider the ethics committee to be often the best source for certain hospital policies (Macklin 1988). Hospitals will have different procedures for establishing how ethics committees receive the charges to develop these policies. IECs should not try to usurp the role of other hospital divisions and committees. Just because a policy involves ethics—and every hospital policy does; health care delivery is at its core a moral enterprise—does not mean the IEC is the place where the policy must be developed. Perhaps the administration or the medical executive committee will ask the IEC to research and develop a policy. Sometimes external agencies, such as the Joint Commission on Accreditation of Healthcare Organizations, will require a policy, as it does in the area of forgoing treatment. Ethics committees may be the best place for these to be written. Or the committee may itself decide that a policy is in need of review. If the IEC is seen not as a policing agency but as an intrinsic part of the hospital community, policy creation and review should not present serious problems, although developed policies will doubtless be reviewed by other divisions of the hospital. New IECs should not try to develop policy. IECs are not ad hoc committees, and trying to short-circuit their own period of self-education will be harmful in the long run.

What authority does the ethics committee have to enforce its developed policy? The best answer is probably none, at least in the direct sense. IECs should submit their proposals to the established chain of authority within the hospital. They should not be another enforcement body. Policies that the IEC are asked to write should be submitted to the division that requested them. Usually major policies, such as on forgoing treatment, will need approval by the medical staff, the administration, and the board of trustees. The IEC does not itself have administrative power. But established and accepted ethics committees do have moral authority. As other hospital divisions come to respect the work of the IEC, its created and redesigned policies will gain authority. Finally, it should be recognized that the IEC will at times report its concerns to the administration if a policy is being ignored or violated. This responsibility of the IEC is no more than that of any other committee or individual aware of a violation of ethics.

Case Review

The third function usually ascribed to IECs is case consultation. Here lies the greatest degree of controversy about the IEC's role. Commentators have noted the seemingly low numbers of consults actually being done (Lappetito and Thompson 1993, 37; Cohen 1988b). Some IECs explicitly reject this function, fearing that case consultation will be seen as an intrusion into the physician–patient relationship. And some physicians and ethicists agree, restricting the role of ethics committees to the creation of policy, and arguing that case consultation be done only by clinically trained professionals, preferably by physicians trained in ethics who may bill for consultations (LaPuma and Toulmin 1989; LaPuma et al. 1988; LaPuma and Schiedermayer 1991). Others, who almost certainly represent the majority, counter this opinion by supporting case consultation by IECs (Orr and Moon 1993; Perkins and Saathoff 1988; Bell 1993; Lappetito and Thompson 1993; Rubin and Zoloth-Dorfman 1994; Hughes 1992; Glaser and Miller 1993, 86; Tulskey and Lo 1992, 344; Fletcher 1990). Some point to the valid role that nonclinicians can and ought to play in case consultation (Thomasma 1991).

Though disagreement persists, it seems clear that properly functioning and properly educated IECs will and should function in this role, although case consultation is better done by teams of committee members than by the IEC as a whole. Ethics committee consultations serve in ways similar to other consultations. They provide written and personal resources to the decision makers. They provide opportunities for collaboration. They contribute significantly to the general ethical education of the hospital community. Properly understood, ethics committee case reviews are helps in mutual decision making.

Initiation and Recommendation

There is a helpful way of clarifying the role of IECs in case review. A distinction is made between the origin of the review and its outcome. That is, under what circumstances are consultations initiated, and how authoritative are the opinions rendered?

Either can be mandatory or optional. Mandatory-mandatory case review is uncommon and unattractive. Here certain treatment options, such as withdrawing ventilation, must be prospectively reviewed by the IEC—the initiation is mandatory—and the judgment of the IEC must be followed—the outcome is also mandatory. This approach is not recommended.

The best way to set up case review is to make it optional-optional. This model appears to be the most widely used, or at least the most widely claimed (Agich and Youngner 1991, 17; van der Heide 1994, 73; Griener and Storch 1994, 469; Randal 1983, 10). Among the Catholic hospitals with ethics committees in the 1993 survey, a full 93 percent claimed either that their ethics committee "advises only" or "advises and makes recommendations" (Lappetito and Thompson 1993, 36). In the optional-optional model, review is voluntary and the final suggestion that the consult team makes is not officially binding on the hospital, patient, physician, or family. IECs are not supposed to be courts. Decisions about treatment are best made by the patient and the physician with the family at the bedside, that is, in the clinical setting. Case reviews and consultations by persons who have educated themselves in these questions are often helpful and are part of the internal clinical process. In most instances, the consultation will enable the patient, family, and health care team to get a clearer idea of what is happening, of what the ethical and legal implications of the situation are, and of what the general ethical agreement is, if there is one. Additionally, individual members of the IEC may be versed in certain religious traditions and may be able to offer knowledge and solace from the patient's faith perspective. But the advice or judgment of the consultation team should not be binding as such.

This is not to claim that such an opinion lacks moral authority or that health care providers will or should easily ignore it (Ritchie 1989). As the IEC and its consult service gain respect within the hospital, its opinions will be perceived more and more as valid helps to proper medicine. It is even possible in some cases that the opinion rendered is so clear and so essential to the institution's well-being that the hospital administration will wish to enforce it. But the consult opinion as such, in a way similar to directly medical consults called from specialists, is not mandatory.

There are two other possible ways of dealing with initiation and outcome. Initiation might be mandatory in certain situations with the outcome optional. For example, if a hospital were to be concerned about the possibility of withdrawing medically induced nutrition from a patient in a persistent vegetative state, it might want to require an IEC review in all such cases. Although the reasons for this kind of policy are in some sense understandable, the approach is generally unhelpful. Certain types of cases may at first be perceived as particularly difficult, and health care providers may call ethics consults. But after experience and education, hospital personnel will become less needful of such consults. There is likely to be a shift in the kind of consults the committee is asked to undertake, from the less to the more complex. This is due to a greater familiarity among physicians and other providers with the basic ethical and legal issues involved—a familiarity that results from previous consults. In any case, mandating ethics consults gives them an aura of external imposition that in the long run threatens to undermine their acceptance and thus their effectiveness.

If the mandatory-optional model is used, it should be restricted to cases where there is no reasonable alternative. We saw in chapter 16 a suggested policy for dealing with incompetent patients who have no surrogates. Since the usual way to deal with this has been to get a court-appointed guardian, and since the suggested policy changes this, that policy does require an ethics consult in those cases.

It is theoretically possible to make initiation optional and recommendation mandatory, but this seems illogical and would probably result in the collapse of case review.

Who Calls the Consult?

It is best when consults can be called by anyone actively involved in the case. This recommendation disagrees with those who argue that the chair of the committee should serve as a gatekeeper for deciding which cases will be reviewed (van der Heide 1994, 73). Experience suggests that the great majority of ethics consults will be called by physicians, but this does not support the argument that only physicians should call them (Andereck 1992). It is rare that consults are initiated against the wishes of the attending physician, but in those few cases there may well be strong reasons for calling them. Indeed, given accreditation requirements now in place for hospitals, where nurses are required to have access to IECs, it seems unlikely that such a restriction would stand. Experience shows that nurses are always central to patient care and therefore to the ethical issues concerned with it. And surely the patients themselves, their families, and social workers must be given access to this procedure. This refusal to limit access to physicians appears to be the position taken by most ethics committees and is supported by commentators (Hughes 1992; Olson et al. 1994, 438; Hoffmann 1993, 688; Freedman 1981, 20; Agich and Youngner 1991, 17).

The perception among some physicians that only they should have the right to call ethics consults is due to a misperception of what an ethics consult is. That misperception may be caused by experience with poorly educated or simply intrusive and arrogant ethicists or ethics committees. But a properly functioning ethics consult service should not be perceived as intrusive. Indeed, there is evidence that physicians support such consults and claim a gain in confidence as a result of them (Perkins and Saathoff 1988, 764-65).

Ethics consults, then, may rightly be called by anyone actively involved in the case. On admission to the hospital, patients should be informed in writing, in accordance with the PSDA, of the possibility of their requesting an ethics consult. If someone other than the attending physician initiates a consult, that person should, of course, attempt to discuss the anticipated consult with the patient's primary attending physician. And it is essential that the attending physician be informed of any consult that she or he does not initiate. The attending is going to be centrally involved in any case.

Composition of the Consult Team

Some IECs provide prospective case consultation by the committee as a whole. This undoubtedly has the advantage of introducing a greater divergence of perspectives and of lessening the likelihood that some relevant aspect will be overlooked. But the process is unwieldy and has significant disadvantages. The entire committee can rarely be gathered at one time on relatively short notice. It cannot meet in the clinical setting; thus, most members will not have seen the patient. Family members are often overawed when asked to appear before such a group. Some IEC members will not wish to participate in consults or will find themselves in some conflict of interest on many cases. Thus, some process using consult teams appears a far better alternative. The team speaks with the attending physician, the staff physicians, nurses, and other hospital personnel. The patient and the family are actively involved, speaking to the team, or to individual members of the team if that is easier for them.

One particularly good approach is to use a team of three persons. None of them may be directly connected with the case. Usually one will be a physician, one a nurse, and one neither a physician nor nurse. In all cases, however, one member ought to be a physician and at least one member a nonphysician. This combination of persons thinking and speaking from differing bases best ensures that relevant aspects of the case will be uncovered and addressed.

It is likely that some members of the IEC will not serve as case consultants. This means that a group will emerge over time of those who do consults. It is strongly recommended that this group attend an extra set of meetings, chaired if possible by an ethicist, for retrospective review of cases and discussion of relevant theoretical and practical concerns. This "quality review" is essential for ongoing education and checkup. If it seems helpful, consults can also be reviewed by the IEC as a whole, especially if a consult involves some critical issue of which the IEC as a whole needs to be aware. When this is done, all names except those of the consult team should be deleted to help ensure confidentiality. Admittedly, in most hospitals many IEC members will already be aware of the details even though names are removed. Especially in light of the Health Insurance Portability and Accountability Act of 1996 (HIPAA), it is incumbent on all who attend IEC meetings to be aware of the confidentiality requirements.

Arbitration and Communication

The role of arbitrator and communicator in ethics consultation is essential (West and Gibson 1992). So is the similar role of offering psychological support to patients, family members, and health care providers (McCartney 1992a, 224). Although the primary role of ethics consultation is not psychotherapeutic as such (Rubin and Zoloth-Dorfman 1994), in a considerable number of cases, ethics consultation smoothes the waters, enhances communication, and facilitates the decision-making process for patients, family members, and health care providers.

Communication within hospitals is notoriously problematic. Indeed, a specialty has developed within communication as an academic discipline to emphasize this issue. Answers to the problem are not easy. Hospitals are sometimes horrifyingly hierarchical, which adds to their other terrors. Morale problems are serious. Various professionals within hospitals come from differing backgrounds and develop different kinds of sensitivity and callousness. Tertiary care hospitals, especially in their more intense units, such as ICUs, are too often technology-driven. Crisis becomes commonplace, and speed and tension the rule rather than the exception. It is not surprising that in such a setting, communication with patients and families and among health care providers is less than optimal.

It is often true that ethics committees are the one place within a hospital where interdisciplinary conversation can take place on a consistent basis. IECs tend to break down interprofessional barriers, affording members from various professions the opportunity for at least some level of egalitarian dialogue.

Ethics consultation enhances this interprofessional communication as well, while also affording the chance for conversation with families and patients. Ethics consults allow families to understand better what it is that various specialists tell them about their loved one's situation. Although their purpose is not to confirm prognoses, ethics consult teams can often help families understand what the prognosis is in lay terms. Ethics consult teams are attuned to these kinds of issues and go to the meetings with the explicit intention of trying to do this—something physicians, in the time-constraints of their workday, may not be able to do as well. Finally, ethics consult teams are often able to alleviate family guilt and anxiety, explaining to them the moral implications of various decisions, setting up meetings with clergy, listening to their grief. It is not that no one else in the hospital does this, or that such work should be referred to the IEC. The entire hospital and all its personnel should be aware of the need for sensitive conversation with patients and families, and IECs are merely one resource among many for carrying out these functions. But they are an important resource.

Other Issues

First, should the process be called a consult? Some have claimed that there may be legal ramifications when IEC reviews are called consults—ramifications that would not arise if the term were not used. This is not a real issue. Although IECs are properly concerned about such legal questions, this sort of problem should not be exaggerated to the point where it paralyzes IECs and their work. Ethical consultations are as much a part of medical practice as any other consultation. The consultation should be charted like any other medical consult.

Some have feared that IECs might increase the possibility of lawsuits by bringing up issues otherwise ignored; however, it is now generally recognized that the opposite is true. IECs are more apt to reduce litigation than to increase it. They allow patients and families an opportunity for dialogue. The right decision is more likely to be made. The presence on the chart of an ethics consult backing up the decision by the physician, after consultation with the patient, the family, or both, can serve as evidence of proper procedure. The bottom line—and this is quoted from a workshop run by the American Society of Law and Medicine—is that "the best way to avoid losing lawsuits is to do the right thing in the first place." Ethics committees and ethics consults can help in reaching the right decision.

Second, what happens when the consult is completed? The conclusion of the consulting team can take many forms. Most of the time everyone involved will come to agreement about what to do, and this will simply be charted by the team. When disagreement persists, the ethics team may be able to help in showing exactly where the disagreement lies. Sometimes a compromise solution is available. Often an agreement is reached to wait for a time-limited trial for a certain course of treatment, after which another meeting is held.

The team's recommendation and how they arrived at it should be charted. Usually one member of the consult team will write this; others may amend it. All members should sign. There is no single accepted way to do this. Some chart entries are very brief, others quite long. It depends on the case. Although not all agree, it may be better to write more rather than less, since this serves as a way to be sure that the IEC is acting carefully when doing consults and it also helps in later review.

Range of Issues

One final question deserves some attention. What kinds of issues are institutional ethics committees likely to get involved in, and what issues should they stay out of? There is no easy answer to this. Theoretically and practically, all policy issues in hospitals have ethical components. The most obvious areas, and these are of great immediate importance, are those involving decisions to forgo treatment. As we have seen, IECs were first suggested to deal with this kind of question and to develop hospital policy for this. But IECs cannot be limited to this question. Policies and practices concerning informed consent, confidentiality, Jehovah's Witnesses, AIDS patients, dialogue among nurses and physicians, hospital discipline, and many other aspects of the hospital's work all have ethical ramifications. The IEC is not the only or even the most important body within the hospital to deal with such issues, but such issues may well come before it for reflection and proposed action.

The IEC also ought to educate itself and the hospital community about the problem of allocation of health care resources, both within the hospital and at the national level. There is controversy as to whether the IEC ought to propose policy for in-hospital allocation, such as whether or not to buy this or that machine, open this or that wing, develop or drop this or that specialty. These are most often issues involving questions of justice and are often of the highest ethical import. But they are just as clearly complex issues, and the IEC may decide it will not focus its own energies on policies of this kind. It should, however, include in its agenda the general education of the hospital community about the importance of hospital and societal issues of this type.

The Joint Commission on Accreditation of Healthcare Organizations now requires that hospitals have mechanisms for dealing with organizational ethics as well as with clinical ethics. It is not clear exactly where this line is drawn because organizational issues impact clinical cases, and often these cases ask organizational questions. It is clear, however, that organizational ethics must not be divorced from the IEC. If a special committee is established to focus on these issues, it ought to be a standing committee within the IEC, not a separate body. Here the focus will be on issues such as the hospital's mission, advertising, managed care contracts, pharmacy formularies, investments, allocation of hospital resources, personnel workloads and benefits, and many more. Clearly, these issues require special expertise and knowledge that IEC members may not have. But the IEC can be of help to those who do have this knowledge and expertise by pointing out the ethical implications of hospital policies and decisions and the principles that ought to govern them.

Conclusion

With interested, knowledgeable, and energetic leadership, and with a hospital community dedicated to good medical care of patients, institutional ethics committees can be of significant help. They must not be the only resource within a hospital where ethics is taken seriously. But good IECs prod, expedite, and make ethics visible. They serve as a reminder that good patient care is central to any hospital's mission. They are integral to good medicine.

CHAPTER 23

RESEARCH ETHICS

RESEARCH ETHICS was one of the original areas of concern for health care ethics as it expanded in the 1960s (see chapter 1). After a series of scandals and classic publications, the ethics of medical research with human beings was at the top of the agenda for researchers, ethicists, philosophers, lawyers, and politicians. An extensive system of review committees was developed in many countries. National legislation was introduced, and international codes, guidelines, and declarations were drafted and accepted. For decades, the general impression was that this area of bioethics was sufficiently well understood that it did not provide further challenges. It was also considered an excellent example of the positive interaction between ethics and health care. In recent years, however, the subject of research has been a renewed topic of heated debate and controversy. One reason for this is the emergence of new technologies and innovations—for example, genetic screening and stem cell technology—that give rise to new ethical issues and questions. Another reason is the growth of multinational research and the globalization of clinical trials that raise questions about the ethical framework for research in developing countries and different cultures.

Development of Research Ethics

Medicine is as old as humanity. As we saw in chapter 1, early physicians and healers in general combined an empirical approach with religious and magical practices. Medical papyri in ancient Egypt provided a supernatural interpretation of diseases together with empirical observations that contain many effective prescriptions. Subsequently, Greek medicine put more emphasis on rational approaches. Hippocrates was the first to argue that medicine should be a science. This implies (1) that empirical observation is the source of knowledge, (2) that the physician must proceed methodically, and (3) that empirical data must be rationally explained. Medicine, according to his contemporary, the philosopher Plato, is the science of the healthy and the unhealthy. The history of Western medicine, however, is not a story of continuous scientific progress. For centuries it was dominated by different theoretical approaches and had little practical impact. The return to empirical observation led to a breakthrough in 1543 when Andreas Vesalius published an anatomical atlas based on dissections. One century later William Harvey combined empirical observation and measurement with experimentation to discover blood circulation. In the eighteenth century scientific analysis produced several major advances: the emergence of morbid pathology (identifying diseases with alterations and dysfunctions of body parts), physical diagnostics (relating symptoms with pathology), and physiology (using rigorous experiments, especially in animals, to study the functioning of body mechanisms). From then on, medicine was primarily interpreted as a natural science. Whereas in the seventeenth century the philosopher Francis Bacon classified medicine as a human science, for the eighteenth-century French *Encyclopedia* it had become a subdivision of the natural sciences along with mathematics, biology, and physics. These advances improved medical interpretation and diagnosis, but they did not produce much therapeutic progress. This started to change at the end of the nineteenth century with the new discipline of bacteriology. Louis Pasteur and Robert Koch each identified microorganisms, demonstrated that microorganisms cause infectious diseases, and showed how vaccinations could make people immune to disease. These findings also promoted antiseptic procedures, making surgery and obstetrics much safer than they had been. The twentieth century is characterized by a "therapeutic revolution." Many discoveries (e.g., vitamins and hormones) generated beneficial treatments. In particular, the discovery and invention of effective medication changed the practice of medicine. For example, the discovery of the antibiotic effect of penicillin by Alexander Fleming in 1928 forever changed the treatment of infections and saved millions of lives (Friedman and Friedland 1998).

Although science in the last few centuries has transformed medicine through discoveries, innovations, new knowledge, and technologies, medical research as systematic investigation and experimentation is rather new. An early exception is the clinical trial conducted by navy surgeon James Lind in 1747. He treated two groups of scurvy sufferers with different remedies and demonstrated that scurvy can be treated successfully by taking citrus fruits. Also famous are the studies undertaken in 1789 by Edward Jenner to inoculate people (including his own son) with cowpox to make them immune to smallpox, a procedure later called "vaccination," the first documented method to prevent the onset of infectious disease.

In the nineteenth century, medicine undeniably became a scientific endeavor, with experiments performed in the laboratory and with the help of basic sciences such as physiology and pathology. The emergence of microbiology encouraged experiments with chemical substances to find a "magic bullet" against diseases (Porter 2006). In 1865 Claude Bernard, the founder of modern physiology, published his famous book, "An Introduction to the Study of Experimental Medicine." This publication signals the birth of modern medicine. Scientific medicine, argues Bernard, can be established only by experimental means. Progress in medicine is only possible through experimentation. This will endow medicine with "knowledge of the laws of healthy and diseased organisms" (Bernard 1957, 2, 197).

The Basic Problem

The growing use of experimentation in medicine has introduced a specific problem that is fundamental in research ethics. In health care, the interests of the individual patient have priority. In experimentation, the primary interest is the acquisition or validation of scientific knowledge. Scientific medicine embodies at the same time two different value systems: the values of science (reliable knowledge, truth, coherence, relevancy, utility) and the values of patient care (human dignity, autonomy, beneficence, nonmaleficence, trust). It wants to realize two moral goods: the individual good of subjects and the social good of obtaining reliable knowledge to improve health. In theory these different values should not conflict. Research is conducted to obtain knowledge; the new knowledge can be used to improve health. But there are different orientations that can easily conflict. First, the starting point is different. In health care, patients enter into relationships with health professionals because they have a concern or a symptom that they want to have examined. Research usually is initiated with a problem or research question that is scientifically challenging and that the researcher wants to address. Second, the aims differ. In health care, the aim of activities, examinations, and tests is to find a specific therapy so that a patient's complaint can be treated. In research, the aim is generalized knowledge, for example, evidence that one treatment is better than another. Third, in health care, the individual patient is the interested party as the ultimate decision maker whose interests have priority. From an ethical point of view, the patient is respected as an end in himself. In research, the interested parties are the researcher and the sponsor of the research; they decide on the arrangements. They only need individuals as subjects for the research, as "research material" for exploring and testing new medication. In research, therefore, the subject is used as a means to obtain knowledge.

These different orientations would not be problematic if they could be separated. It is sometimes argued that the roles of scientist and health care provider should be clearly demarcated. However, in practice they often overlap. Now that modern health care itself has become a scientific enterprise, it is often the case that practitioners are at the same time researchers. In this context patients will be regarded as potential research subjects. In medical research new drugs are eventually tested in clinical trials. This can imply that the relationship between doctor and patient coincides with the relationship between research and subject. In can be unclear in these conditions which interests and values are given priority. Scientific curiosity, the drive to solve urgent problems, and the desire to contribute to scientific progress as well as mundane factors such as reputation, publication pressure, or commercial interests may override the interests of the patient and the need to provide the best care available. The basic problem in research ethics is in fact an example of the tension in ethical theory discussed in chapter 8: deontology and consequentialism. Some of the more simplistic approaches to consequentialism and utilitarianism, which we reject, might ask: What is wrong with research if it can deliver results that may save many lives? "The results justify the research" is an argument often used by researchers. But the ends do not justify an otherwise wrong means, as is stipulated in a deontological argument and by some more sophisticated versions of consequentialism; even very useful research needs to respect human beings and cannot sacrifice some individuals for the benefit of others.

This basic tension in contemporary medicine explains why the history of research ethics is characterized by so many scandals. One of the first notorious cases happened in 1900 in Prussia (later included in Germany), at a time when it was one of the leading countries in medical science. Dr. Albert Neisser, a famous professor of dermatology and the discoverer of gonococcus, the bacteria that causes gonorrhea, deliberately injected syphilis materials into eight minors without giving any information or asking permission. He argued that they would contract syphilis anyway because they were prostitutes. The Prussian authorities responded with a condemnation and with directives; they prohibited experiments with minors and stipulated the need for informed consent. But the German medical profession supported Neisser.

Public indignation increased in 1930 with the first large-scale lawsuit against medical doctors in the North German city of Lübeck. In a few months' time 76 babies had died after the use of an oral vaccine against tuberculosis (among 244 babies vaccinated). The physicians regarded the vaccination as normal medical treatment and were convinced that it was beneficial and harmless while in fact it was an experiment because the scientific evidence was inadequate. The case accelerated the issuing of national directives in 1931 that regulated scientific experiments and the introduction of new treatments. Again the importance of consent and information was underlined. In fact, Germany was the first country to regulate scientific research (Bonah, Lepicard, and Roelcke 2003).

Ethics and Regulation

For a long time most countries did not have any ethical regulation of scientific research. The medical profession argued that external regulation is unnecessary, claiming that it is the duty of the profession to regulate itself. The argument is that the public could have confidence in the moral virtues of individual physicians and researchers. Perhaps from time to time cases might emerge due to the transgressions of some doctors and researchers, but these were rare incidents. In principle there is nothing wrong with the system of the scientific enterprise itself. This ideology of self-regulation has been seriously questioned since World War II.

The Nuremburg Code

In 1946 the Nuremberg Medical Trial accused twenty-three Nazi physicians and administrators of war crimes and crimes against humanity. The medical doctors were on trial for atrocious experiments on prisoners in concentration camps. Prisoners had been subjected to experiments involving malaria, typhus, freezing temperatures, mustard gas, sterilization, bone transplantation, and the drinking of sea water. Individuals were sacrificed for the sake of society, the state, and a political program of racial hygiene. In fact, the German medical profession was on trial since the atrocities reflected attitudes to science that were broadly shared despite the existing regulations. About 50 percent of all German physicians were members of the Nazi party. The atrocities were committed in the name of medical science (Weindling 2004).

At the close of the trial in August 1947 the Nuremberg Code was promulgated by US judges. The code is the first international document to protect the rights of research subjects. It is based on human rights principles that have universal application. The code clearly articulates the principle of informed consent. A necessary condition for medical experimentation is the voluntary, competent, informed, and understanding consent of the subject.

However, the impact of the code was rather limited. Many physicians argued that it was primarily a code for uncivilized professionals. Civilized doctors did not need regulations that deal with such colleagues. Even in Germany, many of the Nazi researchers kept their influential positions, the victims of the experiments were marginalized, and Nazi research continued to be cited in the literature. The emphasis in the code on informed consent was also peculiar given the fact that all research subjects had been prisoners with no choice at all. But at least the code insisted that respect for human dignity and self-determination should set limits to the utilitarian argumentation used to defend these immoral experiments.

Declaration of Helsinki

In 1947 national medical associations established the World Medical Association (WMA). Concerned with violations of human rights, the WMA started working on medical ethics, which resulted in the adoption of the Declaration of Helsinki in 1964, which set forth ethical principles for medical research involving human subjects. This declaration has become the most influential international guidance document on research ethics. It has been revised six times, most recently in 2008. The 1964 declaration makes a distinction between therapeutic research (research that may improve diagnosis and therapy for the patient) and nontherapeutic research (research that has no therapeutic value to the person involved in the research); but this distinction was dropped in the revision of 2000. The declaration furthermore articulates two basic principles:

- Risk assessment: The expected benefits of the research should be in proportion to the possible risks to the subject: "Every clinical research project should be preceded by careful assessment of inherent risks in comparison to foreseeable benefits to the subject or to others" (Declaration of Helsinki 1964, I.4).
- Informed consent: Each subject must be adequately informed of the aims, methods, anticipated benefits and potential hazards of the study.

In contrast to the Nuremberg Code, however, the Declaration of Helsinki allows for substituted consent: "In case of legal incapacity consent should also be procured from the legal guardian; in case of physical incapacity the permission of the legal guardian replaces that of the patient" (ibid., II.1). The requirements for informed consent were more elaborated in later revisions of the text.

The 1974 revision added a third requirement, independent review: The research proposal should be clearly formulated in a protocol that should be submitted to "a specially appointed independent committee for consideration, comment and guidance" (Declaration of Helsinki 1975, I.2). This requirement of advance review led to the establishment of institutional review boards (IRB) in the United States and research ethics committees in other countries.

These three requirements for medical research would remain the cornerstones for the development of research ethics. Later revisions of the declaration, especially since 2000, became increasingly controversial due to the globalization of health research.

The Declaration of Helsinki initially differs from the Nuremberg Code in that it puts more emphasis on the responsibilities and duties of physicians toward patients and research subjects, rather than underlining the rights of patients. The Nuremberg Code is more focused on protection of individuals; hence, the central role of informed consent. The Helsinki Declaration is concerned with the need to balance scientific interest and patient interest, underlining the central role of the physician, for example, in judging whether benefits and risks are in proportion. Informed consent is only one principle among others. Over time, subsequent revisions have shifted the emphasis more toward the interests of human subjects.

Henry Beecher

In 1966 Henry Beecher, a professor at Harvard Medical School, published a paper on clinical research in the *New England Journal of Medicine*. He presented twenty-two cases of clearly unethical research, all published in leading medical journals. Experiments involved injecting live cancer cells, feeding subjects with the hepatitis virus, and withholding antibiotic treatment from subjects whose health and well-being were thereby endangered but who did not even know they were included in research. The cautious conclusion of Beecher was that unethical procedures were "not uncommon." He was not convinced that new or more rules were needed; he continued to believe in the integrity and responsibility of the individual researcher (Rothman 1991).

Beecher's publication caused an outcry in the public media. It contributed to the emergence of the new discipline of bioethics. But it also troubled the authorities responsible for funding medical research. In 1966, the National Institutes of Health (NIH) in the United States issued for the first time ethical guidelines for all federally funded research involving human experimentation. One of the requirements was that research institutions document evidence of informed patient consent. The other was that they set up a mechanism for peer review to assess the potential benefit and risk of the research undertaken. For the first time, the individual judgment of investigators was subjected to required collective surveillance.

The Tuskegee Study

In the first few decades after World War II, researchers were completely autonomous, free from external constraints; ethical considerations were left to the investigators. It became increasingly clear to the public and to policymakers that there was a fundamental conflict of interest between research and health care. What might have been in the interest of investigators might not also be in the interest of the research subjects. There were crucial differences between the doctor–patient relationship (governed by the best interests of the patient) and the researcher–subject relationship. Professional self-regulation was no longer sufficient for protecting research subjects. The need for outside intervention was propelled into action with the revelation in 1972 of the Tuskegee syphilis experiment conducted by the US Public Health Service, a federal government agency. Between 1932 and 1972 more than four hundred black men from Alabama who were suffering from syphilis were left untreated in order to study the natural progression of the disease. Treatment was even withheld after the discovery of penicillin. The study was only ended when newspaper articles created a public scandal. The US Congress started hearings. In 1974 the National Commission for the Protection of Human Subjects of Biomedical and Behavioral Research (hereafter, "National Commission") was established in order to develop policies for human experimentation.

The Belmont Report

The creation of the National Commission signaled that research policies were no longer to be determined by physicians alone. The monopoly of the medical profession in medical ethics was over (Rothman 1991). In 1978 the commission published the Belmont Report, which is essentially a statement of a general framework of moral principles of research (see chapter 8). The report identified three basic principles, each of which has implications for the practice of research. The first principle is respect for persons, including respecting their rights as autonomous persons to decide whether to participate in research. The requirement for informed consent means that researchers must disclose information, and the research subject must comprehend the data and volunteer to participate. The second principle is beneficence. This principle applies to risk–benefit assessment. The possible benefits of research need to be maximized and the possible harms minimized. Risks and benefits should be presented to research participants but also assessed by an institutional review board. The third principle is justice, which applies to the selection of research participants. Too often research has been conducted with vulnerable and disadvantaged populations. These groups were carrying the burdens of research without being able to receive its benefits. With these three principles the National Commission intends to counteract a justification of research based only on the sort of utilitarianism and consequentialism we rejected in chapters 8 and 10. The Belmont Report has a tremendous impact on bioethics because it focuses not only on the moral principles underlying medical research but also on the regulation and oversight of research that in many countries resulted in legislation.

Ethical Framework

In many Western countries the ethical framework regulating research with human beings has been consolidated since the 1980s. In the United States, federal regulations established a process for systematic review, approval, and oversight of all human subject research that is supported, conducted, or otherwise regulated by the federal government. These legal requirements came into effect in 1981; they were codified as The Federal Policy for the Protection of Human Subjects, known as the "Common Rule," in 1991. France enacted special legislation in 1988, creating forty-eight Committees for the Protection of Persons in various regions. Although the first research ethics committees were established in Germany in the 1970s, committee approval of clinical trials became mandatory there only in 1994.

The comprehensive framework to guide clinical research and to protect research subjects comprises a set of interconnected principles (Emanuel, Wendler, and Grady 2008). The first is collaborative partnership. Clinical research involves people who are participants rather than subjects. The second is social value. Clinical research should contribute to improvements in health for society; therefore, it is important to assess the potential value of the research undertaken. The third principle is scientific validity. If a research protocol is not designed to produce valid and reliable data, then the research is hard to justify ethically. Fair participant selection is the fourth principle. In the past, research subjects were often selected among poor and uneducated populations or among special vulnerable populations, such as prisoners, children, and the elderly.

Selection of the study groups should only be based on scientific reasons related to the frequency of diseases, the harms caused by diseases, or high transmission rates of an infection. The fifth principle is a favorable risk–benefit ratio. Since all research implies uncertainty and risks, a careful assessment of risks is necessary. Risks should be minimized. At the same time, the benefits of the research should be evaluated, especially the potential benefits to the individuals who participate in the research itself. Finally, risks and benefits should be compared to assess what is an ethically justifiable balance. However, there is no exact standard to determine when potential benefits are proportionate to risks (see the discussion of proportionalism in chapter 10). The sixth principle is independent review. An ethics committee should review and approve the protocol before the research starts. The committee and its members should be independent, that is, not involved in the research or affiliated with the researchers or sponsors, and without financial interest in the outcome of the study. The committee's composition and procedures are usually specified in the relevant legislation. Informed consent is the seventh principle. This expresses respect for the dignity and autonomy of the persons involved. Participants should be competent, that is, they should have the capacity to understand and make decisions. Information should be disclosed orally and in written form so participants will fully understand. Participants then need to give explicit permission, voluntarily and without coercion. They should be aware that they have the right to refuse participation and that they can withdraw from research. Finally, the eighth principle is respect for participants. This emphasizes that even when informed consent has been obtained, certain obligations exist. For example, researchers should monitor the health of participants and treat harms that result from adverse reactions. They should also protect confidentiality and make sure that data are secure. Furthermore, they should provide new, relevant information when this is gained.

Challenges of Globalization

Important changes in research ethics started to take place around the turn of the millennium. The increasing reliance in health care on drugs has magnified the search for new medication. In 2007 total drug sales amounted to $712 billion; 50 percent of these sales were in the United States. New products are marketed continuously. Expenditure for pharmaceutical research and development has increased from $1.1 billion in 1975 to $44.5 billion in 2007. No one knows exactly how many clinical trials are conducted. As a result of these pressures, clinical research has been "offshored." During the 1990s a great deal of clinical research was transferred from the United States to Eastern Europe, in the 2000s to Latin America, and more recently to developing countries in Asia and Africa. Various motives have exacerbated this trend. One is cost reduction. Conducting large-scale clinical trials is much cheaper in India than in North America or Europe. Another motive is fast-track execution. It is much easier to enroll participants in a research project in developing countries; there, being included in a trial is often the only opportunity for many people to receive basic health care. A third motive is more suspicious: less regulation. Many developing countries do not have legislation regulating research; they lack oversight, and ethics review committees are often weak (Petryna 2009).

Globalization of medical research has given a new drive to the debate on research ethics. Controversies have emerged concerning the use of placebos. In clinical trials a new substance is usually compared with a standard treatment or a placebo. Many scientists argue that methodologically a comparison with placebo controls is preferable. However, the use of inactive substances such as placebos is ethically only justified if there is no known effective therapy. The principle of respect for participants implies a moral duty to care. The concern to provide the best therapy for the patient should override the concerns for scientific evidence. In 1997 two studies were published in the *New England Journal of Medicine*. Both studies were conducted in developing countries, both focused on HIV transmission, and both were sponsored by NIH. One study used placebos in the control group, and the other simply observed research subjects even though effective antiretroviral treatment was available. In the same journal, both studies were condemned as unethical. They would never have been approved in the United States. However, NIH defended the withholding of effective treatment because in their view the application of ethical principles can vary according to the social and economic context. The argument was that in a country such as Uganda, the standard treatment that is available in the United States does not exist, is too costly, and cannot be applied for logistical reasons. This argument introduced double standards. What is ethically permissible in one country may not be permissible in another. This approach has seriously undermined the existing framework of research ethics, but it also led to pharmaceutical power politics attempting to facilitate the conduct of clinical trials in poor and low-income countries. Western research sponsors subsequently tried to revise the Declaration of Helsinki to restrict the use of placebos. Revisions in 2000 and 2008 did not produce the desired relaxation. Later, in 2008, the US Food and Drug Administration announced that it would use new standards for human clinical trials, and that it would no longer recognize the Declaration of Helsinki. The journal *Nature* criticized this decision, calling it "a message that ethical considerations are expendable when research subjects live half a world away" (Editorial 2008, 428).

A similar controversy concerned the so-called Trovan case in Nigeria. In 1996 the city of Kano was devastated by a deadly meningitis epidemic. Humanitarian organizations provided assistance. Pfizer, one of the world's largest pharmaceutical companies, sent a team of researchers to conduct a trial with Trovan, a new drug that had never before been tested on children. After having successfully included two hundred children over two weeks, the researchers went back to the United States. In 2000 the *Washington Post* broke the story that described how Pfizer used the African children as guinea pigs. The children's families brought suit against the company in the United States. The major argument focused on informed consent. The parents pointed out that they were not aware that their children were included in an experiment or that alternative treatment was available. Pfizer argued that informed consent was impossible because the parents were illiterate. They also argued that the research had been approved by the hospital ethics committee (but in fact no committee was in existence at that time). Pfizer claimed that informed consent is not a universal norm that can be imposed on other cultures. The outcome of the lawsuit, however, reiterated the tradition of research ethics. The court found that the informed consent requirement is a universal norm that should be enforced in courts and practices all over the world (Annas 2009).

Globalization of research has reactivated the debate on the moral status of ethical principles (see chapter 9). Will respect for cultural diversity and the application of ethical principles in diverse research settings result in diverging standards and ethical relativism? The general view in bioethics is that the framework of ethical principles is universal (Emanuel, Wendler, and Grady 2008). The principles apply in all countries and contexts. But the principles require practical interpretation and specification. This can only be done within specific cultures and social contexts, but this does not make the principles less universal or entirely determined by the context (see chapter 30). A distinction should be made between substantive and procedural ethical requirements in research. The substantive requirements are based on the fundamental principles of bioethics: respect for persons, justice, and beneficence. They constitute ethical standards that should be applied universally. They imply requirements such as obtaining individual informed consent and disclosing information about expected risks. The procedural requirements, on the other hand, may vary according to cultural and other differences in multinational research. For example, some countries have requirements that informed consent forms must be signed. But in other cultures, asking for a signature can be a sign of mistrust. Also, when people are illiterate, special efforts have to be made to inform them properly and to make sure that they give permission to proceed. How the ethical principles are applied in different settings demands ingenuity and variable approaches, but this does not imply ethical variability of the principles themselves (Macklin 2004).

Clinical Research as Business

Another phenomenon that has influenced the recent practice of research is the growth of commercial interests. Before 1990 almost 90 percent of clinical research with human beings was conducted in universities. Now most clinical trials take place outside of academia (Petryna 2009). The process of clinical research is increasingly based on the business model of outsourcing. Currently 70 percent of pharmaceutical sponsoring goes to contract research organizations (CRO), companies that develop the research design, recruit subjects, monitor the implementation of the research protocol, and collect the data. This clinical trials industry now comprises more than one thousand CROs whose sales have more than doubled over the last ten years (Shuchman 2007). But there are also other types of companies focused on only one component of the clinical research process: site management organizations that supervise the execution of a trial in a private practice, patient recruitment agencies that specialize in developing countries, and sophisticated advertising agencies that specialize in publishing information about the research trial. An ethical review industry has emerged with for-profit research ethics committees. CROs and pharmaceutical companies have established their own ethics review committees, or they increasingly use committees not affiliated with universities, hospitals, or research centers (so the name institutional review board has become obsolete). These committees are commercial enterprises commissioned by the pharmaceutical industry. The number is unknown since there is no duty to register, but it is estimated to be between three thousand and five thousand (Petryna 2009).

These developments raise serious ethical concerns. How ethical are for-profit research ethics committees? It is clear that they embody a serious conflict of interest.

The system of independent ethics committees was created to prevent the interest of science from overruling the interest of the patient or subject. It seems that there now is another basic conflict due to the commercialization of research and ethics review: the conflict between the value of protecting the rights and health of research subjects and the value of financial benefits from scientific research. Patients' interests can be endangered by the profit motive. The US Governmental Accountability Office (GAO) demonstrated that this danger is real (2009). It carried out undercover tests with fake IRBs that were receiving assignments from the industry, and with fake research protocols that were rapidly approved by real IRBs. The GAO concluded that the current system of ethical review is susceptible to unethical manipulation. The system of ethical regulation of research that was developed in the 1970s and 1980s is now outdated. The CROs, for example, are operating below the radar, and the level of monitoring and auditing is minimal. Physicians who are contracted for the trials are not primarily hired as scientists to conduct clinical trials but first of all as practitioners to execute trials, preferably in their own practice. They use their patients, but their professional autonomy is restricted. The drive to develop new pharmaceutical products has furthermore exposed vulnerable populations. The majority of clinical trials in the United States are carried out today with uninsured and impoverished persons (Fisher 2009). This focus on money rather than science has produced new ethical problems.

Scientific Conduct

The last decade has witnessed a long series of embarrassing cases of scientific misconduct: fabrication and falsification of data, plagiarism, and fraud. In 2006 Vermont professor Eric Poehlman, a well-known expert on menopause, aging, and metabolism, was sentenced to jail for falsifying data in fifteen federal grant applications and seventeen publications in prestigious journals. Jon Sudbø, a Norwegian specialist in oral cancer, was exposed in 2006. His publications in *The Lancet*, among others, were based on completely fictional patients; the mistake that uncovered his duplicity was that he forgot to vary the birthdates of 250 patients. The same year saw another high-profile case: groundbreaking publications on human cloning turned out to be based on embryonic stem cell lines fabricated by South Korean scientist Woo Suk Hwang. A related phenomenon is so-called ghost management of publications. There are now medical publication companies that produce complete manuscripts and recruit the requested "authors," preferably famous academic experts on the topic who for a payment lend the publication scientific status. Data from lawsuits indicate that up to 40 percent of all publications on a specific drug can be managed by the producing company and written by publication agencies (Sismondo and Doucet 2010). It is therefore unclear what "authorship" of scientific publications means.

These examples of misconduct were initially regarded as exceptions; many argued that there are always some bad apples in the barrel. But it has become clear that only a low number of cases are reported. People who do detect fraud and misconduct and make it public (so-called whistle-blowers) are usually blamed so that reporting is risky. Falsification and fabrication of data in scientific research actually is rather common. One in fifty scientists has used falsified data; 34 percent of researchers have deleted contradictory data; and one in seven scientists know a colleague who has falsified and fabricated data (Fanelli 2009). This situation has caused governments and academies of science to take action. The Office of Research Integrity in the United States (created in 1992) investigates allegations of research misconduct. The government of Denmark established the Committee on Scientific Dishonesty, and the German research organization established a research ombudsman. These efforts intend to rearticulate the importance of ethical principles in the conduct of research. Scientific activity should be guided by honesty, integrity, reliability, and critical, impartial assessment. Obviously, the ethical framework of scientific inquiry is itself seriously compromised.

Conflict of Interest

One of the fundamental reasons for loss of scientific integrity is conflict of interest. Health professionals have a professional responsibility to give priority to the best interests of their patients. Medical researchers have a professional responsibility to obtain reliable knowledge to advance patient care. However, these professional responsibilities may be overridden by other interests, such as personal gain and profit that primarily promote the personal interests of the health professional and researcher. A recent example is orthopedic surgeons who receive bonuses from companies producing orthopedic devices. How can their patients trust that the treatment in is in their best interests? Another example is the case of the editor of the *Journal of Spinal Disorders & Techniques* who has received almost twenty million dollars in exchange for favorable publications on devices produced by the donating company. International outcry occurred when it became public that many of the scientific advisors of WHO during the 2009 pandemic of avian flu had financial ties with vaccine manufacturers. Conflict of interest is now a major subject of concern in ethics. If it is no longer certain that scientists produce reliable data or that the interests of the patient come first for health professionals, how can the public trust researchers and health professionals?

The first response to conflict of interest is transparency. Physicians and medical researchers have to disclose possible conflicts of interest. But this remedy of self-reporting is limited insofar as it is voluntary, without any sanctions for those who do not disclose competing interests. There is often no possibility of verification. And if verification is possible, it turns out that there is no disclosure in one of three to four cases. Self-reporting is unreliable, particularly if individuals are not convinced that there is anything wrong with conflicting interests. Another approach suggested is zero tolerance. Conflict of interest is not necessary; financial conflict is the result of choice and is thus avoidable. One can be an excellent scientist without being paid by pharmaceutical companies. However, others argue that competing interests cannot be eliminated. In the current climate, universities encourage scientists to be entrepreneurial. Most research funding in universities today is based on competitive grants. And experts may have multiple connections to enhance the impact and outreach of research, even if it increases the risk of conflicting interests (Macrina 2012).

Systematic promotion of a scientific culture of integrity is necessary. To achieve this, several things are needed. First, there needs to be more emphasis on training researchers in science and research ethics. As of January 2010 the National Institutes of

Health and the National Science Foundation in the United States have required that researchers funded by their grants must received ethics education focused on promoting research integrity. Education in ethics is seen as a remedy against deficiencies in professional behavior. Second, some limits need to be set against commercial interests. This is currently debated with regard to sponsoring medical education. More than 50 percent of postgraduate medical education in the United States is sponsored by the pharmaceutical industry. It is sometimes difficult to distinguish between education and commercial promotion. Medical schools must take their responsibility and must provide objective and critical education. Several centers and schools have now decided to stop external financing of educational activities. Grassroots organizations have emerged to stop industrial sponsoring.[1] Third, new guidelines will be necessary. Scientific societies are developing codes of ethics. The majority of universities and research institutes do not have policies regarding conflict of interest or "ghostwriting," and medical students want more transparency and policy. Scientific journals are enacting more stringent rules concerning data and authorship in publications.

Restoration of Trust between Science and Society

In medical research as well as in health care, the well-being of the patient or the individual person should be the primary consideration. The dignity of the human person must not be violated for the sake of science, society, or commerce. The relatively recent history of research ethics shows that there is a continuous risk that scientific considerations will override the need of protection of individual dignity and rights. This is an inherent risk because scientific research is the only way to contribute to medical progress. The health and life expectancy of present-day populations have increased tremendously due to scientific advances. However, the significant value of scientific research can be jeopardized if research is regarded as an end in itself, and if medical experiments are conducted in unethical ways that do not respect research participants. This was exactly the concern of Henry Beecher in 1966: the legitimacy of research would be undermined if it did not follow strict ethical principles. But contrary to what Beecher advocated, the history of research ethics has demonstrated that the integrity of the individual researcher as such does not provide sufficient guarantees. For society to maintain trust in scientific research, effective regulation is also necessary. Protection of research participants cannot rely only on conscientious researchers but should be guaranteed by enforceable regulations.

Furthermore, concerns have emerged concerning the social value of medical research. Now that research is a global enterprise, protection of research participants is no longer enough to justify research activities. If the rationale for research is that it contributes to medical progress, conducting clinical trials in poor and low-income countries should contribute to ameliorating and improving health care in these countries. Otherwise populations will feel that they are guinea pigs for Western companies. The ethical principle of justice, one of the basic principles of the Belmont Report, requires that research must be focused on the needs of the countries in which it is performed. Since 1996 the World Health Organization has exposed the fact that 90 percent of the economic resources spent annually on research target the health needs of the richest 10 percent of the world's population. This gap is not diminishing even though more and more clinical trials are now conducted in developing countries. It is clear that the debate on research ethics from a global perspective is only beginning.

Note

1. See the website of No Free Lunch, a group of "health care providers who believe that pharmaceutical promotion should not guide clinical practice"; www.nofreelunch.org.

CHAPTER 24

ORGANIZATIONAL ETHICS

Introduction

THE AREA GENERALLY KNOWN AS "organizational ethics" is related to but distinct from the clinical issues that have thus far concerned us. The recent increased interest in organizational ethics has been due in some measure to the apparent chaos in health care (Lee and Mongan 2009) and to the many scandals that have compromised public trust in health care organizations over the past few decades (Shore 2007), including widespread malpractice and fraud in Medicare and the difficult problem of conflict of interest (Fernandez-Lynch 2008). Health care must be held more accountable (Morreim 2001) as its organizations pursue a continuing quest for excellence (Pearson, Sabin, and Emanuel 2003), and market forces must be more responsive to moral inquiry (McDonough 2007).

It is not surprising that many practical topics are considered under the rubric of "organizational ethics." These involve all levels of health care institutions, from the general oversight of the boards of trustees (Jennings et al. 2004) to the daily organizational interactions of the various professionals who work in them (Purtilo 2005). Many of these specific topics can be explored by referring to the literature cited in this chapter (e.g., Boyle et al. 2001; Field 2007; Hall 2000; Spencer et al. 2000), but we do not attempt here to discuss them in detail. We instead adopt a more general approach. The purpose of our analysis is to explain the moral concept of stewardship as providing a foundation for organizational ethics. We apply this concept to two major debates of recurring interest in organizational ethics: first, patient safety and medical error within health care in general; and second, the dispute within Catholic health care concerning the provision of services such as abortion, contraception, and sterilization as well as including such procedures in insurance offered to employees. We pursue these topics in four sections: stewardship as the foundation for organizational ethics, patient safety and medical error, cooperation with proscribed services in Catholic health care, and the development of Church teaching on cooperation with proscribed services.

Before discussing these topics, it is helpful to mention a question that often arises in organizational ethics related to moral agency. In clinical ethics, it is usually clear which person or group of persons is responsible for a specific action. When a doctor makes a clinical mistake that injures a patient, for example, it is usually easy to determine who is responsible, even though there is significant debate about how best to address that responsibility to prevent its recurrence (we return to this question later in this chapter). However, it is not always clear in organizational ethics where the moral responsibility lies. Is it with individuals or with institutional policies and procedures?

The following points can help to clarify the meaning of moral agency in an organization. An individual's conduct can represent an organization when enacting its policies. When this occurs, such as when purchasers in the business office avoid disreputable but cheaper vendors of products, those individuals engage in moral conduct: they are individually responsible not only for their own behavior but also for the reputation of the organization. Here the issue of moral agency is quite clear: the reputation of an organization can be developed based on the responsible moral agency of its individual employees. In contrast, an organization can also develop a positive reputation by fostering the trust of the surrounding community. An example might be when a health care organization is responsive to its nonprofit status by having a robust and transparent community benefit program (e.g., Magill and Prybil 2011). However, here the issue of moral agency is less clear. The organization can be construed as being involved in moral agency only by analogy. That is, while individuals engage in moral agency for which they are responsible, it is only by analogy that an organization has moral agency. That occurs insofar as an organization's policies and procedures foster a sense of integrity across the community it serves. Hence, it is legitimate to ascribe to health care organizations a level of moral responsibility, albeit analogously. The next section further explores this matter of analogous moral agency by suggesting that the foundation for organizational ethics can be found in the moral concept of stewardship.

Stewardship as the Foundation for Organizational Ethics in Health Care

The American Society for Bioethics and Humanities explained the concept of organizational ethics in health care in its 1998 edition of *Core Competencies for Health Care Ethics Consultation* (1998). The society referred to an organization's positions and behavior regarding individuals (such as employees and patients), regarding groups (such as the medical staff), regarding other organizations (such as the American Hospital Association), and regarding the communities served. In the original 1998 edition, a section of the manual was dedicated to organizational ethics. However, in the revised 2010 edition of the manual, this section was removed; the Society explained that it had decided against distinguishing organizational ethics from clinical ethics, based upon the wide divergence of opinion regarding the meaning of these terms and the recognition of their increased integration in health care (American Society for Bioethics and Humanities 2010). But this does not mean that organizational ethics cannot be distinguished from clinical ethics. The change in the manual is meant to be seen in the specific context of ethics consultation, and the meaning of the decision seems to have been to integrate the less widespread practice of consultations in organizational ethics with the far more extensive practice of consultations in clinical ethics.

The discussion of organizational ethics here extends beyond this specialty of ethics consultation. The broader approach to organizational ethics in this chapter includes issues related to business ethics, corporate ethics, and regulatory compliance, although these can all be defined in a variety of ways. The discussion considers issues in organizational ethics that pertain to all health care arenas; however, the analysis is especially attuned to the realm of Catholic health care.

In the Catholic tradition there is a rich understanding of the meaning of stewardship that can be adopted as a foundation for organizational ethics, pertaining as much to secular health care as it does to religious health care. We have discussed the theological bases for stewardship in part 1, especially chapters 2 and 3. A biblical understanding of stewardship is presented in Catholic theology in terms of God's creation: we are called to respect God's gift, to enable it to flourish, and to conduct ourselves in a manner that is consistent with it. The relationship between these concepts, as indicating the moral meaning of stewardship, can be interpreted in organizational terminology as the relationship between mission, vision, and practice (Magill and Prybil 2004). Hence, stewardship calls upon an organization to respect its mission (we respect what we have received in the gift of creation), to pursue a bold vision (we enable creation to flourish), and to enact practices consistent with that mission and vision (we conduct ourselves in a manner that is consistent with the gift of creation). This understanding of stewardship within an organization adopts a view of moral agency by analogy—an organization is responsible for its mission, vision, and practices in a manner that is analogous to individual moral responsibility.

Of course, stewardship can be understood much more narrowly as referring to prudent allocation of limited resources—that approach is mentioned in the *Ethical and Religious Directives*, such as in directives 4 and 6 (USCCB 2009a). While this narrower view has validity and is widely adopted, the deeper meaning of stewardship suggested here provides a foundation for organizational ethics that is pertinent for both secular and religious discourse. The moral concept of stewardship enables organizational ethics to focus upon the mission, vision, and practices of health care in an integrative manner. When specific actions are being reviewed, they need to be understood within the context of the mission and vision of a particular organization or health care enterprise. Within that context, more particular issues in organizational ethics can be pursued, such as resource allocation.

This understanding of the moral concept of stewardship as the foundation for organizational ethics is developed in the next three sections in the following manner. The widespread problem of medical error calls out for a renewed focus upon the mission of health care to provide patient care in a safe manner. To effectively address this problem a bold vision is needed—a comprehensive program for patient safety—and organizational policies and procedures must reflect this mission and vision to inspire appropriate practices in conduct and behavior. Here, the moral concept of stewardship highlights this integration of mission, vision, and practices.

The subsequent sections discuss organizational cooperation with forbidden procedures in the context of government regulations as well as doctrinal development of the moral principle of cooperation in Catholic teaching. This debate on moral complicity and cooperation has significant secular implications (Kutz 2000) as well as far-reaching religious repercussions (Watt 2005). In each section the concept of stewardship helps to focus upon the relevant mission, vision, and practices of Catholic health care to distinguish between licit and illicit organizational cooperation. The mission of Catholic health care clarifies its values that involve the prohibition of specific services; its vision seeks to provide health care in a secular and pluralistic context, at times requiring material cooperation with procedures it considers wrong while avoiding moral complicity; and the practices of Catholic health care have to be meticulously planned and managed to respect this mission and vision in a practical and consistent manner.

In sum, the moral concept of stewardship provides a robust foundation for discourse in organizational ethics that enlightens complex dilemmas in both the secular and the religious realms of US health care.

Patient Safety and Medical Error

Increasing concerns with patient safety and preventable medical error have escalated over the past decades and are volatile issues related to organizational ethics in health care. Medical errors and injuries constitute a serious problem in organizational ethics in this sense. While medical errors typically occur as mistakes, the injuries they cause need to elicit a response that not only informs the patient but also prevents recurrences. When that response is lacking, there is a fundamental moral compromise of professional and organizational integrity whose basic mission is to support patient care. This compromise involves health care professionals who cause the error yet cover up the mistake when possible or explain the injury away in one way or another. It also involves the health care organization that either discovers the error and does nothing, or does not create mechanisms to accurately trace errors in daily practice, especially in light of the national trends on these matters.

At the turn of the millennium, the Institute of Medicine (IOM) published a harrowing report, *To Err Is Human: Building a Safer Health System*, on the astounding number of deaths and serious injuries caused by medical error in US health care (IOM 2000a). This report was applauded as a much-needed breakthrough that generated a series of related studies to improve patient safety, including studies by the National Coalition on Health Care (National Coalition on Health Care 2000), by the American Hospital Association (Spath 2000), and by the National Patient Safety Foundation (National Patient Safety Foundation 2001). Until the IOM report, the routine way of dealing with theses errors was on an individual basis through malpractice lawsuits. But the enormous penalties in those lawsuits had little impact on preventing or reducing the escalating trend in medical error. With hindsight, we can now see that the reason for that failure was rather straightforward: although medical errors typically result from the individual actions of a clinician upon a patient, the underlying causes tend to be systemic problems that have little or nothing to do with medical malpractice. The insight that we have gained over the past decade is to realize that avoiding medical error occurs by creating systems and processes that enhance patient safety. The outcome in this arena of organizational ethics in health care has been to develop preventive systems rather than to pursue contentious lawsuits.

To understand the significance of this topic it is helpful to grasp its scale. The IOM report suggested that there could be as many as ninety-eight thousand deaths per year in the United States caused by medical error. These results were extrapolated from other studies stretching back to the mid-1980s. This shocking number of annual deaths is the equivalent of a 747 jet crashing every day in the country. If there were that many aircraft crashes each day, year after year, one wonders how frequently anyone would fly. Given these statistics, it seems confounding that a grassroots backlash against medical error has not occurred. Again, there seems to be a simple rationale: patients have little understanding of the statistics underlying medical error because patient deaths occur one at a time, not in large numbers as occurs in an airplane crash. Moreover, there is no central database or mandatory reporting system to track the medical errors and near misses that occur every day across the nation. Because there is no centralized documentation of these errors, it is difficult to extrapolate reliable data from small-scale studies. However, just a few years after the IOM report, another prestigious study was published that suggested the original statistics underestimated the scale of the problem: in reality, the number of US deaths caused by medical error annually may be twice as high as estimated by the IOM report (Health Grades Quality Study 2004).

Fortunately, progress is being made because of the continuing focus of the IOM on this problem. A year after its original report, the IOM published another study, *Crossing the Quality Chasm*, to relate medical error to the problem of quality in patient care (IOM 2001). This report emphasized the need to develop more reliable systems and processes that enhance patient safety in order to reduce medical error. That insight led to an investigation of government roles in the improvement of health care, which in turn generated yet another report, *Leadership by Example* (IOM 2002). This report encouraged government-funded health programs (Medicare and Medicaid) to promote patient safety by focusing upon better quality standards across the continuum of health care delivery.

Significant progress also has been due to the efforts of the Joint Commission on Accreditation of Healthcare Organizations. Most hospitals in the United States receive accreditation (on a voluntary basis) through this organization. Two aspects of this accreditation process have been especially effective: its requirements for "national patient safety goals" and its standards for reporting "sentinel events" as unexpected occurrences involving death or serious injury, such as the loss of a limb or significant function (Joint Commission 2011). The word "sentinel" is used to indicate the need for immediate investigation and response. However, it is important to note that sentinel events are not the same as medical errors: not all sentinel events result from a medical error, and not all medical errors lead to sentinel events (Joint Commission 2008). In the wake of the IOM's original report, the Joint Commission has developed several widely used resources to address the root causes of medical error (e.g., Joint Commission 2004; 2010) in order to foster patient safety.

The major accomplishment in the problem of medical error has been the shift from a so-called professional sanctions approach to a patient safety model (Magill 2006). Instead of assigning blame to individuals when medical errors occur (the professional sanctions approach) such as via malpractice lawsuits against clinicians, the emphasis increasingly focuses upon systems and processes to enhance patient safety. A closer look at these contrasting approaches helps to enlighten the debate in organizational ethics about medical error. On the one hand, the professional sanctions model punishes individuals for carelessness or incompetence leading to the error in order to prevent future occurrences. Of course, there will always be the need for malpractice lawsuits when negligence clearly occurs. But the professional sanctions model tends to generate a climate of fear and shame that causes professionals to hide mistakes or gloss over the widespread problem of preventable injury. This approach focuses upon *who* caused the error.

In contrast, the patient safety model focuses upon *what* has occurred and tries to trace the error back to inadequate systems or unreliable processes that underlie preventable medical errors. The focus here is to foster quality improvement of these systems and processes to enhance patient care by emphasizing the prevention of medical error. Several examples from other industries have been able to shed light on the systemic approach that is advocated. In road safety, when a particular site is prone to accidents, barriers are constructed in an effort to avoid future trouble. In the aviation industry, extraordinarily high standards of safety have been developed based upon this systems-oriented approach. The process of confidential incident reporting enables pilots to reports errors or near misses in a manner that avoids recrimination or punishment. These reports enable the aviation industry to design and implement preventive measures quickly and efficiently. This combination of confidential reporting and preventive intervention has led to a major increase in pilot cooperation and to one of the safest travel records in the world. We need a similar approach to develop an environment of patient safety in US health care, such as by establishing a centralized reporting system and database at the National Institutes of Health.

The widespread problem of medical error presents a profound cultural challenge in US health care. We need to shift the focus from the reactive and punitive measures in the outdated professional sanctions approach to a more effective emphasis upon proactive and preventive measures in the patient safety model. There are several related ways whereby discourse on organizational ethics can support the patient safety model.

First, greater attention needs to be given to pursuing the root causes of medical errors that occur (Joint Commission 2010). The point here is to examine the systems and processes connected with medical errors, sentinel events, or adverse events (Joint Commission 2008), rather than to fixate upon the personal performance of the individual clinicians involved—hence the widespread colloquialism about seeking to fix systems and not to fix blame on individuals. In other words, the goal is to avoid assigning blame (moral or legal) and to clarify underlying causes so that they can be changed to avoid future errors (Runciman, Merry, and Walton 2007). Illustrations of these systems and processes occur daily in hospital care, such as when different nurses check a patient's identification in a variety of ways before the patient undergoes surgery, or when surgeons mark a patient's limb in creative ways to avoid wrong-site amputation. To facilitate the patient safety approach, it behooves a health care organization to appoint a team or group, empowered with appropriate resources, to be responsible for the oversight of medical errors and sentinel events in order to develop preventive processes to avoid future occurrences. Standard quality improvement processes for root cause analysis can be adopted, including how to gather and record information in an appropriate manner that accommodates requirements of patient confidentiality, legal discovery, and peer review; developing risk reduction strategies and action plans for improvement; and designing assessment measures and communicating results across the organization in a proactive manner.

Second, greater attention needs to be given to developing a culture of safety in health care organizations based on nationally established recommendations (Vincent

2010; Wachter 2008). Nurturing this culture involves a moral commitment from various constituencies within an organization to collaborate. There are several guiding principles that foster this culture: providing leadership from the top within the organization to foster effective team empowerment and functioning, such as by preparing and compiling written plans and policies; understanding and adhering to the limits of design processes that shape jobs for safety, such as being attentive to work hours and fatigue, staff ratios, and so on; and designing a sophisticated learning environment that encourages training for safety, confidential reporting of errors, and open communication across all levels of the organization.

Third, greater attention needs to be given to the controversial matter referred to as no-fault compensation, in contrast to tort-based malpractice (Wachter 2008). This endeavor requires the involvement of the organization's executive leadership and the board of trustees as well as the organization's senior counsel or risk management personnel, or both, to address a variety of controversial components. To develop a viable no-fault compensation program requires attention to different layers of moral discourse that include these related components: the need to respect patient autonomy that provides the foundation for clinical ethics; the demands of professional ethics that honor the standards and codes of the professions involved; the requirements of virtue ethics that shape and reflect the character of the participating clinicians; and the expectations of business and corporate ethics that uphold the mission and reputation of the relevant facilities or institutions. In this context, it might seem straightforward to expect, from the perspective of organizational ethics, that health care providers would undertake the following steps after a medical error has occurred: to explain to the patient (or the patient's representatives) the relevant details of the medical error and to apologize for it; to identify what measures have been enacted to prevent recurrence with other patients; and to compensate the patient victim for the pain and suffering involved. But these are not straightforward issues. Talking with patients and families about medical error and injury is not an easy undertaking (Truog et al. 2011).

Efforts to design no-fault compensation programs seek to address these steps, but many concerns continue to create roadblocks for progress on this significant moral matter. These concerns, and possible responses to them, include the following. On the one hand, there is concern that the process of providing an apology and disclosure that admits the medical error can be construed as exposing the offending individual and the organization to legal jeopardy, thereby increasing malpractice lawsuit penalties. In response, there appears to be scant evidence of this outcome. Patients often are quite satisfied when they receive an apology with a reasonable compensation settlement for the medical error and injury, especially when there is an accompanying explanation that the root cause has been identified and remedied to prevent recurrence with others. For patients who opt not to accept the compensation and seek external legal remedies, courts appear to be sympathetic to organizations that deal with the matter in an honest, transparent, and proactive manner (Truog et al. 2011). On the other hand, there is an additional concern that adopting a no-fault compensation program can be construed as undermining incentives to address the systemic issues that underlie and often cause medical errors. In response, the opposite appears to be the case. When an organization adopts a no-fault compensation program, the typical result is a close alignment of quality improvement that connects compensation for injury with patient safety objectives, including increased error reporting. This alignment fosters the culture of patient safety, which is widely recognized as the best way to proactively prevent medical errors (Joint Commission 2008, 189) and which typifies high performing health care systems (Vincent 2010).

The related issues of medical error, sentinel events, and adverse events, combined with the proactive and preventive efforts to alleviate these issues by focusing upon patient safety programs, constitute ongoing concerns for organizational ethics in health care. To the extent that a health care organization or institution knows of medical errors and covers them over, or does nothing to prevent them by developing patient safety programs, there can be moral complicity in the wrongful occurrences that injure patients. There is a technical term for this type of organizational complicity, "formal cooperation," which we will discuss in greater detail in the next section.

Institutional Cooperation with Forbidden Procedures: Health Care and Government

Insofar as Catholic health care in the United States functions within a pluralistic and democratic society, dilemmas frequently arise that pit Catholic mission against health services provided in the public forum, especially when mandated by government. Abortion is legal in all states, assisted suicide in some, and for most of the nation the practice of sterilization and contraception is widespread. Yet abortion, assisted suicide, sterilization, and artificial contraception are forbidden by official Catholic teaching. The dilemma that arises is whether Catholic organizations can work with other institutions, or the government, when these proscribed services are involved. Some religious denominations uphold their teaching so strictly that they will not compromise their principles by any form of cooperation; for example, the Mennonites refuse to enlist in military service. In contrast, the Catholic tradition seeks to live its principles in the murky morass of daily life. Hence, the famous ethical theory of just war was developed within the Catholic tradition to justify killing in some circumstances while upholding its ethical principle against violence.

In health care, perhaps the most common guide for dilemmas connecting Catholic values with secular practice is the principle of cooperation. The principle of legitimate cooperation is likely the most commonly used principle in the daily lives of individuals and organizations (Watt 2005). The distinction between formal and material cooperation is discussed in chapter 12. Formal cooperation involves the cooperator intending the perceived wrongdoing of another: this is always wrong. Immediate material cooperation was explained as being so inseparable from the forbidden procedure as to be implicitly tantamount to being formal cooperation: typically this also is wrong and the US bishops forbid it in the 2001 and 2009 editions of the *Ethical and Religious Directives*. However, the subsequent discussion explains how there appears to be a change in the bishops' teaching on the legitimacy of immediate material cooperation, apparently permitting it in the 1995 edition of the directives but forbidding it in subsequent editions.

For centuries the Catholic tradition has routinely permitted mediate material cooperation, which means that the cooperator undertakes an action (construed as being either morally good or neutral) that is connected with the perceived wrongdoing of another person or organization. To justify this connection, the cooperator must not intend the perceived wrongdoing, and there must be sufficient distance from the evil being perpetrated: that distance determines whether the act of cooperation constitutes remote or proximate material cooperation. These forms of material cooperation can help to clarify a significant dilemma that Catholic health care encounters in our secular society: being involved with health insurance plans that mandate proscribed services such as contraception.

To illustrate how the principle of cooperation can illumine this sort of dilemma, it is helpful first to consider another widespread practice that regularly causes Catholic conscience to conflict with secular practice: voting for candidates who support forbidden procedures such as abortion. If Catholics can vote for regulations or legislators that support abortion, then perhaps they also can cooperate with situations that involve contraception coverage.

Catholic Voting That Permits Forbidden Procedures, such as Abortion

One of the clearest official Catholic teachings is the prohibition of direct abortion as an intrinsic evil of the most serious type. Yet, surprisingly, Catholic teaching permits Catholic legislators to vote for laws that permit abortion. This astounding "arrangement" on voting helps to clarify how important the principle of cooperation can be for upholding Catholic values in a secular, pluralistic society (Magill 2012).

This principle helps to implement the mission of the Church. In a pastoral letter, *Forming Consciences for Faithful Citizenship*, the US bishops explained the mission of the Church as shaping society, transforming the world, and promoting the common good (USCCB 2009b, nos. 9 and 14). This reflects the teaching of Vatican II that the saving and eschatological purpose of the Church is to be a leaven for God's renewal of society (Paul VI 1965, no. 40). However, this noble quest involves both hope and realism, as noted by the US Bishops' pastoral letter on the economy, *Economic Justice for All* (USCCB 1986, no. 55), requiring prudential judgments in different historical and cultural contexts (ibid., nos. 20, 56). The principle of cooperation has been adopted by the Catholic tradition to guide these prudential judgments that implement the mission of the Church in secular society.

The US bishops emphasize this need for prudence in voting and legislating. To understand how far prudence can reach using the principle of cooperation, two related Church teachings can shed light on the complex circumstances of voting for legislation that permits the continuance of abortion services. In the pastoral letter on forming consciences, the US bishops explain:

> Decisions about political life are complex and require the exercise of a well-formed conscience aided by prudence. . . . Sometimes morally flawed laws already exist. In this situation, the process of framing legislation to protect life is subject to prudential judgment and "the art of the possible." At times this process may restore justice only partially or gradually. Pope John Paul II taught that when a government official who fully opposes abortion cannot succeed in completely overturning a pro-abortion law, he or she may work to improve protection for unborn human life, "limiting the harm done by such a law" and lessening its negative impact as much as possible. Such incremental

improvements in the law are acceptable as steps toward the full restoration of justice. (USCCB 2009b, no. 31)

The second quotation that clarifies the reach of prudence using the principle of cooperation is the passage that the US bishops allude to in the encyclical of Pope John Paul II, *Evangelium vitae (The Gospel of Life)*:

> A particular problem of conscience can arise in cases where a legislative vote would be decisive for the passage of a more restrictive law, aimed at limiting the number of authorized abortions, in place of a more permissive law already passed or ready to be voted on. Such cases are not infrequent. . . . In a case like the one just mentioned, when it is not possible to overturn or completely abrogate a pro-abortion law, an elected official, whose absolute personal opposition to procured abortion was well known, could licitly support proposals aimed at *limiting the harm* done by such a law and at lessening its negative consequences at the level of general opinion and public morality. This does not in fact represent an illicit cooperation with an unjust law, but rather a legitimate and proper attempt to limit its evil aspects. (Emphasis added; John Paul II 1995, no. 73)

Here, Pope John Paul II explicitly uses the principle of material cooperation to justify a Catholic legislator voting for a law that permits abortion, conditional upon the legislator being pro-life and limiting the harm of previous legislation on the matter.

Likewise, Catholic citizens may vote for legislators who support forbidden procedures such as abortion, conditional upon the voter supporting the other good that the legislator can accomplish while opposing the legislator's defense of abortion. As Prefect of the Congregation of the Doctrine of the Faith, Joseph Cardinal Ratzinger (now Pope Benedict XVI) specifically stated that a vote of this kind would be a licit material cooperation. He did so in an official instruction to Theodore Cardinal McCarrick to assist him as leader of the Conference of Bishops on domestic policy. On the one hand, Cardinal Ratzinger explained: "A Catholic would be guilty of formal cooperation in evil . . . if he were to deliberately vote for a candidate precisely because of the candidate's permissive stand on abortion and/or euthanasia." On the other hand, he clarified: "When a Catholic does not share a candidate's stand in favor of abortion and/or euthanasia, but votes for that candidate for other reasons, it is considered remote material cooperation, which can be permitted in the presence of proportionate reasons" (Ratzinger 2004, final note).

This use of the principle of material cooperation to justify voting by Catholics (either as legislators or as citizens) in a manner that permits abortion services can be applied to other dilemmas in Catholic health care. In 2011 a highly controversial example of the standoff between Catholic values and secular practices occurred over the mandating of contraceptive services in health insurance programs. The principle of material cooperation can be used to illuminate and defuse the controversy.

Health Insurance Supporting Proscribed Services

In 2010 a far-reaching health care reform act was signed into law by President Barack Obama, achieving a goal of extending health insurance to most of the US population, many of whom lacked health insurance. This reform had been beyond the reach of all too many preceding US presidents. The Patient Protection and Affordable Care Act (HR 3590) was a federal statute signed into law on March 23, 2010, by President Obama along with the Health Care and Education Reconciliation Act of 2010 (Pub. L. 111–152), signed on March 30, 2010. Together these constituted the health care reform accomplishment of the Democratic 111th Congress. This achievement of extending health care insurance and access to more than thirty million citizens who previously had none appeared to be consistent with Catholic social teaching on justice, which had for generations insisted on the right of each person to "adequate health care" (USCCB 2009a, part 1, introduction; USCCB 1981). Yet the Catholic bishops opposed the legislation, fearing that it would increase federal funding for abortion and not provide sufficient conscience clause protection. The supporters of the legislation insisted that no additional federal funding for abortion would occur. To confirm that stance, the president signed an executive order, "Ensuring Enforcement and Implementation of Abortion Restrictions in the Patient Protection and Affordable Care Act" (White House 2010). Although the US bishops did not support the legislation, the Catholic Health Association offered its support.

Closer scrutiny of this legislative process can clarify the important contribution of the principle of cooperation in this pivotal issue in US health care. It may appear that the US bishops opposed the legislation because it permitted abortion. In reality, the bishops accepted the fact that abortion was included in the legislation; that was not the rationale for their opposition. The bishops were willing (as permitted by the principle of cooperation to justify legislative endeavors) to preserve the status quo on US abortion legislation; on the one hand, they recognized the difficulty in overturning the 1973 Supreme Court ruling on *Roe v. Wade*; on the other hand, they were willing to continue the 1976 Hyde Amendment even though it supported some federal funding for abortion via the annual appropriation bill in the US Congress. As the legislation was being prepared, representatives Bart Stupak, a Democrat from Michigan, and Joseph R. Pitts, a Republican from Pennsylvania, proposed an amendment to the act (Stupak and Pitts 2009) that elicited the support of the US bishops. Specifically, their amendment prohibited using federal funds for abortion except in cases delineated in the 1976 Hyde amendment (which provided an exception for rape, incest, or danger to the mother's life). The Stupak-Pitts amendment did not succeed, although the Hyde amendment continued to be operative. However, Representative Stupack eventually supported the legislation, satisfied by the executive order that abortion funding would not be increased by the legislation. Nevertheless, the bishops remained firm in their opposition. In addition to their fear about insufficient conscience protection, they remained convinced that federal funding for abortion could be increased. Assuming that their assessment of future developments over abortion was accurate, presumably it was because the principle of cooperation could only permit them to live with or to limit the status quo dealing with abortion in the legislation; the principle could not justify extending abortion. Of course, the crucial issue here was whether their assessment of future developments about abortion funding, despite the president's executive order to the contrary, was accurate.

Nonetheless, disagreeing with the bishops, the Catholic Health Association as well as many Catholic legislators offered support for the legislation. On what basis, then, could they provide support when the bishops could not? Again, the explanation is found in the principle of cooperation. Presumably, like the Catholic representative Bart Stupak, they construed the president's executive order as a sufficient assurance against extending federal funding of abortion. In that case, continuing the status quo on abortion while extending health insurance and access to more than thirty million citizens justified their support for the legislation using the principle of material cooperation, just as had been articulated in the encyclical of Pope John Paul II. It is interesting that the US bishops, despite their opposition to the legislation, did not make a public statement against the Catholic legislators who supported the legislation, presumably recognizing their right to do so based on Catholic moral theory about the principle of cooperation. Nonetheless, the battle was far from over. With the passage of the legislation, another controversy quickly ensued that also involved the principle of cooperation: mandating health insurance to provide artificial contraception.

In January 2012 the US Department of Health and Human Services (HHS) indicated that the implementation of the 2010 Patient Protection and Affordable Care Act would follow the guidelines recommended by the independent IOM (issued in July 2011), based on scientific evidence and empirical analysis, to provide contraceptive services without charging a copay, coinsurance, or deductible. Several months previously, in August 2011, HHS adopted additional guidelines (issued in an interim final rule) for women's preventive services including contraception to be covered free of charge in new health plans from August 2012 onward. At that time, it appeared that a sufficient conscience protection for religious bodies would be provided. The announcement in the final rule on preventive health services in January 2012 made it clear that only a narrowly construed exemption would be provided to religiously affiliated institutes, fulfilling these four criteria: first, the organization must have religious values as its purpose; second, the organization must primarily employ persons who share its religious tenets; third, the organization must primarily serve persons who share its religious tenets; fourth, the organization must be a nonprofit entity under the Internal Revenue code. However, the narrowly constructed exemption did not cover most Catholic organizations, including Catholic health care, education, and social services. The final rule provided an additional year, until August 2013, for religious organizations to comply with the new law, meaning that Catholic organizations would have to provide the contraception coverage in their health plans.

The ruling elicited massive reaction among Catholics, including strenuous opposition by the US bishops and the Catholic Health Association, based on arguments that the law compromised the constitutional principle of religious liberty and conscience rights. Within a matter of weeks, the White House pivoted over the controversy and announced a compromise or accommodation. In the revised plan, religiously affiliated employers could decline contraceptive coverage, but insurance companies had to provide that coverage free of charge to the employees of those religious organizations. The compromise sought to avoid mandating that religious institutions acting against their organizational convictions must provide or subsidize contraceptive coverage or refer employees for those services elsewhere. The Catholic Health Association welcomed and supported the compromise, but the US bishops continued their opposition, explaining that they wanted HHS to rescind the mandate altogether.

What explains this dissonance between the Catholic bishops and the Catholic Health Association on this compromised mandate? The principle of material cooperation can clarify the matter. On the one hand, the bishops opposed the government mandate upon society of an act that is deemed to be an intrinsic evil (see chapter 11 on the controversy over the morality of contraception). However, this opposition alone does not prevent the bishops from reaching a working agreement with government policy. If the bishops can do so regarding abortion (such as by acceding to the status quo of the Hyde amendment, which annually provides some—albeit restricted—federal funding for abortion services), they may be able to do so regarding contraception coverage. It should be emphasized that opposition to a perceived wrongdoing is a crucial component in the use of the principle of material cooperation: otherwise the cooperator may be perceived to intend the wrongdoing. Hence, just because the bishops oppose contraception does not mean that they cannot agree to arrangements involving material cooperation with contraceptive coverage. On the other hand, the support of the Catholic Health Association for the president's compromise suggests that it recognizes how the principle of material cooperation can justify Catholic organizations dealing with the legislation in the manner suggested by the president's compromise.

A brief explanation of how the principle of material cooperation can function in this situation might suggest a way forward. Two situations seem to be pertinent. There are Catholic organizations that provide their employees a health plan through an insurance company, and there are Catholic organizations that are self-insured, although they may use external companies to service their health plan and insurance claims. In both cases, there are several conditions that seem to be met to justify using the principle of material cooperation. First, there is external duress: the government in our secular society is mandating that contraceptive coverage must be available free of charge; without duress that forces cooperation with perceived wrongdoing, there is no rationale for enacting the principle. Second, there is clearly no intention of doing what is wrong: Catholic organizations are being forced to cooperate with coverage that conflicts with official Catholic teaching. Third, there is proportionality insofar as great good is accomplished by Catholic organizations providing health plans, despite having to cooperate with the government mandate with which they disagree. Finally, there appears to be little or no widespread scandal: if the bishops can reach a working agreement with government policy on the much more serious evil of abortion, it seems that they can do so for contraceptive coverage. However, there is one important difference in applying the principle of cooperation for these two distinct sets of Catholic organizations. For Catholic organizations that provide their employees a health plan through an insurance company, it seems that their material cooperation is remote: the circumstance justifies applying remote, mediate material cooperation. For Catholic organizations that are self-insured, it may be that their material cooperation is proximate insofar as contraceptive coverage is provided not through another insurance company but through the insurance component of the Catholic organization itself: the circumstance justifies applying proximate, mediate material cooperation. However, in a further accommodation, the White House exempted religious organizations that were self-insured. Hence, the argument of proximate cooperation may not pertain. In either case, the grand principle of mediate material cooperation sheds light on possible pathways to resolve the standoff over such a crucial matter of health care access across the nation. As this book goes to press, the controversy continues.[1]

The principle of material cooperation is not only helpful for arrangements involving government-related matters such as voting or mandated health services such as contraception coverage. The principle is also very helpful for understanding how Church teaching develops on justifying cooperation with proscribed services such as direct sterilization. The topic of doctrinal development in this aspect of organizational ethics is discussed in the next section.

Institutional Cooperation with Forbidden Procedures: Developing Church Teaching

We have now seen the importance of the principle of cooperation. But in recent years that principle has itself undergone changes that are often not recognized and that cause some difficulties and inconsistencies in medical ethics. The discussion in this section considers the development of Church teaching on the principle of cooperation in the 1995, 2001, and 2009 editions of the *Ethical and Religious Directives for Catholic Health Care Services*. To trace the development of doctrine on the principle of cooperation (adopting the distinctions discussed in chapter 12 and in the previous section) there are two directives that are especially important in the 2001 and 2009 editions of the directives. First, immediate material cooperation is prohibited with regard to intrinsically evil actions: "Catholic health care organizations are not permitted to engage in immediate material cooperation in actions that are intrinsically immoral, such as abortion, euthanasia, assisted suicide, and direct sterilization" (USCCB 2001; 2009a, no. 70). Second, mediate material cooperation may be permitted: "If a Catholic health care organization is considering entering into an arrangement with another organization that may be involved in activities judged morally wrong by the Church, participation in such activities must be limited to what is in accord with the moral principles governing cooperation" (USCCB 2001; 2009a, no. 69).

These directives help to identify significant changes from previous teaching. First, a change with regard to immediate material cooperation can be identified by comparing the 2001 and 2009 editions with the 1995 edition that included an appendix on the principles governing cooperation. Second, another change can be traced in the directives by examining official communication between the Vatican and the US bishops in the 1970s on using mediate material cooperation to justify sterilizations in Catholic hospitals.

The first point for discussion is the appendix on cooperation that appeared only in the 1995 edition of the directives and was removed from the 2001 and 2009 editions. The bishops provide a general rationale for its removal. However, there appears to be a much more specific reason that the bishops do not mention: the 1995 appendix permitted immediate material cooperation in some circumstances, whereas the 2001 and 2009 editions of the directives forbid immediate material cooperation with actions deemed to be intrinsically immoral. The 1995 appendix makes this statement: "Immediate material cooperation is wrong, except in some instances of duress. The matter of duress distinguishes immediate material cooperation from implicit formal cooperation" (USCCB 1995, appx, para. 2). We do not know what sort of duress was considered here. However, in 1995 the bishops were certainly aware of one form of duress—the threat of closing a Catholic hospital—as possibly justifying cooperation with direct sterilization. That was mentioned in a document from the US bishops in 1977, which is discussed further under the next point. In contrast, in the 2001 and 2009 editions of the directives the Bishops unambiguously removed this justification of immediate material cooperation: "Catholic health care organizations are not permitted to engage in immediate material cooperation in actions that are intrinsically immoral" (USCCB 2001; 2009a, no. 70). Undoubtedly, these teachings are clearly in sharp contrast and appear contradictory.[2]

The second point for discussion is the change that can be traced in the directives by examining two official documents in the 1970s on mediate material cooperation being used to justify sterilizations in Catholic hospitals. Before discussing these two documents, it is important to emphasize that the prohibition of immediate material cooperation with sterilizations in the 2001 and 2009 editions of the directives is absolute and without exception. It can only be assumed that by "immediate" the bishops mean material cooperation with proscribed services within Catholic facilities. After all, the 2001 and the 2009 editions of the directives remain open, as discussed later in this section, to mediate material cooperation with other organizations that provide proscribed services such as direct sterilization.

However, by prohibiting immediate material cooperation with perceived wrongdoing in a manner that interprets the meaning of "immediate" as occurring in Catholic facilities, two difficulties arise from the perspective of doctrinal development of Church teaching. On the one hand, the prohibition of immediate material cooperation conflicts with its justification in the appendix of the 1995 edition of the directives, as discussed earlier. On the other hand, the prohibition of material cooperation with direct sterilizations in a Catholic facility (which seems to be the meaning of the bishops' prohibition in directive 70) conflicts with two Church documents in the 1970s that specifically discussed permitting direct sterilizations in Catholic hospitals using mediate material cooperation. These documents are the "Reply of the Sacred Congregation for the Doctrine of the Faith on Sterilization in Catholic Hospitals" and the "Commentary on the Reply of the Sacred Congregation for the Doctrine of the Faith on Sterilization in Catholic Hospitals."[3]

The substantive point under discussion in these two documents was that direct sterilizations could be justified in Catholic hospitals under circumstances of external duress. What lay behind this justification of direct sterilizations in Catholic hospitals using the principle of mediate material cooperation? The text of the Vatican's 1975 reply sets the context for interpreting the 1977 commentary by the US bishops. The Vatican reply stated:

> Insofar as the management of Catholic hospitals is concerned:
>   a) Any cooperation . . . directed to a contraceptive end, . . . is absolutely forbidden. . . . Any cooperation so supplied . . . would be contrary to the necessary proclamation and defense of the moral order.
>   b) The traditional doctrine regarding material cooperation, with the proper distinctions between necessary and free, proximate and remote, remains valid, to be applied with the utmost prudence, if the case warrants.

c) In the application of the principle of material cooperation, if the case warrants, great care must be taken against scandal and the danger of any misunderstanding by an appropriate explanation of what is really being done (CDF 1976, sec. 3).

Three comments are needed to clarify the meaning of this quotation. The Vatican's reply clearly deals with the use of mediate material cooperation, referring to its specific distinctions in item "b." Also, item "c" indicates that the Vatican justified the possibility of applying the principle in some circumstances ("if the case warrants"). Finally, the issue under consideration for using mediate material cooperation "if the case warrants" is identified explicitly in the title of the Vatican's reply, "Sterilization in Catholic Hospitals." In other words, what is not being discussed is either immediate material cooperation or partnership arrangements with other organizations that provide sterilizations. The focus is upon using mediate material cooperation in some circumstances to justify direct sterilizations in Catholic hospitals.

The 1977 commentary of the US bishops further specifies the circumstances when such an application of mediate material cooperation could justify direct sterilizations in Catholic hospitals: "Material cooperation will be justified only in situations where the hospital because of some kind of duress or pressure cannot reasonably exercise the autonomy it has (i.e., when it will do more harm than good)" (USCCB 1983, "Guidelines," sec. 2). To elaborate on what might constitute the type of duress that would warrant the justification of direct sterilizations in Catholic hospitals, the bishops explained in their 1997 commentary: "Direct sterilization is a grave evil. The allowance of material cooperation in extraordinary cases is based on the danger of an even more serious evil, e.g., the closing of the hospital could be under certain circumstances a more serious evil" (USCCB 1983, 7). In other words, the external duress of the hospital having to close could be sufficient cause to justify direct sterilizations in the Catholic facility using the principle of mediate material cooperation.[4]

A contrasting teaching occurs in the 2001 and 2009 editions of the directives. The bishops explain that directive 70, referring to the prohibition of immediate material cooperation with actions that are intrinsically immoral such as direct sterilization, replaces the official teaching in the earlier documents: "This directive supersedes the 'Commentary on the Reply'" (USCCB 2009a, note 44). Directive 70 appears to forbid direct sterilizations in Catholic hospitals (interpreting the use of immediate material cooperation as referring to the procedures occurring in Catholic facilities, as discussed earlier). This shift in official Church teaching highlights a fascinating aspect of organizational ethics in health care that is replete with significance about the development of moral doctrine in the Catholic tradition.

A third point for discussion is the consistent stance by the bishops regarding the use of mediate material cooperation to justify partnership arrangements between Catholic facilities and other organizations that provide proscribed services. However, there are sophisticated nuances that need to be explored on the prohibition of abortion and of other proscribed services such as direct sterilization.

Let us begin with the prohibition of abortion. Directive 45 explains that "Catholic health care institutions are not to provide abortion services, even based on the principle of material cooperation." However, the meaning of this directive needs to be clarified in the following manner. On the one hand, directive 45 and directive 70 make the same point: "Catholic health care institutions are not to provide abortion services" (no. 45), and "Catholic health care organizations are not permitted to engage in immediate material cooperation in actions that are intrinsically immoral, such as abortions" (no. 70). The point here is that abortion services must not be provided in a Catholic organization (construing "immediate" cooperation as meaning within Catholic facilities, as discussed previously). If this interpretation is what the bishops mean, then directive 45 could benefit by including the word "immediate" (as occurs in directive 70), to be stated in this manner: "Catholic health care institutions are not to provide abortion services, even based on the principle of immediate material cooperation."

On the other hand, directive 45 may be intended by the bishops to present a broader prohibition, forbidding "abortion services, even based on the principle of material cooperation"—including both immediate and mediate material cooperation. If so, the prohibition of abortion services based on mediate material cooperation appears to refer to a Catholic organization partnering with another organization that provides abortion services. A case example illustrates what is involved here.

A rural Catholic hospital that provides health care for a large population with no other hospital in its remote region is threatened with closure due to market pressure. To survive and continue its healing ministry to the rural population, the hospital decides to join a secular health system that includes other Baptist, Jewish, and secular hospitals. One of the secular hospitals provides abortion services. May the Catholic hospital partner with this health system, assuming there is no direct involvement with the provision of abortion services (such as profit sharing)? In this case, the Catholic hospital does not provide abortion services in its own facilities—doing so would constitute immediate material cooperation, which is forbidden both by directive 45 and by directive 70. Nonetheless, the Catholic organization is materially connected via its partnering arrangement with the provision of abortion services in another facility in the health system. The Catholic facility does not intend the forbidden procedure, is distant from it, and is under duress through threat of closure to partner with the health system that provides the abortion services.

Technically, the principle of mediate material cooperation could justify such a partnering arrangement. However, it may be that in directive 45 the bishops intend to forbid this type of partnering arrangement even when using mediate material cooperation. If this interpretation is what the bishops mean, then directive 45 could be revised to make the prohibition clearer, such as in this manner: "Catholic health care institutions are not to provide abortion services or participate in arrangements that involve abortion services using the principle of mediate material cooperation." In other words, further clarification of the meaning of directive 45 is needed.

This distinction between immediate and mediate material cooperation helps to understand when the principle, in circumstances of duress, can justify partnership arrangements between Catholic organizations and others that provide direct sterilizations. The absolute prohibition of immediate material cooperation with direct sterilizations in directive 70, construed as occurring within a Catholic organization, suggests that mediate material cooperation remains permissible. That permissibility seems to be the purpose of directive 69: "If a Catholic health care organization is considering entering into an arrangement with another organization that may be involved in activities judged morally wrong by the Church, participation in such activities must be limited to what is in accord with the moral principles governing cooperation" (USCCB

2001; 2009a, no. 69). Two examples illustrate how mediate material cooperation might be justified, including the use of the distinction between remote and proximate cooperation.

On remote cooperation we can consider a rural Catholic hospital that is forced under threat of closure to join a secular health system in which other partner organizations provide direct sterilizations. The Catholic facility does not intend the forbidden procedure, is distant from it insofar as the proscribed services occur in other facilities in the health system, and there is no direct involvement with the provision of the proscribed services (such as profit sharing). This would be an example of justified mediate material cooperation that is remote insofar as the forbidden procedure occurs in other (albeit partner) health care organizations.

In contrast, another example sheds light on the principle of mediate material cooperation that is proximate. An outdated and inefficient Catholic hospital closes when it reaches an agreement with a recently built community hospital to merge the two facilities in a lease-management arrangement with the new name "Catholic/Community Hospital." The Catholic organization manages the services of the previous Catholic hospital and the services of the Community hospital, now integrated to save costs and maximize efficiency in the new community hospital building. The agreement mandates that the Catholic organization must continue the reproductive services—including direct sterilization but not abortion—that were previously available in the community hospital. In other words, direct sterilizations must continue in the community hospital under the management of the Catholic organization. The Catholic organization moves the suite for sterilization services to the top floor of the hospital building with separate elevator access from the ground floor. No other patient services are provided on the top floor. Upon entering the suite, its affiliation is clearly indicated as being only "Community Hospital": everywhere else in the building, the hospital's identity logo appears as "Catholic/Community Hospital." Also, the staff members providing the sterilization services are not employed by the Catholic organization: the original community hospital outsourced those services to another organization but insisted that the sterilizations continue to occur in the hospital building to maximize access for the patient population. This arrangement could constitute an example of justified mediate material cooperation that is proximate in this sense: the Catholic organization does not intend the forbidden procedure, is distant from it insofar as the proscribed services occur on the top floor clearly associated with "Community Hospital," the staff providing the services are not employed by the Catholic organization, and there is no direct involvement with the provision of the proscribed services (such as profit sharing). However, the provision of the proscribed services constitutes proximate cooperation because of being in the same hospital building that is managed by the Catholic organization.

There is one final point to note regarding the use of mediate material cooperation, whether proximate or remote, with regard to the provision of proscribed services such as sterilizations. Some argue that making any arrangements to create distance between the Catholic organization and the provision of proscribed services actually constitutes formal cooperation insofar as the Catholic organization can be accused of planning—thereby necessarily intending—the forbidden procedure. This is an odd argument that misunderstands how the principle functions in practice. The principle requires creating maximum distance from the forbidden procedure, which necessarily involves planning arrangements to accomplish that goal. The necessary condition for the principle to function is that the Catholic organization does not intend the forbidden procedure and that there is duress that requires cooperation with it. Hence, planning arrangements to create maximum distance from the forbidden procedure can be a necessary component of the principle. It stretches credulity to argue, for example, that the Catholic organization in the previous case is formally complicit with providing direct sterilizations when it moved the sterilization suite to the top floor of the hospital to maximally separate the proscribed services from all the other legitimate hospital services.

It should be clear by now that the exact specifications and applications of the principle of cooperation are complex and variable. Succeeding editions of the directives have changed these specifications and applications. In some cases only cooperation with abortion seems prohibited; in later editions certain kinds of cooperation with sterilization, formerly permitted, seem now forbidden as well. The reason for the difference is never explained. The exact meaning of "immediate" as opposed to "mediate" is not always easily determined. It might mean "in the hospital" as opposed to "outside the building," as we have interpreted it here, but that may be the difference between "proximate mediate" and "remote mediate" instead. It is never really clear. How much distance must be present before "proximate" becomes "remote" is also unclear. And finally, since Catholic moral theology is supposed to be based on the natural law and not on episcopal and Vatican decree, it is unclear whether these changes are intended to represent changes in natural moral law or in its interpretation, on the one hand, or simply to be new disciplinary rules, on the other. All of this leaves Catholic health care institutions in a quandary when it comes to making the difficult decisions with which they are faced in the real world. All too often it comes down to the interpretation of the local bishop.

It will be truly unfortunate if Catholic institutions decide that the only way out is to stop being "Catholic," something that seems sadly already to be happening. In January 2012 Catholic Healthcare West, based in San Francisco, restructured its governance: it ceased to be a sponsored ministry of the Catholic Church and became a secular nonprofit health care system with a dominantly secular board of trustees. San Francisco's archbishop George Niederauer approved the arrangement. He initiated discussions over the arrangement in part because of his concern that Catholic Healthcare West's non-Catholic hospitals provided direct sterilizations, a procedure that is contrary to official Catholic teaching. The twenty-five Catholic hospitals and the fifteen non-Catholic hospitals remain part of the new health system called Dignity Health, with the Catholic hospitals continuing to follow the *Ethical and Religious Directives* (Niederauer 2012).

In this chapter we have examined two of the major issues in organizational ethics: the problem of medical errors and how best to prevent them, and the complex issue in Catholic health care of cooperation with forbidden health care services. We have noted that the best basis for examining these, as well as other organizational issues, is to put them in the context of stewardship, a theological concept well based in Catholic theology. Catholic health care organizations have served our nation and our world well. We must all try to ensure their continued prosperity.

Notes

1. It is also important to note that American law must be religiously neutral. Were the law to make an exception for Catholic opposition to contraception, it would likely also have to exempt any organization run by Jehovah's Witnesses from covering blood transfusions and perhaps any organization run by religious groups claiming opposition to medical treatments and preference for faith healing from covering surgery or other medical procedures. These complexities are too often forgotten in the public debate. Some may use the debate here as a convenient cover for their opposition to government-sponsored or government-mandated health insurance as such—insurance that is, as we have seen, consistently supported by the Catholic tradition. However, this opposition may stand against official Catholic teaching on the human right to basic health care.

2. The rationale provided by the bishops appears in the introduction to part 6 in the 2001 and 2009 editions of the directives: "This new edition of the Ethical and Religious Directives omits the appendix concerning cooperation, which was contained in the 1995 edition. Experience has shown that the brief articulation of the principles of cooperation that was presented there did not sufficiently forestall certain possible misinterpretations and in practice gave rise to problems in concrete applications of the principles." The "articulation of the principles of cooperation" in the 1995 appendix included the justification of immediate material cooperation that the 2001 and 2009 editions of the directives repudiate. Naturally, it would be interesting to know the theological basis for the bishops in 1995 justifying immediate material cooperation in some instances of duress. Perhaps they were aware of a view in the Catholic tradition that immediate material cooperation can be justified in extraordinary circumstances of duress, illustrated in this case: "a person in great need may lawfully ask a Sacrament from a minister who is unworthy and who will sin by conferring it" (McHugh and Callan 1929, 614–15). It may be that the US bishops were influenced by that stance. Of course, we do not know their reasoning insofar as they did not provide an explanation. It would be helpful to have an explanation from the bishops of their specific decision to change their teaching from permitting immediate material cooperation in some cases in the 1995 appendix to prohibiting it outright in subsequent editions of the directives. Significant questions about ecclesial process and doctrinal truth arise, including the following: what was the historical precedent in the Catholic tradition to justify defending immediate material cooperation with wrongdoing in some instances of duress; and in light of that historical tradition and official teaching, what was the doctrinal rationale for the subsequent prohibition of immediate material cooperation by the US bishops; was the doctrinal teaching in the 1995 appendix construed to be erroneous, thereby requiring its removal; if erroneous, on what basis, using what criteria, and what implications result for understanding the authority of the official teaching of the Bishops in documents such as the directives?

3. The documents are identified in the 2001 and the 2009 editions of the directives in endnote 44 that accompanies directive 70: "This directive supersedes the 'Commentary on the Reply of the Sacred Congregation for the Doctrine of the Faith on Sterilization in Catholic Hospitals' published by the National Conference of Catholic Bishops on September 15, 1977, in Origins 7 (1977): 399–400" (USCCB 2001; 2009a, note 44). In this endnote the bishops also cite the original text from the Vatican to which the "Commentary on the Reply" refers, as follows: "See also 'Reply of the Sacred Congregation for the Doctrine of the Faith on Sterilization in Catholic Hospitals' (Quaecumque Sterilizatio), March 13, 1975 Origins 6 (1976): 33–35" (USCCB 2001; 2009a, note 44). These documents also appear together in a pamphlet published in 1983 (USCCB 1983).

4. To emphasize that cooperation in this situation is material and not formal, the bishops emphasized that the justification must be external to the reasons for sterilization: "If the cooperation is to remain material, the reason for the cooperation must be something over and above the reason for the sterilization itself" (USCCB 1983, p. 7, sec. 4).

CHAPTER 25

EMBRYONIC STEM CELLS AND THE BEGINNING OF PERSONHOOD

I N AUGUST 2001 President George W. Bush announced his decision concerning the federal funding of human embryonic stem cell research (Cohen 2004, 97–98). Reaching what was both applauded and condemned as a compromise, Bush said that he would permit federal funding only for further research on embryonic stem cell lines already established, and would not fund the creation of more cell lines or, apparently, further research on any cell lines that might be privately created after the date of his announcement.[1] He left all privately funded researchers alone, presumably free to continue their research as they saw fit. Although this announcement did not please the more strict among his pro-life supporters, it was in a way a perfectly Republican decision. Government's role would be limited. Private enterprise would continue free of restriction. Indeed, while the Bush policy was in effect, private institutions and individuals created new stem cell lines, and state governments and universities started stem cell institutes to bypass the ban on federal funding (Kalb 2004). More recently the Obama administration has changed the Bush policy, removing some of the restrictions. At this writing, however, legal challenges have been brought to the new policy, resulting in uncertainty as to the final outcome. Stem cell scientists have claimed that this uncertainty has caused delays in stem cell research (Austriaco 2011a, 353).

Why Stem Cells?

Human stem cells are of interest to scientists and to physicians because of their ability or potential to differentiate into many different types of cells, and thus into different tissues and possibly even into complete organs. Once retrieved, stem cells can be cultured in such a way that an "immortal cell line" is derived, as the cells reproduce themselves over and over, giving researchers and physicians an unending supply. The ability of stem cells to differentiate is often broken down into three categories: totipotency, the ability or potential to become any kind of cell in the human body, and also to become the cells of the extraembryonic tissues of the placenta; pluripotency, the ability to become any kind of cell in the human body (there are 210 types of these cells) but not to become extraembryonic cells; and multipotency, the capacity to become certain kinds of cells but not others (Mirkes 2001, 167–68). Only totipotent stem cells can become embryos and potentially grow into new human persons. Totipotent stem cells are found only in the one- to three-day-old embryo; thereafter, embryonic stem cells have differentiated sufficiently that, although they are still able to become any of the cell types of the human body, they can no longer become the cells of the placenta and thus are called "pluripotent" (ibid., 167). It is the pluripotent stem cells that are sought for their ability to become other kinds of cells, and a basic source for these cells is the early human embryo. Harvesting them kills the embryo.

Because of the obvious moral problems associated with this destructive harvesting of human embryonic stem cells, other sources for pluripotent stem cells have been sought. The claim has been made that fetal cells, possibly derived from spontaneously aborted (miscarried) fetuses, are also good sources and are actually better than embryonic stem cells (Michejda 2002), but some research suggests that these are not good sources (Austriaco 2003c, 790–91). Postnatal stem cells, often called "adult stem cells," are found in bone marrow, blood, body fat, and some organs (Cohen 2004, 101). These cells are multipotent; they do not have the ability to differentiate into all the various types of cells in our bodies, though it seems they can be manipulated into becoming cells they had not been prior to manipulation. "In other words, [scientists] have de-differentiated and then re-differentiated them" (Mirkes 2001, 168n14). Although some claim that adult stem cells offer promise similar to that of embryonic stem cells (Catholic Organization for Life and Family, and Catholic Health Association of Canada 2002, 2–3; Austriaco 2002a; 2003a, 180; 2003c, 790; Conner 2002, 649; Gómez-Lobo 2004, 76), others claim that they are not as desirable (Ford 2003, 699; Faden et al. 2003, 15; Knoepffler 2004, 57). Multipotent adult stem cells "often lose their ability to differentiate into a desired mature cell. For example, stem cells harvested from brain tissue lose the ability to produce the neurotransmitter dopamine, which is desired in the treatment of Parkinson's disease. As a result, the perceived risk would be the development of cancer originating from transplanted stem cells that failed to complete the differentiation and maturation process" (Ahmann 2001, 148–49). Some studies have shown that adult stem cells may not in fact differentiate into other kinds of cells, thus limiting their potential (Austriaco 2003b, 574; Cohen 2004, 101–2). Recent studies have suggested that these induced pluripotent stem cells (iPS cells) may be inherently abnormal, while other studies suggest that at least some of them are equivalent to embryonic stem cells and that further manipulation in the laboratory can correct some of their defects (Austriaco 2011a, 347–48).

In any case, many scientists consider embryonic stem cells better for the purposes that are envisioned for this type of research (Cohen 2004).[2] Research on pluripotent embryonic stem cells is proposed with three aims: a better knowledge of how cells specialize, leading possibly to a better understanding of certain diseases such as cancer and birth defects; a better and quicker way to test drugs by using stem cell lines; and "the development of 'cell therapies,' a renewable source for debilitating diseases such as Parkinson's, Alzheimer's, arthritis, and spinal cord injury" (Mirkes 2001, 168). Pluripotent embryonic stem cells might also be used in the creation of embryos and of healthy children (Parens and Knowles 2003, S13). It should perhaps be noted here that some stem cell therapy attempts for the treatment of Parkinson's disease have been far less successful than was hoped; indeed, some patients seem to have been harmed by the treatment (Caplan and McGee 2001).

The usual source of embryonic stem cells is "extra" embryos, that is, embryos resulting from in vitro fertilization (IVF) that are not implanted into the woman's uterus. The stem cell lines approved by President Bush for federal funding were derived from this source (Cohen 2004, 97). Because the process of retrieving eggs is costly, uncomfortable, and even dangerous—the drugs used to stimulate ovulation can cause harm to the woman—and because unfertilized eggs cannot be frozen as successfully as embryos, physicians usually try to fertilize as many eggs as possible with the man's sperm after they are retrieved. Some eggs will not be successfully fertilized. But usually enough eggs are fertilized that there are too many embryos for one attempt, so only some are implanted and the others are frozen for later use if the first attempt does not succeed at producing a pregnancy. It is these "extra" embryos that are seen as a good source for stem cells.

Naturally aborted early embryos might also be sources, and in this case the embryo, already dead, need not be killed in order to harvest cells and create a cell line. But for various reasons, these may not be good sources of stem cells. Early embryos are not usually detected when they miscarry. And since the embryo has failed to mature, there may be some anomaly. Or one might use embryos created specifically for this purpose, either through IVF or by therapeutic cloning. This last method would duplicate the genetic material of one existing person to provide stem cells identical to her or his genome, thus ensuring complete compatibility. One successful attempt at this has been reported (Knoepffler 2004, 55).

The distinction between embryonic stem cells and adult or postnatal stem cells makes a major difference from the perspective of ethics. This chapter focuses on the ethics of embryonic stem cell research. It does not deal with adult stem cell research since there are no particular ethical issues connected with research on adult stem cells as long as they are not manipulated into being the equivalent of nascent human life. Gathering them does not result in harm to the donor. Nor is there any particular Catholic ethical issue in the use of adult stem cells. Donald Wuerl, then bishop of Pittsburgh, is cited in an interview as saying "that the Catholic Church does not see a moral problem in using adult stem cells for scientific research because it does not destroy human life. He added the caveat that as long as basic ethical guidelines for this research are followed, the Church does accept the benefits of this scientific use" (Esposito 2001, 1).

Some claim that there are ethical problems with adult stem cell research having to do with what is produced when these cells are "reset" to accent or increase their multipotency. John Ahmann states that "when encouraging 'adult stem cell' research, the water becomes morally murky if the definition includes those cells having the capability of being rejuvenated to a state that is equivalent to inner cell *mass-like* cells (in other words, into embryoid bodies)" (Ahmann 2001, 149, emphasis his). The question here is whether these embryoid bodies are human persons or should be treated as such. They are different from the cloned human intended for live birth in that they cannot develop in that way. They are not totipotent. But is this difference sufficient for one who argues against all embryonic stem cell research as the destruction of human life, as Ahmann does, to permit this kind of research as morally right? Ahmann says the answer is not clear. Norman Ford claims these embryoid bodies are not embryos and thus not human persons (Ford 2003, 701).

In this chapter we distinguish between the creation of stem cell lines by the destructive use of embryos, on the one hand, and the further use of stem cell lines already created, on the other. The first of these is generally considered the more ethically problematic, although the second is also opposed by many. Most of the chapter concerns the first of these procedures, the creation of stem cell lines from living embryos, by which creation means the destruction of the embryo as a living being. Then, in a briefer second section, we consider the question of research on stem cell lines already created.

Creation of Stem Cell Lines from Human Embryos

Concerning the ethics of creating stem cell lines by the necessarily destructive use of human embryos, we deal with two issues: the question of who gives consent, and the question as to when human life or human personhood begins. This second question is the more important one, perhaps the essential question. It is a difficult question to answer, and much of this chapter deals with it.

The Question of Consent

As we have seen in earlier chapters, American bioethicists tend to emphasize the question of consent. Some seem to imply that once proper consent is given for a procedure, the ethical issues connected with it are largely or even completely settled. American bioethics arose in the context of response to some unethical medical experiments performed in American institutions and in response to the paternalism of physicians who consistently refused to allow families to stop medical treatment that was doing no more than prolonging the process of dying. In this context it was understandable that American bioethics emphasized (and still does emphasize) the individual right of choice based on the principle, or value, of individual freedom and autonomy. This fits in quite well with the value most often attributed to the American way of life, individual liberty. Catholic medical ethics is less likely to worry about this, and, as we have seen in considerable detail, puts far more emphasis on the rightness or wrongness of what is done. As has been noted often already, this approach is generally correct. Consent alone is not sufficient to make a procedure morally right.

Some authors suggest that the living embryo from which a stem cell line is to be derived must somehow be said to give consent. To what degree must the fetus or embryo give its consent to this procedure, or for that matter, to any procedure to be done upon it? Since it is clear that no actual consent can be given, the issue turns to presumed consent or consent because of membership in a common humanity. This argument suggests that since the fetus or embryo shares humanity with those to be helped by the research, it can be presumed that the fetus would give consent were it able to do so.

This seems bizarre. That is not to say that the entire question of presumed consent from children (and perhaps, therefore, from fetuses) is bizarre. That is, we do not mean here to reject Richard McCormick's claim that children, who are presumed not to be able to give their own free and informed consent even though they may be able to give "assent," may be made the subjects of experimentation even when it will not benefit the children themselves, but only, he stresses, when the experiment is "risk-free, pain free, inconvenience-free" (McCormick [1972] 1981, 412). It seems that McCormick is right. In the present case, however, the issue does not revolve around something that is risk-free. It has to do with certain death. The whole notion of fetal or embryonic consent to being killed in order to help others seems strange. It is bizarre whether the fetus or embryo is being killed for this purpose or, as is often the case, is killed or allowed to die for other reasons. To speak in this context of the obligation of the now-killed fetus or the about-to-be-killed embryo to contribute to the benefit of others seems to misplace the substantive issue to the kind of issue American bioethics likes to talk about: individual autonomy and consent. It completely misses the ethical importance of the larger question.

Similarly, some theorists claim that the consent can come from the aborting mother or from the genetic parents of the embryos. To this, of course, others respond that this is like allowing a murderer to give consent to organ donation from the corpse of the victim. Neither of these answers is helpful because both avoid the real question here. In the American context, permission to take embryonic cells from an embryo (or cells from an aborted fetus) will likely be required of the "parents" or gamete providers of that embryo or fetus. Such a requirement of consent is necessary, and the consenting couple in the case of embryo donation (or the consenting woman, in the case of tissue to be taken from an aborted fetus) should be fully informed as to the use of the cells and the purposes of the research. This information is especially necessary when the embryos donated are to be used by commercial organizations that stand to profit from the cell lines they can establish from them (Holland 2001). However, even though this kind of consent ought to be required, the giving of it does not as such justify the procedure. Claiming that it does badly misplaces the ethical question.

The Question of the Beginning of Human Life

In November 1998 President Bill Clinton asked the National Bioethics Advisory Commission (NBAC) to advise him on the ethical issues concerning embryonic stem cell research (Mirkes 2001, 163). The commission's report, submitted in September 1999, stated that the early human embryo, while not yet a human person, is nonetheless human life and thus deserves respect (ibid., 164). In doing this, the commission tried to avoid what it saw as two extremes sometimes proposed: one, that the early embryo is a full human person and thus must be treated as such; and two, that it is merely a cluster of ordinary cells deserving no moral consideration (ibid., 164–65). The NBAC thus suggested requiring (1) that embryonic stem cell research be done only for important goals; (2) that informed consent be obtained from the parents; (3) that donors of embryos not be allowed to name the persons who would receive possible therapies; (4) that payment or sale of embryos be prohibited but not, it seems, that sales of cell lines be banned; (5) that the creation of embryos for the purpose of research be banned, thus limiting this to embryos left over after in vitro fertilization; (6) that other sources of stem cells be used when possible; (7) that the use of embryos created by human cloning be prohibited; and (8) that a review panel be established to monitor that these restrictions are followed by anyone receiving federal funding and to urge private companies to do the same. This set of recommendations was seen by some as too restrictive, by others as too lax, and by still others as a legitimate answer to a difficult and divisive issue.

The NBAC deserves support for at least recognizing that the issue hinges on the status of the early human embryo. Catholic medical ethics agrees that the status of the embryo is central to this question. To that problem we now turn. No simple answer is given here. The purpose of this section is more to lay out the issue and the approaches to it than to attempt a resolution. Some answers are, however, rejected, and some approaches are defended as better than others.

What is the precise question that is being asked here? Usually it is stated as trying to determine when human life begins. In some sense, however, the answer to this question must be that human life began many millennia ago and has not stopped since. Sperm and eggs are alive, and they are forms of human life (they are not, after all, lion or giraffe life), but no one claims today that they are in themselves persons. It was held for a long time that the "little man" or "homunculus" was present in human semen, but this is now known to be false. In any case, the real question here cannot be when human life begins.

Perhaps the technically best way to ask the question is to ask when human-life-with-full-basic-human-rights begins. This is a properly phrased ethical question. And this is, as we show, the way it must be phrased if one is to make coherent sense out of official Catholic Church teaching on the matter.

Another way to phrase the issue is to ask when a new human person begins. Properly understood, this way of phrasing the question is also valid, although it seems that in official Catholic teaching the two ways of putting the question are not synonymous since official Church documents explicitly refuse to claim that human personhood is present in the early embryo while claiming that this human life must be treated as if it were a human person, that is, that it must be accorded the full basic rights of a human person. But because the phrase "human personhood" is a proper way to ask the question, and because the alternative phrasing—"When does human-life-with-full-basic-human-rights begin?"—is so awkward, we use the "human personhood" way of asking the question.

All approaches to answering this question start by attempting in some way to recognize what it is that makes humans different from other animals. Personhood, after all, is an attribute of human beings and not—or at least most claim that it is not—an attribute of other animals, even somewhat smart ones like dolphins and apes, although personhood may be said to characterize intelligent extraterrestrials, if such are found to exist.

What Do We Look For? Three Approaches

Among the possible approaches for what we should look for in deciding whether an entity is a human person, three are commonly proposed.[3]

1. Some philosophers require the actual capacity to exercise the behaviors we generally classify as human, such as reason and choice. Sometimes called "moral individualism" (Walker and King 2011, 285), this might seem the most obvious

approach. But if we begin by insisting that certain actions or the capacities for them be actually present, we end up, as philosopher Peter Singer does, by saying that infants and possibly very young children are not persons since they cannot yet reason and choose, so they are less deserving of moral respect than are adult animals such as pigs, dogs, and chimpanzees that have more actualized capacity than human babies (Singer 1992; 1993). On this view, if we need to decide whether to sacrifice an infant or an adult animal, the infant is less worthy of life. Few have accepted this view; the authors of this book certainly do not. But Singer insists that the rejection of this view is based on "emotionally moving but strictly irrelevant aspects of the killing of a baby" (Singer 1993, 171). Infanticide is acceptable unless it hurts the parents or other adult human persons. And some adults with severe mental disabilities would not qualify as persons either. If we insist on actual capacities, it is difficult to refute these claims.

2. The second approach is to look to potentiality and to claim that human infants, and perhaps also fetuses and embryos, have the potential to become free, rational, autonomous beings (here theologians would add "spiritual" or "self-transcendent") and thus are human persons. The problem with this approach is that people are divided about how much potential and what kind of potential are needed. In a sense, human sperm and human eggs, which are certainly alive and certainly human, have a potential to become free, rational, autonomous human beings if mixed together properly, but no one thinks of them as persons. So there are significant differences of opinion about what kind of potential is needed. Some distinguish between passive potentiality and active potentiality (Ashley and O'Rourke 2002, 125; 1997, 231–32; Austriaco 2002b, 675–76), or between preparatory and expressive potentiality (Naumov, Wilberger, and Keyes 1991, 40–42), and require active or expressive potentiality for there to be a human person. But even here there is not agreement about what constitutes active potentiality or when it arrives. And what does this mean for the severely mentally disabled human individual whose capacity for reason and free choice is severely limited? Does this mean that she or he is not a person? Few would reach that conclusion.

3. The third approach is simply to claim that membership in the human species is enough to make a person. But that has its own problems. The formal problem here is that it merely pushes the question back one step; we still have to ask what constitutes membership in the human species. When is it that we can correctly say that a new member of the human species comes to be—when is it that we have a new human-life-with-full-basic-human-rights? And why is it that we ought to grant this kind of moral standing only to humans and not to some of the higher animals? Is this not simply an unjustified "speciesism"? Materially, the problem is that perhaps sperm and eggs qualify as human persons. We are not likely to think of them as members of the species, but to simply say that and conclude that we are done with the problem would reduce the issue to what society happens to think, which is inadequate. And what would we want to say about newly dead bodies? Why are these no longer members of the human species? Life still exists in them, for a short time at the organic level (or for a longer time if we are going to transport organs and then transplant them), and

for a much longer time at the tissue and cellular level. And these cadavers are human, after all, not dolphin or tiger. Yet they are not human persons; they are not what we mean by "members of the human species." They have lost something they used to have. And so the question must inevitably be "What have they lost?" This brings us back either to actual capacities or to potentiality for such capacity.

Thus, the three general approaches for what should be looked for in deciding whether an entity is a human person each have their own difficulties. This difficult set of issues is intricate and complex, and perhaps at times a bit boring. It is certainly frustrating. After all, we know a human being when we see one. But we can turn to history where we find many examples when human beings have denied membership to blacks or "Indians" or whomever else they wanted to see as somehow less than human. And, of course, this is precisely what the defenders of fetal personhood say that many are doing to the unborn child. So the question, complex as it is, has to be thoughtfully asked and the answers to be critically examined.

Three Schools of Thought

Philosopher Daniel Callahan proposes what has become a widely used starting point when he suggests that there are three schools of thought about when human personhood (or human life with full basic human rights) begins. There are, he says, the geneticist school, the social consequences school, and the developmental school (Callahan 1970, 377–401). We could call them the firm, the free, and the fickle.

We begin with the free, the social consequences school, which Callahan (1970, 400–401) and just about all Catholic medical ethicists reject. This school of thought, by denying any possibility of attaining objective evidence, simply claims that human personhood begins when adult humans choose to say it begins. The adult members of society make a decision based on the consequences of that decision for themselves. Presumably, they will agree that human adults are members. Philosophers will require that they decide "under a veil of ignorance" about their own gender, race, and ethnicity to avoid a decision rejecting the personhood of other races or clans, but philosophers who support this approach do not require that they attempt to discover when human personhood begins. The human adults who make the decision simply posit when it begins, and they do so based on their own needs and desires.

To our knowledge, no Catholic theologian holds this, but at least one Catholic feminist author, Marjorie Maguire, has argued that personhood begins when the woman carrying the fetus accepts it as a person (Maguire 1983). Even she admits, however, that at some point in time the fetus becomes a person regardless of whether the woman accepts it. This "relational school" has not been accepted by many Catholic scholars (Curran [1973] 1996, 250–52). And the "free" social consequences approach has no theological defenders that we know of and seems utterly inadequate.[4]

That leaves the firm and the fickle. And here we do find significant disagreement among Catholic thinkers. Official Catholic Church documents have explicitly refused to resolve when human personhood begins. In theological language, this is to say that the Church's magisterium has explicitly refrained from stating that the human rational spiritual soul is infused into and thus present within the human material body from the moment of conception. In its "Declaration on Procured Abortion," the Vatican Congregation for the Doctrine of the Faith states:

> This declaration expressly leaves aside the question of the moment when the spiritual soul is infused. There is not a unanimous tradition on this point and authors are in disagreement. For some it dates from the first instant, for others it could not at least precede nidation [implantation]. It is not within the competence of science to decide between these two views, because the existence of an immortal soul is not a question in its field. It is a philosophical problem from which our moral affirmation remains independent for two reasons: (1) supposing a later animation, there is still nothing less than a *human* life, preparing for and calling for a soul in which the nature received from parents is completed; (2) on the other hand it suffices that the presence of the soul be probable (and one can never prove the contrary) in order that the taking of life involve accepting the risk of killing a man, not only waiting for, but already in possession of his soul. (CDF [1974] 1999, 37n19)

Note the moral conclusion drawn from the premise that we may not really know when human personhood begins. The moral conclusion is that the potentiality present from the moment of conception means that the human embryo, even the very early preimplanted and predifferentiated human embryo, must be treated as if it were a human person because it is "a *human* life, preparing for and calling for a soul" that will make it a full human person. But one can ask whether that moral conclusion is necessarily drawn from that premise. It can be drawn. It is not contradictory to draw it. But does it necessarily follow that a not-yet-person must be treated as if it were a person? That debate continues even within Catholic medical ethics, the debate between geneticists and developmentalists. And some Catholic authors also dispute the second reason given by the "Declaration on Procured Abortion" for its conclusion that abortion is always wrong, the claim that it cannot be proven that the early embryo is not a person. They claim that it can be proven. And even if it could not be proven, some might reasonably argue that a certain human person would take precedence over a possible human person, thus allowing at least some cases of "direct" abortions where the woman's life is truly at risk, procedures which, as we saw in chapter 12, are forbidden in official Church documents.

It may be of interest to note why the official Church has decided not to claim human personhood for the zygote and the preimplanted embryo. It comes mainly from the long Thomistic tradition, from Thomas Aquinas, that there must be some organization of the material principle, the human body, before it could be ready for the formal principle of humanhood, the human immortal soul. Thomas claimed that three "animae"—souls if you will, but life principles may be better here—come into the human body successively: a vegetative life principle, an animal life principle, and finally a rational life principle, the spiritual human soul (Ashley and Moraczewski 2001, 200). Increasing levels of organization, each more complex than the one preceding, are required in the body for these to be present. Now Thomas was unaware of what we know from present biology. He thought that for some time after conception there was a kind of diffuse liquid that only later gained organizational complexity (ibid.). He claimed that boys get their souls at forty days after conception and girls at ninety. He was wrong, of course. From the moment of conception, there is indeed a new entity of some considerable complexity. But the question is still asked as to whether this organizational complexity is sufficient for us to claim that this is a human person. This is the debate between geneticists and developmentalists.

The geneticist school argues that everything is present even in the very early preim-planted human embryo—indeed even in the one-celled zygote formed by the union of human sperm and human egg—to enable us to be sure that this is a human person. That is, in theological terms the geneticist school claims that everything is present in the zygote to be sure that indeed a human soul is present. The developmental school argues that at least some development of the body of the embryo is needed before one can rightly claim that human personhood has been attained, in theological language, that a spiritual soul is present. At the very least, "developmental individualization" must have occurred, and this means that the very early embryo or "pre-embryo" from which stem cells are derived is not a human person (Shannon and Wolter 1990; McCor-mick [1989] 1993, 112–14). And the developmental school claims that this means we need not treat the pre-personal entity as if it were a human person. Thus, the develop-mental school is likely to agree with the NBAC, at least in its central claim that the early embryo deserves respect but that stem cell creation is morally right under certain guidelines because the destruction of the not-yet-person is permissible for certain purposes.

We can pass over the complex details of each school's position and look at the major arguments made by the developmental school and at the answers given to them by the geneticist school. It seems true—perhaps not to anyone's satisfaction—that the case is not yet proven by either side, though some of the arguments are better than others.

First, developmentalists claim that until the possibility of twinning has passed, that is, until approximately two to three weeks after gestation, with implantation and the formation of the primitive streak, there cannot be a human person (Shannon and Wolter 1990). A human person must be an individual, not a group of potential individ-uals (McCormick [1989] 1993, 115). As long as one can become two or more persons, a human person cannot be present. This argument seems a strong one. But geneticists answer that what happens in twinning is caused by a disruption in the development of the already existing human person rather than by any intrinsic drive within it. A new embryo-person is added to the original one, and the original continues on its own trajectory (Hurlbut, George, and Grompe 2006b). This is similar to what would happen in human cloning. In adult human reproductive cloning, if such ever becomes possible, a new human person emerges from one cell of an existing human being. Surely the human adult who is cloned was an individual prior to the taking of the cell used for the clone. Thus, say the geneticists, so too is the early human embryo from which a cell is taken to form a new one (Mirkes 2001, 177; Ashley and Moraczewski 2001, 195–98). Developmentalists might respond that one would not call the individual cloned cell a human person, only the more complex human person from which the cell was taken. Thus, the "new" zygote is more like the cloned cell than like the human person from which the cell was taken. It cannot be a human person until it achieves individuality, and it does not do that as long as it can be split into two or more individuals. The blastomeres (early embryonic cells) do not therefore constitute one human person but constitute a potentiality for a number of human persons (Ford 2001, 160). To this claim geneticists have answered that there is in fact some sort of organization among the cells of even the very early preimplanted embryo (Austriaco 2002b, 671), and, as just noted, that embryos do not in fact split into two or more individuals, but continue on their own trajectory as a disruption causes a new embryo to be added (Hurlbut, George, and Grompe 2006b). Thus, they claim, the early embryo does resemble the human person from whom a cell is taken more than the cell that is taken (Ashley and Moraczewski 2001, 196–98). Developmentalists answer that the organization of the early embryo is insufficient to prevent any of the cells from forming new complete embryos, and thus is not enough to make a human person.

Second, and more easily understood, is the developmentalist claim that since a large percentage of preimplanted embryos are discarded and never implanted—figures are given as high as 90 percent (Zoloth 2002, 70)—it is unseemly to claim that these are human persons with immortal souls. Indeed, as Edward Vacek notes, if they are persons, then normal sexual intercourse without contraception would seem to lead to the deaths of four or five persons a year, making noncontracepted sex an arguably immoral practice (Vacek 1988, 122)! Why would God do this? The geneticist answer is that God kills us all in the end anyway, as Paul Ramsey once said, so this cannot be a proof that the early embryo is not a person. In addition, it is certain that at least some, perhaps many, of the discards are not early human embryos at all, but terata (monsters), or hydatidiform moles or other "pseudo-embryos," and thus not human persons (Austriaco 2002b, 667–70). But, the developmentalists answer, the number of true human embryos that do not survive the first few weeks of gestation still makes it unlikely that they are indeed human persons.

Third, and finally, developmentalists hold varying judgments on when there is sufficient potentiality in the embryo or fetus for it to claim human personhood. Some therefore suggest that human personhood begins when the neural system is sufficient for some neurological or even rational activity, perhaps at twenty weeks or so of gestational age (Shannon and Wolter 1990, 620), but perhaps earlier depending on how much integration and complexity are required. To this geneticists respond by saying, quite correctly, that there is no magic moment after conception. Developmentalists must inevitably be unsure as to where exactly to place the beginning of personhood. Developmentalists respond that even conception is not a single moment but a process, and that, while it is true that there is no one obvious moment after conception, this does not refute the claim that some level of complexity is needed for there to be a person. The fact is, complex issues require complex answers; the best we can do here is approximate. The difficulty of determining precisely when human personhood begins does not refute the judgment that the early embryo cannot be a person. The geneticist answer is that there is sufficient complexity and thus sufficient active potentiality at conception.

It is now possible to conclude this section with the simple observation that if one holds that the early embryo is a human person, one will quite rightly conclude that the creation of stem cell lines by the destruction of this person is morally wrong. If, on the other hand, one holds that the early embryo cannot be a person, or even that it probably is not a person, one may rightly conclude that its destruction is right under certain circumstances and for certain purposes. Most developmentalists therefore seem to support the NBAC guidelines and allow for the creation of embryonic stem cell lines.

One further complication arises from the use of "spare" embryos left over from IVF procedures. A reasonable argument can be made that since there is usually no chance of "saving" them—they can be frozen and stored, but only if they are implanted can they become adult persons, and there are not enough women who want to bear them—it is better to use them to help others than simply to let them disintegrate. Perhaps this option might be a valid compromise for national and international policy: we could allow this use but forbid the creation of new embryos for the purpose of harvesting stem cells (Knoepffler 2004, 71). But those who hold that any direct killing of a person is always morally wrong will consistently require that it is better to turn off the freezing mechanism and allow them to die than to kill them directly in stem cell research.

Use of Already Established Stem Cell Lines

Those who permit the destruction of the early embryo in order to create stem cell lines, claiming that the early embryo is not human life with full basic human rights, naturally enough have even less of a problem with the use of cell lines already established. On the other hand, many but not all of those who forbid the destruction of the embryo in order to create embryonic stem cell lines also reject as morally wrong the use of cell lines already established (for example, Ford 2003, 699). This is the approach taken by many Catholic moral theologians who agree with official Church teaching that the early embryo must be treated as if it were a human person. But it is not the only approach possible, even for those who forbid the destruction of the embryo (Moraczewski 2003).

The traditional principle in Catholic medical ethics that may be applied here is the principle of cooperation, discussed in chapter 12. Based on the principle of double effect, the principle of cooperation permits a person to cooperate in some way in a wrong procedure as long as certain conditions are met. A trackman who throws switches may be allowed by this principle to throw the switch for the train to Dachau without being guilty of the crime of genocide. A cleaning woman in a building with a doctor's office where abortions are done may clean the office without being guilty herself of the abortion.

We saw that Catholic tradition distinguishes between formal and material cooperation. If the trackman agrees with the murder of the Jews, and intends his role to be a part of that murder, then he is indeed himself morally a murderer. This is formal cooperation. But all of us are at one time or another caught up in some form of cooperation with actions we consider morally wrong. We pay taxes even though we disagree with some of our government's actions. We work for corporations even though we may not think that everything they do is morally right. And so on. It is true that we have an obligation to use reasonable means to get the government to stop (we vote for a change of officials) or to get the corporation to stop (we tell our bosses and perhaps we vote on stockholder proposals). But we are not morally obliged in all cases to refuse to pay taxes or to quit our jobs. We do not formally cooperate, but we have to admit that our actions, along with those of other people, make possible the procedure we know to be wrong.

Catholic tradition says that material cooperation is morally right if it is mediate, and if the good effects to be realized by our actions outweigh the bad effects, including the bad effect of scandal. As we saw in chapter 12, mediate material cooperation may be proximate or remote, with as much distance as possible being necessary from the wrongdoing. However, there is never any clear dividing line between proximate and remote mediate material cooperation. This judgment is made on a case-by-case basis.

This principle can be applied to the use of embryonic stem cell lines already established. Those who oppose the killing of the embryos might still do research on the established lines not to support the original destruction of the embryos but to enable healing.

Perhaps an analogy might be made to the use of vaccines. In the early development of some common vaccines, including one for chicken pox, human fetal tissue from induced abortions was used (Doerflinger 1999a, 145; Kahlenborn 1996). For decades now, there has not been a need to use new fetal tissue to continue production of these vaccines. It seems that most, though not all, Catholic bioethicists, including many of those who consider the fetus to be a human person, permit the use of these vaccines (Furton 2004). There has not been an official magisterial pronouncement against their use. At some point, the use of a technology becomes morally right, even though that technology may in the beginning have been developed with immoral procedures. We use steel even though the early American steelworkers, on whose backs the steel industry was created, were immorally exploited. We live on land that, many argue, was wrongly stolen from its prior inhabitants (who may, of course, have stolen it from people before them, for all that we know).

It seems reasonable to conclude, therefore, that the use of already established cell lines is morally right. Kevin O'Rourke, who accepts the claim that the very early embryo must be considered a person (or at least treated as if it is), and that thus the destruction of a human embryo to obtain stem cells is unethical, allows for the use of the principle of cooperation to permit the use of lines already developed (O'Rourke 2004, 292–95). Those who oppose the creation of such lines would, of course, want to avoid giving the impression that they thought the destruction of embryos was right. And if they thought that their use of the established lines was giving reason for the creation of new lines, they would want to distance themselves from that and might decide that their cooperation, while material and not formal, was too proximate to be morally right. This is, in fact, the position taken by the Pontifical Academy for Life (Walters 2004, 27).

Conclusion

In this chapter we have examined the problem of the beginning of human personal life in the context of an issue that is now being hotly debated, the creation and use of embryonic stem cell lines. No single position is compelling.[5] While it is clear that the morality of abortion—and thus of the creation of embryonic stem cell lines by the destruction of an embryo—cannot be determined simply by the choice of the woman or the researcher, it is not clear that a new human person exists from the moment of fertilization. This does not, of course, give us permission to go ahead and do what we like with even very early human embryos. Even if these are not full human persons, they are more than ordinary clusters of cells. But this does not mean that it is absolutely wrong to use spare embryos that would otherwise be discarded to develop what might well become a source of significant human good. If other adequate sources of pluripotent cells were to be available, these ought to be used instead, and scientists ought to try to develop such sources.[6]

Notes

1. After President Bush's announcement, scientists and others involved in stem cell research complained that the number of cell lines available for federally funded research was too small, and that many of these lines were unfit for developing cells and tissues for human transplant because they were grown with mouse feeder cells, not human feeder cells, which resulted in the risk of cross-species contamination (Cohen 2004, 98–101).

2. Technology in this area changes almost daily. In addition to multipotent (adult) stem cells reset to become pluripotent, and gonadal cells retrieved from aborted fetuses, some claim that "parthenotes" (the result of parthenogenesis without the need of a male factor) might work, thus providing an alternative source and alleviating the need for embryos. On parthenotes, see Austriaco (2002b, 677–80), who argues that these are not embryos but pseudo-embryos, and thus are morally acceptable sources of stem cells. See also Cohen (2004, 104–5), who notes that some commentators consider them ethically the equivalent of embryos, while some scientists question their availability and usefulness. See also Huarte and Suarez (2004), who claim that proof of personhood is that a human entity will be able to develop to the stage where spontaneous motion is possible. Hence, a parthenote is from the beginning a person if development to the point of fetal movement is possible, and not otherwise. The International Association of Catholic Bioethicists rejected this approach in a 2007 statement (International Association of Catholic Bioethicists 2008, 337).

Umbilical cord blood is also sometimes proposed as a source for stem cells (Austriaco 2003a, 181). On embryonic gonadal or germ cells, which might be retrieved from spontaneously aborted fetuses or from fetuses removed in indirect abortions in cases of ectopic pregnancy, see Ford (2003, 701–5), who claims that these are even better than embryonic stem cells. But many scientists continue to claim that embryonic stem cells are better (Cohen 2004, 101). Another proposed source is embryo biopsy. Instead of destroying the embryo, only one cell is removed from it as a source of stem cells and the embryo is then replanted in the woman's uterus. But the risk to the embryo by this procedure is unknown and probably significant, and women are certainly unlikely to consent to it (Hudson 2006).

Finally, a number of procedures are under development to produce entities from which pluripotent stem cells can be derived ("induced pluripotent stem cells" or iPS cells), which entities might for one reason or another be said not to be human persons. This "altered nuclear transfer" (ANT) might be done by cloning an adult stem cell (somatic cell nuclear transfer or SCNT) from which a gene has been removed, and then replacing the gene in the derived stem cells. The claim made by those who support this as moral is that this entity, without the necessary gene, is similar to hydatidiform moles and other similar terata (monsters), which cannot develop into persons and which are not considered persons (Hurlbut 2005; Hurlbut, George, and Grompe 2006a). Thus, the entity is not a human embryo. On the other hand, some claim that this is morally wrong because perhaps a mistake will happen and the gene will not be removed so that the entity is really a true human clone and thus a person, or that the entity, even without the gene, is a person and is unlike a hydatidiform mole (see Byrnes 2005). For a defense of "direct reprogramming" as a moral method of ANT see Byrnes (2008). For a defense of unaltered SCNT as a source of pluripotent stem cells, based on the claim that human SCNT produces entities that are not true human embryos even without any alteration, see Hyun and Jung 2006.

A second technique of altered nuclear transfer, called oocyte assisted reprogramming (ANT-OAR) is to change the somatic cell from which the entity is to be derived by SCNT not by subtracting a gene needed for it to develop into an embryo, as described earlier, but by reprogramming it so that, before it is transferred into the egg cell, it already expresses factors characteristic of pluripotent stem cells that are not characteristic of the totipotent cells of the zygote. Alternatively, the egg could be reprogrammed so that, when the somatic cell's DNA is introduced into it, the resulting entity immediately expresses these factors. Thus, it never is and never can be an embryo. It directly becomes a pluripotent stem cell. In a widely distributed statement, thirty-five Catholic scholars generally identified with traditional Church teaching on these issues proposed this approach as a moral alternative, provided it becomes technically feasible (Arkes et al. 2005). For a defense of the moral rightness of ANT-OAR against the claim that it in fact would produce and then destroy human embryos, see Brugger (2005).

The ontological status of iPS cells themselves is also controversial because scientists can now develop iPS cells into a fetus if provided with an artificial placenta (using a procedure called tetraploid complementation) and implanted in a womb. Of course, the zygote makes its own placenta whereas iPS cells must be provided with one. But the placenta (natural or artificial) does not contribute to the developing structure of the fetus itself. That is, the fetus develops only from the iPS cells or the blastocyst's inner cell mass. This means that the same embryogenesis potential exists for iPS cells and the cells of the inner cell mass of the blastocyst formed by a zygote. This process has been shown in mouse studies to generate cloned offspring (Magill and Neaves 2009; Nagy et al. 1990). As of this writing, the debate continues concerning the scientific feasibility, the scientific value, and the moral rightness of these alternate sources for human pluripotent stem cells (Austriaco 2008, 2010, 2011a).

3. One further approach is to argue that somehow human personhood depends on an interaction or relationship between the new entity and (other) persons. For the claim that personhood is a narrative identity that involves interaction among persons, such that a severely handicapped infant is a person because of her family's interactions with her, whereas a fetus may or may not be a person, depending on its ultimate acceptance by others, especially by the woman carrying it, see Nelson 2002.

4. A "social presumptions" approach, now gaining some prominence in American policy debates in Washington, is similar to the social consequences approach. It tries to surmount the problems and the controversy in determining the moral status of the fetus by turning to the presumptions that American society seems to have accepted as these are reflected in present policies and community values (Cohen 2004, 105–7).

5. For a helpful listing of various positions ranging from the most restrictive through the most permissive, see Knoepffler 2004.

6. This chapter has concentrated on issues specific to embryonic stem cell research. The question as to whether research projects like this one are ethically right must also consider issues that are common to all expensive medical procedures and research initiatives. One might claim that until basic health care is available to all, projects like stem cell research are unethical. Although this kind of argument is problematic for a number of reasons that are developed in chapters 28 and 29, it is clear that justice does require of us that we spend more on preventative care than we now do and that we establish basic access to health care. This is of far greater ethical priority than stem cell research and other similar projects. The claim that all research that might be of benefit is morally imperative is simply false. Perhaps if scientists decided to close down all such initiatives as a protest against the present unjust American system of health

care, this would prove to be a powerful social force for change. Similarly, one might claim that government funding provided by tax dollars should not be allocated to stem cell research and other similar projects but to improving basic health care, which is more important for the common good. This claim seems valid, but it must be seen in the perspective of what would happen if only private corporations were to be involved in this kind of medical research. There might then be less regulation and less transparency and more likelihood that the research would be driven solely by the desire for profit (Frankel 2003). For these reasons, a working group at the Hastings Center recommended public funding with true governmental oversight (Parens and Knowles 2003). This may be especially important in this area because in addition to the justice issues common to all costly research, there are questions particular to stem cell research. Stem cells come from human sources, and the therapies derived from them will most benefit those who most genetically resemble the original sources (Faden et al. 2003). If we develop cell lines from white Americans, for example, white Americans will benefit most. Private industry is likely to do just that, since that is where the most profit can be anticipated. Correcting this lack of diversity would require developing lines from other groups, something requiring federal regulation and probably federal funding. As this book goes to press, given the current acrimonious debate over the federal debt and federal spending, it appears unlikely that Congress will provide such funding.

CHAPTER 26

GENETIC ENGINEERING

Ethics and Anthropology

Introduction

THIS CHAPTER FIRST LOOKS BRIEFLY at the general ethical issues that are commonly raised concerning genetic engineering, and then concentrates more directly on issues that concern the kind of theological anthropology detailed in part I of the book. Anthropology—hence, theology—plays a special role in genetics because this area asks directly the question of who we are as human beings (Chapman 1999). Thus, we return in a practical way to the questions we asked in chapter 5 about how theological principles work and ought to work in bioethics. In the following chapter we turn to the ethical aspects of some specific areas of genetics.

In his book *Body Parts: Property Rights and the Ownership of Human Biological Materials*, E. Richard Gold (1996) describes what he calls "property discourse." Although Gold's own metaethical theory appears to be antifoundationalist in the strong sense of that term—there seems to be no basis for verification of right and wrong other than our own decisions—his concern about property discourse is also important within a more foundationalist metaethics such as the natural law metaethics supported in chapters 9 and 10. Gold argues that property discourse in American law affects how we value objects that we consider as property—in this case, how we value the human body. He defines "property discourse" as "the sum of the assumptions, conceptions, and language used by judges, lawyers, and legislators in allocating the rights of control over goods" (ibid., 7). He argues that since legal professionals are specialized in confined areas, and focus on specific practical issues, they seldom worry about the underlying basis of that law and that practice. The result, he says, is that "legal practitioners are led, without examination, to certain results rather than to others. This has its effect on which modes of valuation are ultimately encouraged through the award of property rights. . . . Property discourse itself leads to the encouragement of certain modes of valuation over others" (ibid., 9). Property discourse tends to be market-based. So the issue for Gold is that the more we use property discourse in the law about the body, the more we will emphasize economic over noneconomic valuations of our bodies. He argues that there is no way we can supplement property discourse about our bodies with other noneconomic discourses because property discourse will drown them out (ibid., 17). He therefore concludes that since noneconomic valuations of our bodies are important to our culture, we should not subject our bodies to property rights (ibid., 166, 177).

This issue is one of two that are at the heart of the moral and anthropological considerations we should give to the problem of human genetic engineering and the inevitable commercial uses that will accompany it, such as the patenting and the ownership of human genes. The other issue is the directly anthropological question of whether human nature is or ought to be open or closed to self-manipulation of a genetic sort.

General Ethical Issues

There are, of course, a number of other important issues, none of them easily answered. Five that are commonly discussed come quickly to mind: privacy; justice; the possible harm, physical or psychological, to a child born with genetic enhancements; the long-term harm to the genetic line; and how we think of the disabled. Before getting to these, a few general descriptions and distinctions are helpful.

The Human Genome Initiative, a scientific achievement funded by the government with some parallel corporate funding, has successfully "mapped" or decoded the human genome; that is, scientists have produced one complete chemical map of the forty-six chromosomes that constitute the genetic makeup of a human person. The hope is that this will help us to discover markers for the genes that cause various traits, and then ultimately to enhance or eliminate these traits by changing the genes themselves. Until now, we have been able to treat the symptoms of diseases that are genetically caused; now we are starting to treat the cause itself.

Some distinctions are helpful. There are two types of genetic engineering: somatic cell and germ line cell. The first of these affects the forty-six chromosome somatic or body cells. If successful, a change of this type could, for example, eliminate cystic fibrosis in a person who has this disease. But it would not change his or her gametes, sperm or ova. Germ line cell genetic engineering, on the other hand, changes the gamete cells. This might be done in the early embryo, by substituting new genes for those in the embryo prior to cellular differentiation, that is, while the embryonic cells are still pluripotent, as we saw in the previous chapter. That would mean that the fetus would develop without cystic fibrosis, or whatever the trait might be. Germ line cell changes would affect not only the person in whom genetic engineering was done but all of that person's progeny as well. A start in this direction—though not genetic engineering in the strict sense, in that the genes are not themselves altered—is "preimplantation genetic diagnosis," in which embryos created for in vitro fertilization (IVF) are each screened for certain traits, and only those with the desired genes are implanted (Guterl 2003; Frankel 2003, 33). Their progeny would inherit the chosen traits and would be free of certain diseases. There is some concern that present research using somatic cell gene transfer risks inadvertently changing the germ line as well (King 2003; Frankel 2003, 33).

The second distinction is between therapeutic genetic changes and enhancement changes. Therapeutic changes are those intended to return a person (or a germ line) to its "normal functioning status." Eliminating Tay-Sachs disease would be an example.

Enhancement changes are those intended to change the person (or the germ line) to enhance that person or germ line beyond normal functioning. Increasing IQs to 200, increasing lifespan to 150 years, and so on, might be examples. Yet the line between therapy and enhancement is not all that clear (Frankel 2003, 33–35). What about changing the IQ of a germ line from 80 to 120? What is the difference between using genetically engineered human growth hormone to treat a deficiency and using it to increase height beyond the "normal range," as is already being done (ibid., 33–34)? What about decreasing the likelihood that members of a given family will die of heart disease? This would be both therapeutic (assuming the family had a high incidence of genetically caused heart disease) and enhancing (assuming the resulting family had less than the "normal" incidence of heart disease). And would not the elimination of heart disease altogether be considered "therapeutic"? We are trying to do that already, by nongenetic means such as diet, exercise, and medication. Yet this would also "enhance" us since we would live longer than "normal."

Still, the distinction has value, and its use remains important (Sparrow 2010, 116–18). Eliminating heart disease is not the same as creating a family with an IQ of 200. And there are concerns about more subtle effects of enhancing children genetically. Children with genetically engineered high IQs, for example, might well miss out on usual processes of gaining human wisdom, processes that would not be lost by nongenetic means of enhancements such as excellent education. Genetic enhancement is not the same as other means of enhancement, even if the intended end results are the same. There are morally significant differences that should not be overlooked (Malmqvist 2011).

Despite the ethical problems with genetic engineering, we are very likely to do it (Shannon 1999, 5). Many who worry about these issues feel better about somatic cell therapeutic genetic engineering, less good about germ line therapeutic genetic engineering, and even less good about germ line enhancement genetic engineering. The problem with worrying about these is that most probably, if the techniques are proven to work, people who can afford them will do them. Daniel Callahan has often remarked that if bioethics American style is to be said to have succeeded, it will have to have stopped something effective that at first almost everybody thought was a bad idea and morally wrong. The track record here is not very good. Technology that works and succeeds at enhancing its patients and its users is quickly accepted. Thus, even germ line enhancement is likely to be done if it is seen to succeed at really enhancing our progeny.

And the question is, why not? Concerning the first ethical issue, the question of privacy, it is clear that we already tell health care professionals, insurers, and employers our healthy and unhealthy secrets. We do so not because we like to give secrets away but because telling them helps us get better. Perhaps we could design a better system, but privacy concerns are quickly forgotten when we are sick and need help. Perhaps genetic knowledge is in some sense more dangerous than other medical knowledge if it gets into the wrong hands. Employers might fire us if they find out we are more likely than the average person to contract a particular disease. Insurers will want to know what we know about our health. Otherwise they are at risk of "adverse selection." The insurers are blind and have to use basic actuarial data, but I as an individual know I am at great risk of serious illness, so I buy more insurance than the average person would. But if the insurers know—and they can validly argue that it is unfair to subject them to too much adverse selection—then they are likely to reject me altogether if they do not like my genes (this is, by the way, an excellent argument for single-payer universal health insurance, where these problems do not arise). But it is unlikely that these risks about privacy will prevent us from exploiting genetic knowledge if we find it beneficial. We might pass laws protecting the data and try to resolve the issue that way. Indeed, a bill passed in the Senate in late 2003 does just this (Hanna 2003). But we are not likely to let the risks of privacy violations impede the technology itself.

Concerning the second issue, that of justice, it is clear that we already have a society in which the advantaged send children to private schools and universities in order to enhance their future, with the full knowledge that most of the poor do not have that opportunity. Perhaps we could design a better system of public education, but justice issues are not seen to forbid those of us who are able to pay for schooling that most cannot afford. Justice does not prevent us from driving cars just because others cannot afford them, yet this transportational advantage gives us an edge over others less fortunate. It is clear that genetic technology poses special problems in the area of justice that require serious attention (Cahill 2003), issues that the free market is unlikely to solve (Crozier and Hajzler 2010, 170–73). But the justice question is not likely to deter us from improving our lives and those of our children by genetic enhancement if it proves feasible to do this.

As to the third issue, many will be unlikely to think that a true enhancement will cause harm to a child. But we are right to worry about certain potential problems. Some may well try to "produce" a child in a certain way so as to predetermine and thus limit the child's future, as is currently the risk in artificial insemination by donor (AID) using sperm banks and in newly available commercial genetic tests claiming to determine intelligence and artistic and athletic ability in children (Inoue and Muto 2011). But not all parents will enhance their children in a way that limits their future, such as by making them one certain kind of person, a duplicate of a famous musician or of a tall athlete. Many parents will use genetic enhancement to open up a better future for the child, not a more limited one.

As to the fourth issue, we will worry about harming the genetic line, but as Gregory Pence points out in his book *Who's Afraid of Human Cloning?* (1998, 129–31), few people are actually likely to have access to this technique, so any harm will be minimal. We cannot at the same time argue that the technique is likely to endanger the entire human gene pool and say that it will be unfairly limited to the wealthy.

Regarding how we think of and treat the disabled, the fifth issue, although this is a real concern, it appears to most that this should not deter us from finding cures for injuries and diseases. Few of us would want to resist advances in birthing techniques in order not to diminish the number of children born with cerebral palsy, even though this decrease might well increase our sense of disquiet or even of aversion when we meet a person with this affliction.

Now there is one obvious way around the probable failure of these largely consequentialist ethical arguments to deter genetic engineering, and that is to simply forbid it deontologically. The act in itself could be said to be intrinsically evil. This, as we have seen, is the official teaching of the Catholic Church in the related area of reproductive technology. Any procedure that physically separates the sex act from zygote formation (the unitive from the procreative) is forbidden absolutely, apart from intention or effect. The magisterium has not to my knowledge done this relative to genetic engineering, even of the germ line enhancement variety, though many of the techniques to do this would likely violate the absolute proscription of separation of sex act from physical conception, as in IVF. In any case, many Catholic moral theologians, including the authors of this book, have argued against a deontology and physicalism of this kind.

But the question remains as to where to draw the genetic line. And here, although it does not give any easy answer to that question, is where the notion of property discourse, "commodification" (Radin [1987] 1992), or, to use language more familiar to theologians, the issue of resymbolization and revaluation of the human body and thus of ourselves, comes in. M. Cathleen Kaveny asks us to move beyond "the harm principle narrowly focused on tangible harms" and "attend to the embodied and social aspects of human nature" (Kaveny 1999, 140). It may be possible to argue that even if the more obvious bad effects can be reduced to where the good effects outweigh them, there remains this risky reduction of the valuation of ourselves to property. This is a kind of intrinsic consequentialism, which is, as we have noted in chapters 10 and 11, probably what most have in mind when they say they are proportionalists and not consequentialists. We need to worry about effects that are not quantifiable. We need to be concerned that certain kinds of human genetic engineering and gene patenting will inevitably change how we think about ourselves in ways that hurt us. There is at present an intuition that this is true, and this is probably why most people do not accept the idea of human reproductive cloning. But the intuition alone is not enough. It needs articulation in public discourse. As we develop our judgments on these issues, we need to think about the problem of property discourse.

Anthropological Considerations

We can turn now to the directly theological and anthropological issue of whether the human person is open or closed to self-manipulation. Each ethicist is likely to have a bias here toward one side or the other, toward "open" or "closed," a bias that he or she probably cannot adequately defend. And it seems true, as is detailed in chapter 5, that our theologizing about this, necessary as it is to the issue, will not lead directly to ethical judgments about specific procedures of human genetic engineering. It does, however, help set an anthropological context for those judgments by giving us herme-neutic themes and hints about how to interpret the meaning of human life. And this is an important start.

As an excellent example of how theology might work in this context, we will examine now in considerable detail two essays by German theologian Karl Rahner, considered by many to be the foremost Catholic theologian of the twentieth century.[1] The essays offer a fascinating look at this theologian's struggle with precisely this ques-tion. And they show how hard it is to be consistent when we try to work with our underlying anthropology in the context of specific bioethical issues.

The first essay, "The Experiment with Man," is largely an essay in theological anthropology (Rahner 1972a). It is cited in the ethical literature by Paul Ramsey, who attacks Rahner's approach to the possibilities of human self-creativity (Ramsey 1970,

139–43). Ramsey clearly thinks that the human person is "closed" to genetic manipulation, while Rahner's first essay sees us as "open." The essay is cited by James Gustafson in his comparison of his own "theocentric" ethic with Rahner's, which he sees as more "anthropocentric" (Gustafson 1984). The second essay, "The Problem of Genetic Manipulation," is unusual for Rahner because it analyzes a particular moral issue: genetic manipulation in the form of AID (Rahner 1972b). The two essays are found side by side in Rahner's *Theological Investigations*. They were both written and rewritten during 1966 and 1967 and are clearly connected; Rahner refers in the second to the first (ibid., 225n1). All this makes them a fascinating source for looking at how Rahner moves from anthropological principles to moral judgments (Modras 1984, 76n21). And that, in turn, sheds light on how theology works in bioethics.[2]

This section explores the anthropological approach Rahner takes to human self-manipulation in the first essay, and then describes the way in which he makes his moral analysis of genetic manipulation through AID, in the second. There is a considerable difference, even a startling difference, between the two essays. In the first Rahner argues that the human person is open to and should not be afraid of technological manipulation. But in the second he rejects as immoral one possible application of this openness, AID. The difference is due at least in part to a subtle change in Rahner's anthropology, which is the focus here. How does this great theologian actually apply theological anthropology to this ethical issue?

It is helpful to note briefly that the difference between the two essays is also due to normative and metaethical positions Rahner takes in the second essay. Normatively, Rahner introduces in the second essay, in which he rejects AID, the deontological normative moral principle we analyzed at length in chapter 11 on birth control, the principle that forbids the separation of procreation from the marital union. And metaethically Rahner notes in the second essay a kind of faith-intuitionist metaethical position he calls a "moralische Glaubensintinct," a "moral faith-instinct." This metaethical position implies that people of faith have some sort of special insight into these issues. Although this is not, for Rahner, the same as ecclesiastical positivism, in which ethical judgments are verified from the official decrees of the magisterium, it is not totally clear what it actually is. It is possible that Rahner, who wrote these essays in the 1960s, was influenced by Church authority, which had condemned AID. In chapter 10 we saw that the 1960s might be called a "transitional" period in Catholic moral theology, when authors changed their methodology from physicalism to personalism but were not yet ready to change their conclusions. One of the causes for this delay was respect for and submission to Church authority and a resulting tendency toward ecclesiastical positivism. Rahner's "moral faith-instinct" is not meant to be a type of ecclesiastical positivism, but this tendency of the transitional period to submit to official Church statements may explain at least in part Rahner's reluctance to carry through the "open" anthropology of the first essay to the issue of AID in the second. Like many other theologians of the time, he moved more quickly in areas of theory, where official pronouncements were less clear, than in actual moral application.

So normative and metaethical issues are among the reasons why Rahner condemns AID. But what we will concentrate on here is Rahner's use of anthropology. It seems that when he is faced with this actual ethical issue, an issue where he has come to judge a self-manipulative procedure to be wrong, there is a shift away from the usual emphasis he gives to the openness of the human person to self-creation and toward a more cautious and restrictive theological anthropology. Perhaps he was not himself aware of this shift. Drawing from this, we propose that bioethics is better served when ethicists know how principles from anthropology ought to be used, and we conclude the chapter by making again the suggestion made in chapter 5 as to how these principles ought to be used in bioethics.

Rahner's First Essay

In "The Experiment with Man," Rahner argues that Christians ought to be "cool-headed" when faced with the future of humanity. He states: "Man is fundamentally 'operable' and legitimately so. If this proposition, which we shall elucidate directly, is assumed, the first thing which the theologian must say to himself, to Christians and to the Church is that one is not to take fright at this self-manipulation of man" (Rahner 1972a, 210).

This sets the general tone of what will follow. Rahner thinks that our basic stance as Christians should be one of openness to the future. He goes on immediately to argue that this does not mean an automatic acceptance of all possible methods of self-manipulation. There are barbaric methods that must be rejected (ibid., 211). But he also argues that this danger should not lead Christians "to simply condemn the approaching age of self-manipulation as such; to break out into lyrical laments on the theme of degrading barbarity, the cold technological rationalism, the destruction of what is 'natural'" (ibid., 211). Rahner states: "And in this coming world man will be the one who, both as an individual and as a society, plans, controls, and manipulates himself to a degree which was previously both undreamed-of and impracticable. He *must do* so; he can do no other. . . . He must want to be 'operable man'" (ibid., 211, emphasis his). Christians need not anticipate this kind of a future either as "hell on earth [or] as an earthly kingdom of God" (ibid., 211). Human self-manipulation, at least considered in the abstract, will guarantee neither hell nor paradise.

Rahner's second theme continues the argument of the first. Self-determination, he says, is "the nature and task of man's freedom as understood by Christianity" (ibid., 212). He refers to Christian teaching on the possibility of ultimate salvation and ultimate loss of salvation. Our final destiny is something we ourselves make. We make it in dialogue with God or against God, and its preconditions are God's free creation and God's free grace, but we make it nonetheless.

Next Rahner tries to show how contemporary methods of self-manipulation are radically new in that for the first time they permit what used to be possible only on the level of transcendence—we choose our final or transcendent destiny and thus create ourselves—to be possible also on the "categorial" or historical level. It is the same thing, he says, but it is now possible more empirically and more visibly, and—at least as seen from within history—more permanently. "To a larger, more comprehensive, radical and tangible extent," Rahner says, "man has become what, according to the Christian understanding, he *is:* the free being who has been handed over to himself" (ibid., 214, emphasis his).

Rahner goes even further. He contends that modern humans who are able to create themselves in this new fashion are not only in accord with the Christian message but are the "*product* of Christianity" (ibid., 214, emphasis his). He says he cannot elaborate, but makes it clear that he is referring to Christianity's belief that humankind is created in God's image to have dominion over the world.

In a fourth section, Rahner treats of the problem of human nature. What is our "normative essence"? Who are we really? Here he again claims that the new methods of human self-manipulation may run contrary to that essence, but they need not do so. These categorial or historical "this-world" kinds of self-manipulation, says Rahner, despite their capacity for newly forming the human person himself or herself, are actually less total than the form of self-manipulation we Christians have always known we possess, the capacity to choose our eternal destiny for good or for evil. Nor is it easy to define precisely what is "natural" for people. There is good reason, then, to be slow in claiming to know what we are. Not everything technological or artificial or new is dehumanizing and unnatural.

In the fifth section, Rahner shows a more cautious side. He points out that historical decisions are serious and can well be irreversible. He argues against the facile notion that humans can undo any evil they perpetrate. He draws on the concept of original sin and insists that it is not abolished by redemption, and that it endures throughout human history. No self-manipulation can abolish the human state of original sin and its effects. There may well be irreparable negative consequences to humankind brought about by our self-manipulation.

In this essay, then, Rahner's emphasis is on the open-endedness of human nature. Since we are fundamentally open to our own self-manipulation on the transcendental, eternal level, we should not fear the new techniques that allow us to do it on the categorial, historical level. Caution is introduced because we might do it badly, but the impression is given that this does not mean we should fear doing it. It is to this that Paul Ramsey objected.

Rahner's Second Essay

The second essay, "The Problem of Genetic Manipulation," has a different tone. Ramsey did not know the second essay, and here he would have found a Rahner more to his liking. We will omit here any detailed analysis of Rahner's normative inseparability principle and metaethical faith-instinct and instead concentrate on his anthropology. In this context, where he wishes to oppose AID, his "man" is less open to categorial, historical self-manipulation. There is one confusing factor in this essay, however. Rahner may not completely understand the procedure he is talking about. He seems to include in it factors that might be, but need not be, connected with AID, such as the problem of sperm banks, the possibility of extramarital use, the legal problem of determining paternity, the issue of an artificial womb, and the question of a widespread use of AID for the genetic improvement of society as a whole (Rahner 1972b, 237). Rahner seems to reject all AID, not only those procedures where these factors are present. But it is not clear that he is aware that these factors might well be absent, and this ambiguity makes analysis difficult.

It is in the fifth and final section of this second essay that Rahner turns to anthropological considerations. Here we find a shift in emphasis within his anthropology.

Rahner begins with the thesis that "man must freely accept his nature as being predetermined. For he has not called *himself* into existence" (ibid., 243, emphasis his). There is a theological truth here. Humanity has not created itself. Nor, as Rahner points out, can it ever manipulate itself without using something already created. But there is also at the very least a shift in Rahner's emphasis within his anthropology. In the first essay, the emphasis was more on the idea that humans do and must manipulate ourselves. We are projects, we are operable, we create our own essence, we have no easily defined essential nature, and so on. Now he suggests that our nature is predetermined and that we must accept this freely. In the first essay we are open and must manipulate ourselves, although, of course, we should not manipulate ourselves in such a way as to leave us less open, less free, less human than we were. Now in the second essay we seem to be more "closed," predetermined.

This does not mean that Rahner is caught here in a contradiction. It is a question of emphasis. In this second essay, he continues to insist that the human person is open. But now there is a tendency to see us as so open that anything we might do, at least genetically, to manipulate ourselves would necessarily be destructive to that very transcendental openness. At the risk of oversimplification, Rahner now seems to be saying that we are so open as to be paradoxically closed to further opening; any attempt at genetic alteration would indeed limit us. As subject, it seems, we are open to transcendence. But we should never be the objects of our own genetic self-manipulation because such manipulation would close us off and would be a denial of our own humanity.

The ambiguity inherent in Rahner's identification of what kind of AID he is judging makes precise analysis difficult. Perhaps he is only saying what he said in the first essay, that any attempt at manipulating humans that does indeed reduce our transcendental openness is an immoral manipulation. If this is all he is saying here, there is no significant change in his theological anthropology. But it seems that he is saying more than this. He seems not to be at ease in the second essay with the anthropology he presented in the first. Here in the second essay the human person is anthropologically, as created by God, less open to self-manipulation than he or she was in the first essay.

Rahner argues that anyone involved in genetic manipulation by AID must hate his own destiny: "If man, when confronted with his child, saw only what he himself had planned, he would not be looking at his own nature, nor would he experience his true self which is both free *and* the object of external [he means divine] determination. Genetic manipulation is the embodiment of the fear of oneself, the fear of accepting one's self as the unknown quantity it is" (ibid., 245, emphasis his).

Now this is too simple. Does a couple who practice AID hate or fear their own free nature? Do they "make" a child as a product of predetermined kind? Not necessarily, as demonstrated by personal experience in Paul Lauritzen's *Pursuing Parenthood* (1993). Must all self-manipulation of this technological sort come from self-fear? If this is Rahner's axiom here, then how is this compatible with his anthropological approach in the first essay, and even in the opening sections of the second essay, where technological self-manipulation cannot be judged a priori since the human person is, as created by God, open to such self-manipulation and self-creation? One can make a similar critique of Rahner's deontological use of his normative principle forbidding the "fundamental" separation of procreation from the marital union. If technological, categorial self-manipulation of the human person cannot be rejected a priori, then how can a principle that does just that, at least in the context of procreation, be accepted? This kind of rejection does not seem to harmonize with the anthropology of the first essay.

From Rahner's essays we are led again to conclude that it is hard to know what to do with anthropological themes when we want to apply them to bioethical issues. Yet, as we saw in chapter 5, it is consistent with the mystery of human life that theological principles and themes from theological anthropology cut both ways (Verhey 1997, 68). They tell us that we are both creatures and coagents, called both to accept suffering and to reduce it. Some of us tend to one side, some to the other. This is the way theological anthropology ought to work. The proper place for anthropological principles in theological health care ethics is not as ethical rules that can answer specific health care questions but as hermeneutic themes that help in interpreting the meaning of the human person. They serve not so much in the context of specific moral issues—is this procedure right or wrong?—as in the context of the "biosignificance question": What is the meaning of human life?

Principles of theological anthropology, when seen as hermeneutic themes within the context of the biosignificance question, serve to confront us with the mysteries that underlie the dilemmas of moral theology. Theological principles cannot solve these ethical questions. Instead, they contribute to theological health care ethics precisely by denying to us the always tempting escape of ethical shortcuts. By refusing to permit facile judgments, theological anthropological principles as hermeneutic themes recall the mystery of humankind.

Conclusion

This chapter reviews some of the general ethical issues and, in a more focused way, the theological-anthropological aspects of genetic engineering. It suggests the need to be cautious in this area.[3] This is both because of the ethical concerns noted in the first section of the chapter and because of the anthropological concerns developed in the second. The bridge between them is the worry about turning ourselves into property. Rahner is surely right when he says we should not manipulate ourselves in ways that will make us less free, less human, less who we are as God creates us to be. This manipulation is most likely if we use genetic technologies for germ line enhancement. It is less likely if we limit these technologies to therapeutic uses for the curing of genetic defects and diseases. There is no reason to condemn all genetic engineering as usurping God's role, as "playing God," and the use of theological themes proposed here would not permit this. But theology does tell us much about ourselves, and this knowledge ought to make us worry about the risks genetic engineering poses to who we are. We can now turn, in the next chapter, to more specific procedures in genetics and to the ethical questions they pose.

Notes

1. For further development of this, see Kelly 1995.

2. For an analysis of the two Rahner essays in the context of a specifically theological assessment of genetic manipulation, see Mahoney 2003, 730–33.

3. For a philosophical analysis critical of the "cautious approach" taken here, see Powell 2010.

CHAPTER 27

SPECIFIC ISSUES IN GENETICS

Introduction

THE PREVIOUS CHAPTER discusses the relation between ethics and anthropology as a foundation for exploring bioethics discourse on genetics. Discussing principles of theological anthropology as hermeneutic themes helps us interpret dilemmas in genetics within the context of the mystery of humankind. This chapter moves from that general approach to a more practical perspective that considers some of the major ethical dilemmas related to genetics. Of course, there is an abundance of specific issues that could be discussed, especially in the wake of sequencing the human genome at the turn of the millennium (Sloan 2000). The topics in this chapter provide a practical introduction to pivotal issues in the fast-moving field of human genetics.

Using Frozen Embryos for Genetic Research

Cell lines developed from spare IVF embryos can be immensely productive for medical research about genetics. The use of spare IVF embryos for research is mentioned in chapter 25. We explain there that cell lines have been developed from embryonic stem cells obtained by destroying these spare embryos. Two points need to be kept in mind. First, a great deal of good can arise from the research undertaken on these cell lines. Also, the principle of material cooperation can be used to justify ongoing research on these cell lines, akin to legitimately developing vaccines from fetal tissue from abortions that occurred decades ago. Second, for those who treat the human embryo as a person from the time of fertilization, killing spare embryos for research is forbidden. Official Catholic teaching defends the human embryo from fertilization and opposes its destruction, even for noble purposes such as medical research. Both of these points can take on new significance in light of recent developments in IVF procedures. This chapter explains that a new standard of practice in IVF procedures can avoid the problem of killing embryos when harvesting their stem cells. Concomitantly, there is no ethical dilemma about ongoing research on the cell lines developed from these legitimately obtained embryonic stem cells.

We suggest that official Catholic teaching may be able after all to support using spare IVF embryos for medical research. The argument is not that great good can result from using these embryos that will otherwise die, although this argument can be made from secular perspectives (e.g., Guenin 2008) and from religious perspectives (e.g,

Peters, Lebacqz, and Bennet 2010). Official Catholic teaching does not permit doing what is perceived to be intrinsically wrong (killing spare IVF embryos to obtain their embryonic stem cells) no matter what good results. Rather, the argument is that the process of procuring embryonic stem cells may be able to occur after the embryo has died. The analogy is that we can licitly procure organs after a patient dies. To understand such an argument, three distinct but related points need to be made (Magill 2008).

The first point is discussed in chapter 25. It is legitimate in official Catholic teaching to let frozen spare IVF embryos thaw to die. The underlying principle here is that patients may be allowed to die when continued life support is morally extraordinary, as we saw in many earlier chapters: extraordinary or disproportionate means are not obligatory to maintain life. This ethical principle is clearly taught by the US bishops in the *Ethical and Religious Directives for Health Care Services*: "A person may forgo extraordinary or disproportionate means of preserving life. Disproportionate means are those that in the patient's judgment do not offer a reasonable hope of benefit or entail an excessive burden" (USCCB 2009a, no. 57). As we have seen in detail in chapter 13, the use of the preposition "or" in the phrase "benefit or . . . burden" is crucial: there may be insufficient benefit OR there may be excessive burden. In contrast, a much higher ethical standard pertains for determining that a treatment is ordinary or proportionate, and hence obligatory—there must be sufficient benefit AND no excessive burden: "Proportionate means are those that in the judgment of the patient offer a reasonable hope of benefit and do not entail an excessive burden" (ibid., no. 56).

In other words, when life-sustaining treatment is deemed to be morally extraordinary, life support such as medically assisted feeding may be withdrawn to let a patient die. In the case of frozen IVF embryos, cryopreservation is their life support. Hence, when it is clear that the embryos will not be implanted in a womb, it is morally permissible to let them thaw and die. Withdrawing life support in such cases, either from the patient or from the frozen embryo, does not constitute killing: the patient or embryo is allowed to die when continuing life-sustenance is morally extraordinary. In situations where consent cannot be elicited from the dying, it is sufficient to obtain consent from the patient's representative or from the parents of the embryo. It is worth highlighting the teaching of the US bishops on the meaning of disproportionate means to preserve life: they permit either insufficient benefit OR excessive burden. In the case of the frozen embryo, it can be argued that continuing cryopreservation would be an excessive burden, not least from the standpoint of cost. After all, when the bishops refer to "excessive burden" they include "excessive expense on the family or the community" (ibid., nos. 56 and 57). In other words, official Catholic teaching can be understood as permitting the removal of spare frozen IVF embryos from cryopreservation to let them thaw and die.

The second point is related to the dying process of the thawing embryo. Organs can be procured (for transplantation or for research) from the body of a person who has died. Similarly, embryonic stem cells can be procured from the embryo after it dies in the thawing process. Of course, the difficulty is knowing when a thawing embryo is dead to justify taking its embryonic stem cells.

There are two issues that need to be noted here. On the one hand, when organs are procured from a deceased patient, it is because the organs remain viable biologically for a limited period after the patient dies. Similarly, embryonic stem cells remain viable biologically for a limited period after the embryo dies. Just as licit organ procurement does not kill the patient, embryonic stem cells can be procured in a manner that does not kill the embryo. On the other hand, it is difficult to determine when an embryo dies in the thawing process. However, it is also difficult to reach agreement about criteria of death for patients, as we saw in chapter 18. A great deal has been written about cardiopulmonary criteria and brain death criteria, especially as they relate to transplant-ation ethics (e.g., Veatch 2000). The national discussion over defining death effectively started in the United States with the Harvard Medical School's definition of death (Harvard Medical School 1968). The policy debate picked up pace with the 1980 Uni-form Determination of Death Act (President's Commission 1981; Gervais 1986; Zaner 1988) and increased over subsequent decades (Lizza 2006, 2009; Lock, 2002; Munson 2002; Potts, Byrne, and Nigles 2000; Wijdicks 2001; Youngner, Arnold, and Shapiro 1999; Youngner, Anderson, and Shapiro 2004). The debate continues robustly today (President's Council on Bioethics 2008). In particular, recent developments in the neu-rological determination of death contribute to the increased interest in neuroethics (Glannon 2007; Illes 2006; Racine 2010). Perhaps the most complex debate on death criteria today for transplantation surgery is the practice of "donation after cardiac death" (DCD), or non-heart-beating organ transplantation.[1] However, the critical issue for our discussion is that in general the legitimacy of organ procurement is based upon identifying the point of irreversibility after which the patient cannot be recovered. Recent developments enable us to identify the point of irreversibility at which the embryo cannot be recovered.

The third point deals with embryogenesis and IVF standards of practice. When IVF started many decades ago, the fertilized egg that was frozen was typically a three-day embryo. Three days is before embryonic stem cells have developed, which occurs in the five-day blastocyst. From the perspective of official Catholic teaching, it would be diffi-cult to justify using these three-day embryos to procure embryonic stem cells. To do so, the three-day frozen embryo would need to be thawed from cryopreservation and then cultivated in a petri dish until it has developed into a five-day blastocyst with embryonic stem cells. This would require cultivating an embryo to then let it die (in the process of procuring its embryonic stem cells).

However, over recent years researchers have discovered that a five-day blastocyst better implants in the womb after being thawed from cryopreservation (Papanikolaou 2006; Schieve 2006; Thurin et al. 2004). Moreover, human embryonic stem cell lines can be more efficiently derived from frozen five-day blastocysts than from cultivating earlier embryos (Cowen 2004). Hence, the new standard of practice in IVF clinics is to let the spare fertilized eggs grow in the petri dish to become five-day blastocysts before being frozen in a cryopreservation tank. This means that when they are subsequently thawed they have embryonic stem cells already developed. In this case they do not need to be subsequently cultivated before being permitted to die. This is an important point. The five-day frozen embryo that is allowed to thaw and die is just like the patient from whom life-sustaining interventions are withdrawn. In each case, life-sustaining measures are deemed to be futile and are legitimately withdrawn to let the blastocyst and patient die. Also, just as the patient has organs that continue to be viable after death, the blastocyst's embryonic stem cells continue to be viable after death.

Given these similarities, the crucial question is what constitutes death for the blastocyst. Obviously, neither brain death criteria nor cardiopulmonary criteria pertain. What is important is to be able to determine the point of irreversibility. Fortunately, the point of irreversibility can be identified in the thawing process of the human blastocyst, the five-day embryo that has embryonic stem cells. A cell marker can be identified as an objective criterion or operational definition (equivalent to brain death criteria) that indicates the irreversible arrest of cell integration in the embryo: the thawing blastocyst has lost its capacity for integrated cellular division, growth, and differentiation (Landry and Zucker 2004). This discovery complements a previous pathway used to determine irreversibility. That previous determination was based upon the natural history of embryonic death: arrested development at the multicellular stage indicates irreversible loss of integrated organic function (Landry et al. 2006). Hence, there are now two ways to determine the point of irreversibility in the dying process of an embryo. At the point of irreversibility, the blastocyst's embryonic stem cells remain viable for a short period of time. This window of time makes the stem cells eligible for procurement (Heng et al. 2006).

Thus, three distinct but related points permit procuring the embryonic stem cells from spare IVF frozen embryos (Magill 2008). First, the ethical principle of justifiably removing extraordinary life-sustaining measures to let a patient die also pertains to the frozen embryo: cryopreservation can be ended to let the embryo thaw and die. Second, the ethical principle of procuring donated organs from a dead patient also pertains to the frozen blastocyst: the embryonic stem cells can be procured legitimately after the embryo dies. Third, there is a molecular marker in a dying blastocyst to identify the point of irreversibility before the embryonic stem cells lose their viability, just as organs remain viable for a limited time after a patient dies.

In sum, these points allow us to conclude that retrieving stem cells is consistent with official Catholic teaching: removing the embryo to thaw and die is not the same as killing it; procuring embryonic stem cells is akin to procuring organs from a patient after death; finally, there are adequate scientific criteria of death in each case, for the patient and for the embryo, that specifies the point at which viable organs or embryonic stem cells can be licitly procured. This argument can make a significant contribution to genetics insofar as official Catholic teaching might be able to permit this use of frozen spare IVF embryos. That permissibility pertains both to procuring the embryonic stem cells and to developing cell lines or colonies from the original cells for future research and therapy.

Of course, this argument does not change the prohibition in official Catholic teaching concerning the IVF process that creates embryos in fertility clinics. It is this prohibited IVF process that leads to the reality of many spare or unwanted embryos after the genetic parents decide not to have other children. Nonetheless, the three points in the earlier argument about using frozen embryos for medical research are consistent with official Church teaching as it currently stands. The argument does not require a development of doctrine in this sense: the current prohibition by the Church is based on the assumption that obtaining embryonic stem cells necessarily involves killing the embryo; the procedure described here does not kill the embryo. Hence, it is licit according to principles currently adopted by official Catholic teaching.

In contrast, a different debate related to spare IVF embryos may require the development of doctrine in Church teaching, the debate over implantation of spare IVF embryos in a host mother as an early form of adoption. It is clear from *Donum vitae* that Church teaching forbids surrogacy (CDF 1987). An example of surrogacy is implanting a fertilized egg of genetic parents in a host womb (not the genetic mother's womb). That process occurs in "embryo adoption," although some conservative scholars argue that the moral meaning of surrogacy is not involved (May 2008; Mayer 2011). The rationale for embryo adoption using spare frozen IVF embryos is that they will otherwise die. The moral context, then, is rescue ethics. This context contrasts with the fertility context considered in the original prohibition of surrogacy (e.g., using a surrogate when the genetic mother is not able to carry the embryo). Despite the different moral contexts, debate continues as to whether a development of doctrine is needed or would occur. Official Church teaching in *Dignitas personae* voices caution on the matter, even though embryo adoption could rescue hundreds of thousands and potentially millions of frozen IVF embryos otherwise destined to die (Furton 2010; Grabowski and Gross 2010; Jamison 2010; Tollefsen 2010).

Another related debate about IVF will be increasingly important as the field of genetics becomes more sophisticated in the years ahead. Just as with embryo adoption, this debate would require the development of doctrine in official Catholic teaching. The debate deals with preimplantation genetic diagnosis and genetic therapy that requires IVF procedures. We have seen that the context of rescue ethics can lead to a development of Church teaching about surrogacy so that IVF embryos can be adopted. Perhaps the context of embryo health can lead to a development of Church teaching on using IVF for genetic therapy, a process that would require preimplantation genetic diagnosis. This is the topic of the next section.

Preimplantation Genetic Diagnosis

The Church prohibits IVF in clear and unambiguous terms, as is clear in *Donum vitae* (CDF 1987). Nonetheless, Catholic moral theologians have disputed aspects of this teaching (e.g., Shannon and Cahill 1988). Perhaps the field of genetics will lead the Church to consider doctrinal development when IVF is undertaken within the moral context of the health of the embryo rather than in the moral context of the infertility of parents. The Church's prohibition of IVF was made in the context of parental infertility.

Official Catholic teaching in *Donum vitae* forbids IVF because of the separation of the unitive and the procreative aspects of marital intimacy (CDF 1987). However, *Donum vitae* (sec. 2) supports prenatal diagnosis as being morally licit provided it deals with therapeutic, medical, or surgical procedures to benefit the future baby. Naturally, this stance assumes there are no disproportionate risks and there is the consent of the parents. Any abortion chosen as a result of prenatal diagnosis, such as aborting embryos that are malformed or that have hereditary illness, is absolutely prohibited. What the Vatican is referring to here is prenatal diagnosis of the fetus as it develops in the womb. In light of this teaching, what would official Catholic teaching say about preimplantation genetic diagnosis that occurs before implantation in the womb?

In theory, because Church teaching supports prenatal diagnosis, it should also support preimplantation diagnosis, adopting the same criteria mentioned earlier. However, the technological difference between preimplantation and prenatal diagnosis seems to prevent the Church from approving the former. This is because preimplantation genetic diagnosis typically occurs in the petri dish using the process of IVF to fertilize the egg, a process that is forbidden by Church teaching. To clarify the moral landscape of preimplantation genetic diagnosis as a topic for the potential development of Church teaching, a case example is enlightening.

The case of Molly and Adam Nash is a classic example of preimplantation genetic diagnosis. This was the first documented success of what is referred to as a savior sibling (Magill 2002). The Nash parents gave birth to baby Adam by using IVF for the process of preimplantation diagnosis to ameliorate the genetic condition of an elder sibling, Molly. This six-year-old girl suffered from Fanconi anemia, a relatively rare genetic disorder that tends to kill by age seven because of the lack of bone marrow. Fortunately, a bone marrow or stem cell transplant from a matching sibling has a high success rate. But Molly had no matching sibling. Hence, Molly's parents opted to have another child, leading to the birth of Adam. The process involved using IVF for preimplantation diagnosis and included discarding some embryos that were not a good match. After Adam was born his umbilical cord blood and stem cells were transplanted to Molly. There was a successful outcome for Molly and no harm was caused to the newborn Adam. In general, ensuring the ongoing welfare of the so-called savior sibling is crucially important in this debate (Wilkinson 2010). More particularly, the moral debate for official Catholic teaching revolves around several dilemmas.

One issue that might seem problematic is not insurmountable—the issue of a child or newborn to assist with the health of a sibling. Provided that no substantive harm occurs to the donating sibling, donation can be justified with parental consent and clinical approval. However, attention must be given to the extent of the sibling's donation: stem cells at birth are less invasive than blood donation as a baby, which in turn is less invasive than bone marrow donation. Of course, when and why parents decide to have children is a related but distinct moral issue, although the crucial matter is that the parents must want to have the baby for its own sake.

There are three dilemmas that must be addressed about preimplantation diagnosis from the perspective of Catholic teaching. The first moral question deals with the likelihood of therapeutic success with the process of preimplantation genetic diagnosis, such as was used in the Nash case. The procedure is called single-cell embryo biopsy at the eight-cell stage. One cell (a blastomere) is removed for genetic testing. The remaining cells in the embryo appear to accommodate this loss of a single cell and the embryo typically develops properly. Since this successful case with the Nash family, many other births involving preimplantation genetic diagnosis have occurred safely. Estimates of successful births now number more than one thousand in the United States, indicating that the therapeutic success of the procedure is well established (Cohen 2007).

The second moral question deals with the fate of the spare embryos created in the process. In the Nash case, the genetic diagnosis at the eight-cell stage was to ensure not only that there was a match for Molly but also that the embryo did not carry Molly's genetic disorder. As a result, some of the embryos that were created were discarded. This raises the question of the moral status of the early embryo in this process (Panicola et al. 2011, 204–8). From the perspective of official Catholic teaching, discarding human embryos is not permitted.

The third moral question deals with the process of preimplantation genetic diagnosis that requires IVF, which Church teaching forbids because it separates the unitive and procreative aspects of marriage (for the origin of and the controversy about this principle, see chapter 11). These three questions highlight the issues that must be addressed if there might be the possibility of doctrinal development in Church teaching regarding preimplantation genetic diagnosis. The development of teaching pertains not only to using current technology to treat a sibling as in the Nash case. The development of teaching also pertains to future technology for repairing or replacing genes prior to implanting an embryo.

Future technology will be capable of genetic therapy on the embryo prior to implantation. It is feasible that development of Catholic teaching may support this because of the medical context of undertaking IVF to treat the embryo for a genetic disorder (Repenshek 2011). However, the standard distinction between somatic cell and germ line gene therapy (Deane-Drummond 2006; Shannon and Kockler 2009; Walters and Palmer 1997) will need to be further explored at this early stage of embryogenesis. Two assumptions might be made: that gene therapy can occur upon the embryo in a reliably successful manner (the first point); and that future technology will avoid the problem of discarding embryos (the second point). In light of these assumptions, the pivotal question for the development of Church teaching will be whether the IVF process may be acceptable in the moral context of the health of the embryo (the third point). This means interpreting IVF within the moral context of embryonic genetic therapy in contrast to the context of parental infertility. However, in each context the separation of the unitive and procreative components of marital intimacy will continue. The crucial question, then, will be whether future technology to provide genetic therapy for embryos will justify doctrinal development in Church teaching on IVF, and therefore on the application of the inseparability principle.

The two topics we have discussed thus far (obtaining embryonic stem cells for research and using preimplantation genetic interventions for therapy) set the stage for many other forms of developments in genetics. These two topics raise important questions about official Church teaching and its doctrinal development to keep pace with breakthroughs in biotechnology. Closely related to the topic of preimplantation genetic diagnosis is another issue in genetics that causes consternation for official Catholic teaching, the practice of selective reproduction.

Selective Reproduction

The ethical debate on selective reproduction has many interrelated components. These are discussed within the context of avoiding genetic disorders or choosing specific traits for offspring such as gender (President's Council on Bioethics 2004). The concept of selective reproduction here refers to the creation of a child through gamete or embryo selection: one child is more desirable than another possible child for a variety of reasons (Wilkinson 2010). Of course, a less sophisticated and less reliable approach is sperm selection. In secular bioethics there is extensive support for using selective reproduction, using preimplantation genetic diagnosis, to avoid genetic disease in the offspring.

We have seen that official Catholic teaching opposes any technology that discards embryos that are not selected for implantation, as often occurs in selective reproduction. Official Catholic teaching also opposes the process of in vitro fertilization to create these embryos, a process that is typically needed for selective reproduction. Because the practice of selective reproduction is pervasive, it is important to consider the controversial aspects of the debate in secular discourse, even though official Catholic Church teaching prohibits the practice. Catholic ethicists may increasingly encounter these requests from patients and should be familiar with the main issues involved.

The controversial debates in secular bioethics about selective reproduction relate to the choice of specific traits for offspring. There are different reasons for choosing traits. A brief look at the major issues can convey the complexity of this reproductive procedure. The ethical concerns are to avoid a subtle form of evolutionary eugenics and the commodification of human beings. With regard to eugenics, the idea of selecting out genetic disorders can be intended for human flourishing. That genetic process can be undertaken in a voluntary manner based on legitimate criteria of health, such as to eliminate diseases or defects. When that occurs, secular bioethics construes this as legitimate and distinguishes it from the malicious forms of eugenics that seek racial purity, such as occurred in the Nazi holocaust. With regard to commodification, there can be no justification for using human beings merely as instruments. Secular bioethics typically recognizes that children should not be treated as commodities in the sense of perceiving them as merely instrumental. They cannot be treated as mere means to other, albeit laudable, ends.

One major category for selective reproduction is the gender of the future child. This aspect of the debate over gender selection can be illustrated by a controversy in Britain, the Masterton case in 1999. The parents had five children, four boys and one girl. Sadly, their girl Nicole died at the age of three in a tragic bonfire accident. The parents approached the relevant British oversight body, the Human Fertilisation and Embryology Authority (HFEA), to request gender selection for their next baby to ensure that they would have a girl. Their petition was denied on the grounds that it involved gender selection for family balancing and not for avoiding sex-linked disorders; only the latter is permissible for selective reproduction via gamete or embryo selection in Britain. There is more flexibility for such decisions in the United States, which has less centralized oversight of selective reproduction. Nonetheless, the case highlights the ethical debate over gender selection for the purpose of family balancing. There are two major concerns in this controversy. One concern deals with causing a population or demographic imbalance based on gender selection. The other concern deals with the potential for gender discrimination that could foster sexist prejudices in society (HFEA 2002, 2003).

Another controversial category for selective reproduction in secular discourse is selecting for disability in which the technology is used to choose a child with a disability. There can be populations with disability in which the parents want their child to be like them, such as being deaf or blind. This option can involve the opposite practice of discarding embryos that have been diagnosed as having genetic disorders. Here, the embryo with a desired disability, such as blindness or deafness, is selected for reproduction; normal embryos are discarded.

The debate in this controversy deals with two contrasting points. First, there is the future claim of a child to be as healthy as possible regarding its quality of life and its capacity to flourish (Glover 2006). This point is often expressed in terms of avoiding a life not worth living, or being better off not being born, or making death preferable (Buchanan et al. 2000). Second, there is the use of biotechnology to cause the cultural disappearance from society of communities such as the blind and deaf. Understandably, these communities resist such interventions (Stark 2006). It is certainly debatable how the traditional goals of medicine can be applied here. The goals of medicine usually are aligned with healing the sick and relieving suffering (Pellegrino and Thomasma 1981). The question is whether those traditional goals can justify the eventual disappearance of these populations or cultures (such as blind or deaf communities) that are characterized as having preventable genetic disorders.

Not all developments in genetics cause such complex controversy. The next topic deals with an issue that elicits widespread support. Nonetheless, there are moral dilemmas involved that need to be resolved as biotechnology enhances the capabilities of newborn genetic screening.

Newborn Genetic Screening

A routine intervention of genetic science in health care today is newborn genetic screening. The World Health Organization has been involved with the practice of newborn genetic screening for a long time (Wilson and Jungner 1968). These screening programs are mandatory across the United States, although only a few genetic disorders are mandated for screening in all states. There is considerable debate about the extent of parental consent needed for public health programs that involve newborn babies. Currently, parental consent is not required. There is no doubt that great good is accomplished by the genetic screening technologies. A brief explanation of the medical landscape can clarify the issues that elicit ethical debate.

Newborn genetic screening programs began in the mid-1960s when a simple blood test was developed for phenylketonuria (PKU). This genetic metabolic disorder that causes mental retardation can be prevented by a special diet started in the first ten days after birth. Dr. Robert Guthrie developed the blood test, and his name has been thereafter associated with these tests, called Guthrie tests. Guthrie cards provide a vast collection of genetic material for the population, and they provide a comprehensive resource to study population prevalence for allele frequencies about genes that interest researchers. The general purpose of newborn screening programs for genetic disorders is to identify conditions for which timely intervention can prevent mortality, morbidity, and disability. These interventions include diagnostic services as well as short- and long-term treatment and management of the diagnosed disorder. Currently in the United States, all states and the District of Columbia mandate newborn genetic screening for PKU, sickle cell disease, congenital hypothyroidism, and galactosemia. In addition, there are proposals to introduce genetic screening programs in all the states for these disorders: cystic fibrosis, Duchenne muscular dystrophy, medium-chain acyl-CoA dehydrogenase deficiency (MCAD), and severe combined immunodeficiency.

There have been several crucial studies of these public health programs to enhance newborn genetic screening nationally, including a comprehensive report by the American Academy of Pediatrics and the Health Resources and Service Administration (Newborn Screening Task Force 2000); an NIH report providing guidelines for oversight of testing procedures (Secretary's Advisory Committee on Genetic Testing 2000); and a report from the American College of Medical Genetics listing the genetic conditions for which testing should occur in all states (American College of Medical Genetics 2006). This report shifted focus of newborn screening programs from the immediate benefit for the child to include the long-term benefit for the family and for society.

An example of the benefit for families is providing genetic information that is relevant for making future reproductive decisions. Another example is avoiding what is known as the diagnostic or treatment odyssey. The treatment odyssey involves a cluster of activities that become expensive and ineffective: parents seek vast amounts of medical information online, they obtain multiple medical opinions, they incur substantive debt, and they surround their child with high-tech medical care; all this occurs only to have their child die early in life. An example of the benefit for society is the identification of subjects for research to study genetic disorders that are currently untreatable.

A multiyear effort by the Hastings Center researched the origin and treatment of genetic conditions (Baily and Murray 2009). The Hastings Center report focused upon four criteria that represent mainstream ethics discourse on public policy for newborn genetic screening. The policy must be evidence-based; it must consider the opportunity cost of the screening program; it must distribute costs and benefits fairly; and it must respect human rights. These ethical criteria are likely to guide public policy about newborn genetic screening programs for the foreseeable future.

One of the most significant policy issues will be the development of a national database that stores and uses the information from newborn genetic screening. In chapter 24 on organizational ethics we discuss the need to develop a comprehensive national program to enhance patient safety by creating a centralized database for the confidential reporting of medical errors and adverse events. The idea is to enhance patient safety consistently across health care. With regard to newborn genetic screening, there is need for a similar type of program with national outreach. This program is in the early stages of development.

At the moment, all newborn babies have a small amount of blood drawn from the heel to create what are known as long bloodspots that can be stored. Tandem mass spectrometry has increased the detection capability for metabolic conditions from these blood samples: this technology is already used in testing for PKU and MCAD. The increased use of DNA-based technologies such as gene chips and microarrays will continue to increase our understanding of the disease-gene relationship from a single blood sample. These bloodspots contain a vast amount of genetic information about each newborn. Some of that information can be helpful immediately when specific genetic disorders can be identified and treated effectively.

But because the bloodspots can be stored for extended periods, the genetic information they carry could be a burden as well as a benefit. The beneficial contribution deals with the population algorithms that can be developed nationally about genetic traits and profiles. These population approaches could be useful for designing health programs decades ahead. For example, future genetic testing on stored bloodspots could become much more sophisticated. That information could enable future health plan-ners to design cost-effective programs that address the emergence of ailments affecting different groups in an aging demographic.

But there are also problems. It is true that newborn blood samples can provide reliable genetic information about future medical conditions. Examples are adult-onset conditions and the genetic predisposition to disease. Often there is no current treat-ment. In such circumstances, the information could impose an emotional burden upon individuals. What should patients do when there is no anticipated treatment for future diseases that they are likely to incur? And there is some doubt whether a reliable guar-antee can be provided that patient identifiers have been removed from this genetic information. Patients fear that they could be exposed to discrimination long after birth, such as by future employers and insurance companies. Significant safeguards are needed to prevent the illicit discovery of health profiles created from newborn genetic screening.

Nonetheless, it should be feasible to develop a national health information system that ensures confidentiality or anonymity of personal genetic data. That system needs to be transparent. It needs to be designed to elicit the public's trust. Such a system could be used to genetically track population health in a manner that generates ade-quate programs for demographic needs across generations. In principle, official Cath-olic teaching can accept newborn genetic screening for this population approach. However, such a system-oriented endeavor toward population health is far from being developed in a reliable fashion. Hence, the current focus in newborn genetic screening programs will continue to be upon providing health interventions for the immediate needs of the newborn. Also, in principle, official Catholic teaching accepts newborn genetic screening to provide treatments and therapies to newborns.

When discussing the previous topics in genetics, we included the official teaching of the Catholic Church. However, it is unlikely that the Church will be able to present a specific teaching on every future discovery and breakthrough. This will be the case especially as the hectic pace of development in the biotechnology world occurs at the molecular level in regenerative medicine. As we consider topics in regenerative medicine in the following section, we do not engage Catholic doctrine insofar as there has been no official teaching on the issues discussed. Nonetheless, the theological anthropology of the Catholic tradition can continue to enlighten these issues in genetics as regenera-tive medicine challenges old assumptions in health care and inspires exciting new biotechnologies.

Regenerative Medicine

The promise and hopes of regenerative medicine have escalated due to the break-throughs in genetics and the human genome (Collins 2010). The science of genetics can be distinguished from the human genome in this manner. The genome within the nucleus of every bodily cell refers to the totality of genetic information contained within the cell. The science of genetics examines mechanisms that enable traits to pass across generations and be expressed in individuals. Based on the classical genetics of Gregor Mendel in the mid-nineteenth century, the basic laws of genetic heredity had been worked out by the mid-twentieth century.

In 1953 the focus on the human genome effectively began with the discovery of the structure of DNA (deoxyribonucleic acid) as a molecule whose intertwined strands constitute the famous double helix (Watson and Crick 1953). The spiraling double helix of DNA is like a twisting rope ladder whose rungs are composed of a series of base pairs folding around proteins in tight coils. The base pairs are A and T, and C and G: adenine, thymine, cytosine, and guanine. A paired set of genes is required for a trait or disorder to be present. This discovery meant that DNA molecules from different organisms could be combined, creating what is known as recombinant DNA (rDNA). This capacity to manipulate DNA led to the Human Genome Initiative that was started in 1990.

By the start of this millennium the sequencing of the human genome was effectively completed. Its success resulted from collaboration between the International Human Genome Sequencing Consortium (including the US government and the Wellcome Trust, a medical foundation in Great Britain), led by Dr. Francis Collins, and the private corporation Celera Genomics, led by Dr. J. Craig Venter (Lander et al. 2001; Venter et al. 2001). Mapping the human genome meant deciphering and arranging the chemical letters of DNA in the correct sequence. Metaphorically, the significance of the map of the human genome can be portrayed in terms of being the "holy grail" of regenerative medicine in this sense: the map will enable science to understand the molecular pathogenesis of disease and disorders and to develop effective treatments and therapies. These anticipated discoveries will focus especially on the interaction between genomics (how genes work) and proteomics (how proteins function).

A decade has passed since the human genome was sequenced. There is now a realistic expectation that within the next five years the sequencing of any individual's genome might be possible at a cost of one thousand dollars. This achievement will complicate ethics considerably. Patients will be able to discover information about their health that could be very confusing. On the one hand, patients will be faced with the complex problem of calculating probabilities of future disorders that are carried in families. If one family member is diagnosed with a genetic condition that is hereditary, the information may be of interest to the entire family. The ethical issues over consent and shared information will be prominent here. On the other hand, the business of predictive genetic testing is likely to mushroom. This will occur despite the lack of effective treatments and therapies for conditions that could arise years later, such as late-onset conditions. The ethical issues concerning the commercialization of genetic information will also be important here. Moreover, the discipline of genetic counseling will have to develop significantly to remain updated with the cascading issues that likely will result from these advances.

Hopefully, regulatory oversight of developments in genetics will continue to advance briskly to keep up with new and popular technologies such as the one thousand genome test. A brief look at the history of this oversight helps us to grasp the ongoing need for policy and ethical accountability as biotechnology speeds forward.

The first step to provide regulatory oversight of genetic research in the United States occurred at a conference in February 1975 at Asilomar in California. The molecular biologists in attendance at the conference voluntarily restricted experiments with rDNA. Their caution was based on safety issues such as the potential to release new organisms. A consensus statement was submitted to NIH. In the previous year, NIH had established the Recombinant DNA Advisory Committee (RAC). In the early 1980s the President's Commission for the Study of Ethical Problems in Medicine and Behavioral Research studied these issues and published a pivotal report, *Splicing Life* (President's Commission 1982). The report called upon RAC to develop ethical protocols for experiments involving gene transfers. Then, in 1994, RAC provided guidelines that, with some subsequent amendments, remain in effect today (RAC 1994). In other words, gene transfer research is regulated robustly, as is discussed extensively in the report by the President's Council on reproduction and responsibility (President's Council on Bioethics 2004).

The first gene therapy experimental protocol was presented to the Human Gene Therapy Subcommittee in September 1990. However, nearly a decade later, the death of Jesse Gelsinger in September 1999 in a gene therapy experiment caused enormous alarm and elicited widespread caution. Gelsinger was an eighteen-year-old teenager with an X-linked genetic disease of the liver caused by a genetic mutation and whose symptoms were being otherwise managed. He died of multiple organ failure within a few days of receiving gene therapy. His death was caused by a severe immune reaction to an experimental adenoviral vector that carried a corrected gene to deliver the experimental therapy. The FDA temporarily closed all gene research protocols at the University of Pennsylvania where the death occurred. The government's subsequent inquiry uncovered three major issues: conflict of interests by the project director who owned stock in the company funding the research; underreporting of adverse events in trials previously related to the research, including the death of monkeys; and lack of sufficient information being communicated to the patient about potential risks of the experimental therapy (Shalala 2001). As a result, the National Bioethics Advisory Commission enacted much stricter regulatory oversight. Previously, in 1995, President Clinton established the commission to provide further protection for human research participants (National Bioethics Advisory Commission 2001).

The increasing association between gene transfer and gene therapy reflects the developing significance of what is called translational research. This concept refers to the connection between research in the laboratory, in this case at the molecular level, and clinical treatment at the bedside. Hence, translational research typically is understood as moving from the laboratory to patient care, from the bench to the bedside. However, there are two systemic difficulties associated with translating gene transfer to effective clinical applications: vectors can be unreliable as they move genetic materials to the relevant cells; and immune systems tend to attack these vectors and their receiver cells. Each of these difficulties will need to be addressed if gene therapies are to be successful. And this research will shed light on the clinical pathway for other treatment strategies like cell and immunological therapies (Kimmelman 2010). As if translational research was not difficult enough for regenerative medicine, another major enterprise is currently under way to further complicate the ethical terrain of genetics. The effort to create totally new cells has initiated a new focus for bioethics discourse, the ethics of synthetic biology.

Protocells and Synthetic Biology

The term protocell refers to a completely artificial cell. The global effort to create protocells is racing forward with large amounts of funding and many companies seeking to claim the patent rights. Of course, the problem of patenting discoveries about the human genome is not new in the age of regenerative medicine (Mirowski and Sent 2002). Predictably, there is significant interest in the media over this new genetic biotechnology. It is anticipated that these efforts will succeed over the next few years.

Protocells will be different from other inert cells, such as artificial red blood cells. Protocells will be alive as self-organizing, regenerating, and evolving entities that are assembled from organic and inorganic substrates. They will involve a simplified genome being inserted into organisms to make them behave is useful ways. Also, they will be similar to single-cell organisms such as bacteria, although they will be simpler than any bacteria we know of today. This research involves the creation of living matter from nonliving matter (Rasmussen et al. 2008). The study of protocells has led to the new field of synthetic biology that seeks to create biological systems by assembling living organisms from nonliving parts.

There are two approaches being explored to create these artificial or synthetic cells (Bedau and Parke 2009). One approach seeks to create new kinds of life by modifying existing forms of life. For example, in 2005 Craig Venter (who helped to sequence the human genome) created a company called Synthetic Genomics Inc., which seeks to commercialize these artificial or synthetic cells as potential biofuels or vaccines. The research process controls the genome of an already existing bacterium. This occurs by synthesizing the bacterium's DNA and designing a new genome without the original, natural functions of the bacterium. The new synthetic genome is passed along to daughter cells, thereby creating a new line of artificial cells. Then the new genome in the cell line is provided with genes to perform different functions, such as capturing carbon dioxide from the environment. In May 2010 Ventor announced success, creating what he described as a self-replicating species. However, because the discovery included an existing natural host, this success in synthesizing a genome was not truly a new creation.

A different approach in synthetic biology seeks to create new kinds of life completely from nonliving materials. This occurs by clustering molecules in a manner that is sufficiently simple to facilitate self-assembly yet sufficiently complex to regenerate and evolve. This research explores the basic mechanisms required for any form of life, helping to solve an enduring problem of evolution: how the first cells reproduced. The goal here is to find a molecule that functions both as a repository for genetic information and as an enzyme that governs regeneration. A breakthrough in this approach was announced in September 2011 by a team of scientists led by Tadashi Sugawara at the University of Tokyo in Japan (Sanderson 2011).

In 2010 President Barack Obama asked the Presidential Commission for the Study of Bioethical Issues to review the emerging field of synthetic biology to clarify ethical guidelines to maximize public benefits and risks. The commission published its report in December 2010 (Presidential Commission 2010). The commission identified five ethical principles that should be addressed when considering the social implications of synthetic biology. First, the principle of public beneficence refers to maximizing public benefits and minimizing public harms. Second, the principle of responsible stewardship refers to having concern regarding safety and security for those unable to represent themselves, such as the environment and future generations. Third, the principle of intellectual freedom and responsibility refers to respecting research by having regulatory parsimony, providing only as much oversight as is truly necessary. Fourth, the principle of democratic deliberation refers to collaborative decision making that embraces opposing views in debates and active participation by citizens. Fifth, the principle of justice and fairness refers to the distribution of benefits and burdens in an appropriate manner across society. The commission also provided eighteen specific regulations to guide research in synthetic biology. These regulations adopted a position of prudent vigilance, striking a balance between two extremes: the extreme of a precautionary stance that is so careful as to risk paralysis; and the extreme of a protechnology stance that seeks to fast-track synthetic biology without appropriate restrictions. The balanced approach also was suggested by an ethical report from scholars at the Hastings Center on synthetic biology published in 2009 by the Woodrow Wilson International Center for Scholars (Parens, Johnston, and Moses 2009).

There are two general goals in the research of synthetic biology. The first goal is to advance science from the perspective of research knowledge. Uncovering these foundations of life and its biochemical systems will be landmark achievements. And there will be many scientific ramifications in other areas. The second goal is to create from nonliving matter mechanisms with the capacities of living systems. These new systems (cells) will have a wide range of potential applications. For example, there will be applications for biofuels and vaccines, as mentioned earlier. And there will be applications for diagnostic and therapeutic purposes in pharmacology and medicine, such as biosensors that can function in the body, vectors to deliver and activate drugs at the molecular level, and cells that ingest atherosclerotic plaque that causes heart disease. When synthetic biology and nanotechnology combine, there will be a very exciting new terrain for genetics with accompanying benefits and risks. Exploration in this new landscape will be made possible by protocells.

Predictably, these high hopes will be accompanied by significant hazards, not only for public health but also for the environment. Ethical scrutiny and policy oversight will be crucial; the precautionary principle will be much needed. However, the paradox of precaution unavoidably involves the calculation and management of risks while trying to avoid paralysis (Morris 2000). There are two extraordinary risks that arise. Because protocells will be able to self-replicate (a characteristic of becoming a living cell), they could proliferate uncontrollably in the environment. And because they can evolve (another characteristic of becoming a living cell), it is possible that their properties could change in a manner that is not expected.

Society globally needs to be extremely cautious in the face of such far-reaching risks. The enormous investments that have been committed, the scientific progress that has been made, and the reluctance of policymakers to stop the endeavor combine in a manner that suggests the genie is effectively out of the bottle. The focus now must be upon calculating and containing risks. For example, like other dangerous cells that already exist (e.g., the bird flu virus), an effective confinement strategy is crucial during the research process. When these protocells are applied to a myriad of functions, there needs to be built-in controls, such as automatically terminating the cell if it extends beyond identified parameters, causing the cell to die at a preestablished time, or stopping the evolution of the cell when a particular change occurs (Bedau and Parke 2009).

In principle the theological anthropology of the Catholic tradition is open to these utterly fascinating and extraordinarily challenging developments in biotechnology. Of course, the proverbial devil will be in the details. While general ethical support can be provided in bioethics for these amazing ventures, extraordinary caution will be needed, and frequent evaluations will be necessary as concrete discoveries and achievements are announced in the future. Also, there is an abundance of other topics in regenerative medicine that will require ongoing moral scrutiny. While it is not possible to list all of the emerging topics in this arena of genetics, a cluster of general themes can set the stage for bioethics discourse: the connection between our human identity as a species and our understanding of the continuum between health and disease. This concluding section of the chapter introduces these themes in a general manner and provides references to recent literature as a roadmap for further study.

Identity, Health, and Disease

The capacity to manipulate the human genome raises the profound question about the meaning of human identity, both as individuals and as a species. It seems that evolution needed five hundred million years for the human species to develop. Given the astounding capacity to manipulate the human genome, we can envision two dramatic, albeit extreme, scenarios. On the one hand, it is possible that the field of genetics could run amok in a manner that endangers our species. We could manipulate the human genome through germ-line interventions that turn out over generations to undermine our evolutionary competitiveness. If that happens, we could compromise the survival of the species. On the other hand, it is possible to alter our genome over centuries to become a super species. We could substantively change the human genome in the following manner: we could eradicate most known diseases, we could dramatically increase physical size and capabilities, we could generate extensive cognitive enhancement, and we could vastly extend our lifespan. If these happen, it may be that the human species is so transformed as to become a different species.

These extremes set the stage for the debate on "transhumanism"—envisioning extensive manipulation of the human genome across the species. In this debate species extinction or transformation becomes imaginable. These extremes can appear like science fiction. After all, the sort of superspecies mentioned may possibly exist on other planets. Nonetheless, these perspectives provide a cautionary context within which we can explore the meaning of human identity and the continuum between health and disease in our species.

In chapter 26 we discuss foundational issues about theological anthropology that help to clarify the meaning of being human. There are also many specific issues that need to be discussed to guide research in regenerative medicine and the human genome (Ip 2009). Not surprisingly, the debate on the moral status of being human applies to when human life begins (see chapter 25), which involves the science of embryogenesis. This is crucial in many discussions about the creation of human life, from human cloning (Cole-Turner 1997, 2008; Cole-Turner and Waters 2003), to germ-line modification (Stock and Campbell 2000), to designing embryos in the petri dish (Green 2008). The debate on the moral status of being human also pertains to when human life can be allowed to expire, which involves the neuroscience of dying patients (Farah 2010).

Furthermore, a very controversial technology that challenges the meaning of human life deals with creating human–animal embryo chimeras for research (Suarez and Huarte 2011). The moral debate on human identity (Murphy and Knight 2010) engages us with meaning we ascribe to human dignity (Briggle 2010; Pellegrino, Schulman, and Merrill 2009), the human body (Gerlach et al. 2011), and the contingent nature of human life (Duwell, Rehmann-Sutter, and Mieth 2010; Habermas 2003). These issues provide the context for clarifying what can be construed as human goods such as happiness (Fukuyama 2002; Kass et al. 2003), human rights (Mitchell, Pellegrino, and Elshtain 2007; Jasanoff 2011), and especially what we mean by genetics-related justice (Buchanan et al. 2000; Buchanan 2011a, 2011b). As we consider altering human nature (Lustig, Brody, and McKenny 2010; Verhey 2010) there must be appropriate caution with regard to associated risks (Munthe 2011). Moreover, as these issues are discussed from the perspective of secular bioethics and public policy (as we have seen in part I and in chapter 26) there is a robust contribution that religious discourse can make (Brock 2010; Cole-Turner 2011; Deane-Drummond 2006; Smith 2011).

Aligned with these issues on human identity is the continuum between health and disease in an age of biomedicalization (Clarke et al. 2010). Understanding this continuum between health and disease helps to clarify another continuum, the one between therapy and enhancement (Gordijn and Chadwick 2010; Nayef 2011; Savulescu and Bostrom 2008, 2009; Savulescu, Meulen, and Kahane 2011). Of course, cognitive brain enhancement is crucial in this discussion (Fangerau, Fegert, Trapp 2011; Gruenler 2008). In bioethics, the meaning of "therapy" typically refers to the avoidance, cure, or prevention of disease. In contrast, enhancement can be perceived as advancing the normal range of human functioning. Not surprisingly, defining these contrasting meanings more specifically can be very complex. However, the general distinction between therapy and enhancement raises the genetic challenge of what constitutes making people better (Häyry 2010). This question is especially urgent as we develop the next generation of medicines that implement genetic technologies (Stockwell 2011), including making patients better as a form of enhancing evolution (Harris 2010). The distinction between therapy and enhancement is especially important in the debate over genetic testing of adults (Arribas-Ayllon, Sarangi, Angus Clark 2011; Betta 2010; Skene and Thompson 2008). Moreover, these distinctions are crucial for engaging the emerging debates on brain-computer interfaces related with artificial intelligence, nanobiotechnology, and neuroscience (Jotterand 2008; Ramsey and Frankish 2010).

The connection between identity, health, and disease sheds light on another subset of topics that shapes bioethics discourse in regenerative medicine: the relation among normalcy (recognizing that it is difficult to specify what normal means), perfectibility (acknowledging that there are many views of perfection), and disability (understanding there is a wide range of interpretations about what constitutes disability). How we understand normalcy in the human condition is by no means self-evident. Genes influence human traits and behaviors, interacting with different environments. This interaction sheds light on, but does not fully explain, complex genetic disorders, such as schizophrenia and autism (Parens 1998; Parens, Chapman, and Press 2006). Also, socially perceived disorders are increasingly eliciting ethical discourse with regard to stigmatization, such as on the relation between genomics and obesity (Korthals 2010), or on the relation between race and diseases such as diabetes (Montoya 2011).

How normalcy is defined in turn affects how we perceive perfectibility as we try to delineate acceptable boundaries for perfecting the human condition (Hyde 2010). We should recognize, of course, that a quest for perfection is assuredly an elusive endeavor

(Sandel 2007). Historically, we recall that it was an urge to perfect the human condition that lay behind the eugenics movement (Bashford and Levine 2010; Turda 2010). This movement can be found not only in the Nazi holocaust (Rubenfeld 2010; Weiss 2010) but also in shameful health practices in the United States, such as enforced sterilization (Lombardo 2011). This quest for species improvement continues today in terms of defending some forms of human enhancement (Agar 2004).

In the context of normalcy and perfectibility, the topic of disability is crucially important in bioethics discourse on genetics. Controversy arises not just over the idea of aborting deformed embryos that are diagnosed via prenatal genetic testing. There is also a substantive debate over what constitutes disability in the context of the new genetics and what should be done (Swinton and Brock 2007). This debate includes religious perspectives that focus upon the meaning of healing, such as dealing with Down syndrome (Young 2007) when remedial therapies do not exist (Edmonds 2011).

Conclusion

This chapter has explored specific issues in genetics. We have considered several topics dealing with the human embryo that elicit official teaching from the Catholic Church. However, most of the emerging issues in regenerative medicine will likely occur at too fast a pace for the Church to provide a specific teaching on each breakthrough. Nonetheless, the theological anthropology of the Catholic tradition can shed light on the developments in genetics over the decades ahead.

Note

1. Here we see a return to cardiopulmonary criteria of death: when the patient's heart stops, a short time is permitted to elapse, such as under the Pittsburgh Protocol (Lynn 1993), before pronouncing the patient to be dead for subsequent procurement of organs (IOM 1997, 2000b, 2006). The purpose of the time lapse is to reach the point of irreversibility, that is, beyond the point at which resuscitation can occur, usually a few minutes after the heart stops. There is a theoretical conundrum here. Technically, after the point of irreversibility in the sense of auto-resuscitation (the point at which a patient's heart might start beating on its own), a patient could still be artificially resuscitated. In such a circumstance, it is most likely that the patient would have extensive brain damage, but the patient would be alive. DCD occurs in a tightly managed environment. Typically the patient or family provides advance directives to prevent artificial resuscitation; then futile life-sustaining measures are removed following the advance directives, a few minutes later the patient is declared to be dead, and only then does the transplant team enter the operating room to procure the donated organs. In these circumstances, theoretically the patient could be artificially resuscitated but will not be resuscitated because the patient's advance directives forbid doing so. The practice of DCD is widespread in US health care, it is legal, and it is deemed to be ethical. In fact, official Catholic teaching does not forbid DCD (Haas 2011). Nonetheless, there continues to be robust critique of the practice of DCD, especially when using the Pittsburgh Protocol of procuring organs only two minutes after cardiopulmonary functions have ceased. For example, some Catholic scholars argue for waiting until total brain death. They want criteria indicating beyond reasonable doubt that the patient is really dead (Lee and Grisez 2010).

CHAPTER 28

ALLOCATING HEALTH CARE RESOURCES

Health Care in the United States

THE ISSUE OF SCARCE RESOURCES and of the quality of health care is related to the problem of allocating, or rationing, scarce medical resources in a just and effective way.[1] That is, the issue has to do with setting up a system of health care for our nation. It is an excruciatingly complex concern. Unlike some other issues in health care ethics, no consensus has arisen about allocation.

To a considerable extent, this is a new issue for Americans. The Roman Catholic tradition, virtually the only source of American medical ethics up until the 1960s, scarcely mentioned the matter. Over the past forty years or so, the governing context for decisions about treatment has shifted, largely due to the growing influence of medical ethics and of the consumer movement, from that of physician paternalism to that of patient autonomy. The emphasis in recent years on informed consent is characteristic of this shift. But no sooner has patient autonomy gained general acceptance than we are confronted with the need for cost containment, which threatens to take decision-making power out of the hands of both physician and patient and place it in the hands of society as a whole, or of government, which in the late 1980s paid for 41 percent of the nation's health care (Dougherty 1988, 16; Morreim 1995, 9), or in the hands of private insurance companies.

Americans do not like the idea of allocating or rationing resources. They want to believe that technology will make it possible to solve health care problems at lower and lower cost. They point to those scientific and technological breakthroughs that have enhanced medical care and have benefitted so many of us. But this proper pride has brought with it hubris and blindness. When Americans are asked if they think every American should have the same health care that a millionaire can buy, they overwhelmingly say yes. When they are asked how much they are willing to pay in increased taxes for this care, they refuse to pay the price: "Read our lips, no new taxes."

Yet the facts are forcing us at last to look at the problem. The United States spends a greater percentage of its gross national product (GNP) on health care than any other nation. In 1929 it was 3.5 percent of GNP; in 1950 it was 4.4 percent. By the late 1980s, it had risen to about 11 or 12 percent, more than $500 billion, and twice what was spent on national defense (Dougherty 1988, 16; Morreim 1995, 8). In 1998, it was 13.6 percent, compared to 9.5 percent in Canada, 10.6 percent in Germany, 8.8 percent in

Belgium, and 8.2 percent in Austria (Cherry 2002, 19). By the turn of the century it was about 13 or 14 percent, about a trillion dollars (Kaveny 2002, 177; Cowley 2003a). By 2007 it had grown to 16.2 percent. The figure for 2008 is 2.3 trillion dollars (Rush 2011, 1). By 2009 it had risen to 2.5 trillion and a new record of 17.3 percent of the GNP (Walter 2011, 120), still more than any other nation. About 10 percent of this is spent on persons in the last year of life (Walter 2011, 120). From 1997 to 2007 more than one-third of the entire increase in per capita income was spent on health care, and projections for the next forty years suggest that this will grow to nearly one half (Chernew, Hirth and Cutler 2009, 1253–54), with increases in health care expenses significantly outpacing general inflation. In the late 1980s, we actually spent eight-tenths of one percent of the entire gross national product in intensive care units (Dougherty 1988, 4). In 1994 that had risen to one percent, about $64 billion (Cherry 2002, 19).

Despite the fact that we outspend all other nations on health care, we have not achieved a quality of health commensurate with these expenses. Although we spend far more per person than any other nation (in 2007 the United States spent $7,290 per person and the next-highest nation, Switzerland, spent $4,417), our life expectancy is significantly lower (in 2007, seventy-eight years as opposed to eighty-two years in Switzerland and eighty-one in Canada, which spent $3,895 per person, or about half what we did). Japan spent a miserly $2,581 per person with a life expectancy of eighty-three years (Walter 2011, 121). In the late 1980s we ranked about twentieth in the world in infant mortality, although the data on which this commonly quoted statistic are based may be questionable (Dougherty 1988, 4; Waldman, Lachman, and Bradburn 1990, 78).[2] In combined maternal and infant mortality at the turn of the century, the United States ranked eleventh (Cowley 2003b). Nor are we getting better. In 2010 we ranked at number 42 in infant mortality (Walter 2011, 121), and the figure released in August 2011 puts the United States at number 43. And all the money we spend does not mean that hospitals are thriving financially. Delayed and reduced payments to hospitals by government and by private insurers, coupled with increased costs, are driving hospitals into the red and out of business. In the Pittsburgh area, for example, thirteen of thirty-six hospitals lost money in 2002 (Gaynor 2002). And this does not include the St. Francis Health System, a seven-institution system that was forced to close in September 2002 after more than a century of serving the Pittsburgh area because it was simply too far in debt to be rescued.

The United States does not provide health care to all its citizens, with often devastating results (Kirschner 2010). In the late 1980s there were about thirty-seven million persons without health insurance in the United States at any one time and tens of millions more who lacked insurance for important periods of time, usually as they changed jobs (Dougherty 1988, 11).[3] By the turn of the century it was forty-one million more or less permanently uninsured with tens of millions more without insurance from time to time (Alter 2003). The latest figure is fifty million (Rush 2011, 1). It is estimated that almost forty-five thousand deaths result annually from this lack of insurance (Walter 2011, 121). Surveys show that many Americans choose not to take prescribed drugs or to have other important medical tests and procedures because they cannot or choose not to pay for them. While it is true, as opponents of government intervention point out in their advertisements, that some other nations have waiting lists for certain surgeries that are more quickly available in the United States, it is also true that effective access to primary care in this country is not available to all our citizens in a way that even approaches equality. Other nations do far better than we do at this. We tend to stress tertiary care at high cost to the neglect of preventive care at lower cost (although it is not clear that shifting priorities to prevention would save money in the long run[4]). The United States simply does not have a coherent national health care policy.

There are historic reasons for this. Probably the basic one is the tension that has always existed in our country between individual liberty and the common good. This tension is often a valuable one, as it has helped us avoid the extremes of anarchy and statism. Our insistence on individual liberty has doubtless been an important influence on our advances in modern medicine, which, from a technological perspective, are unparalleled. But when the stress on individual freedom is not counterbalanced by insistence on the common good, the common good suffers, and individual freedom is compromised.

Recent attempts to extend health insurance to a larger number of Americans have given rise to contentious political debate. In 2010 Congress passed and President Obama signed the Patient Protection and Affordable Care Act (PPACA), often called "Obamacare" by its opponents. One of the provisions of this act is a mandate that many of those who do not have health insurance must purchase it for themselves, with federal aid if they qualify, a provision that is ethically and economically justified.[5] The legal status of that provision was for a time disputed (Gostin 2010). Various state and federal courts, often by split decisions, approved or disproved the constitutionality of the mandate. In June 2012, by a 5–4 decision, the US Supreme Court upheld its constitutionality, reasoning that Congress has the power to tax those who refuse to buy insurance. Republican candidates for national office are virtually unanimous in their promise to repeal the PPACA if they gain a majority. In any case, although the health care reform enacted by the PPACA, if it is not repealed, will add to the numbers of the insured, it will not achieve universal health insurance and it will not cut costs to the degree necessary. Its supporters claim that costs will be reduced, but it is clear that this reduction, even if it is fully realized, will be insufficient to control increasing health care costs. Allocation will still be needed (Callahan 2011, 25).

Americans have tried a number of ways to avoid the issue of rationing. For example, when were faced with the problem of deciding who should have access to scarce hemodialysis machines in 1972, the federal government added dialysis and kidney transplant, even for those under sixty-five, to Medicare (Beauchamp and Childress 2001, 208; Callahan 2011, 24). This arguably proper decision allowed us to avoid facing that particular issue of allocation. We socialized our kidneys but left the rest of our organs to the mercy of the market. Similarly, we have tried to avoid the issue of government health insurance by setting up a system whereby employers pay for health insurance for their employees. This seemed to protect the right of individual freedom, keep the government out of medicine, and at the same time provide decent medical care for working Americans. But this approach is now in jeopardy, as employers claim they cannot afford to continue paying for it. Economists say that global markets make this approach impossible, since American companies cannot compete with others whose nations provide tax-funded health insurance and who therefore need not shoulder the burden of health care for their workers. Strikes are now as apt to be about health insurance as about salary. With large numbers of Americans lacking health insurance, health care costs are the most frequent cause of personal bankruptcies (Walter 2011, 121).

There are a number of experts who continue to claim that allocation within health care is unnecessary. The main argument here is that the United States is a rich and powerful nation. Statements are often made to the effect that if we can land a man on the moon or build another aircraft carrier, we can afford all the medical care we want. While it is easy enough to show that health care resources are in fact limited, it is harder to show why they cannot be extended. Why can't we double our health care expenditures and spend $6 trillion instead of $3 trillion? Are we not ethically obliged to do so? Surely the needs of the sick outweigh our desire for gadgets and entertainment. That would solve the problem.

It would be nice to think that this is true, but it is not. There are serious difficulties with the argument. Ethically, it suffers from theoretical and practical problems that are explored later in this chapter and in more detail in the next. And there are economic problems as well. Economists tell us that we could increase the share of our wealth and productivity that goes to health care, but they add the all too obvious warning that we would have to reduce the monies and energies spent on other pursuits that we also value and that serve to sustain American productivity. At some point such an increase becomes logically and economically impossible. The global economy also restricts the portion of economic energy that our nation can afford to devote to any one sector.

Nor would shifting allocation within the federal budget solve the problem. Even if we were to reduce those portions of the federal budget that go to other areas, to the military, for example, we would still not be able to absorb the growing health care portion of the budget. Other cost-containment mechanisms, such as health maintenance organizations (HMO) and diagnosis-related groups (DRG), which are already in place, are not doing the job. These measures are themselves ethically problematic, and the savings they realize have probably reached their peak and are now flattening out. Health care costs are rising so fast that these measures are inadequate (Morreim 1995, 14–15). As baby boomers enter the Medicare system, "either a doubling of the tax rate or a 50 percent cut in benefits will be necessary" (Callahan 2011, 25). Thus, a constellation of factors, including international economics and the ever-expanding portion of the United States economy devoted to health care, when seen in the context of other services also required in a just society, force us, despite our reticence, to face the fact that some limitation of and allocation within health care is needed.

Allocation is already a major factor in the way we deliver health care. We are already rationing health care resources, but we lack the political courage to do it openly. We engage in a form of "soft" or "covert" rationing (Callahan 2011, 27), and often this is not done in an ethically justifiable way. Present allocation mechanisms restrict access for the poor, deemphasize prevention and education, and often fail to be cost-effective. African-Americans and women continue to be underserved and discriminated against (Beauchamp and Childress 2001, 237–39; Berteaux 2002). We simply must do better.[6]

It is clear that there is no one perfect way to allocate health care resources, and those who make the claim that there is are simply unaware of the complexities involved and of the deficiencies apparent in the attempts made by various nations thus far toward dealing with this problem. However, despite the fact that no one perfect system is apparent, or perhaps in some way because of it, it is clear that ethical principles and moral virtues must play a central role in the national debate regarding the construction of a system of health care resource allocation.[7]

Allocation and Forgoing Treatment

Allocating or rationing scarce resources means that certain treatments are withheld or withdrawn. They are forgone because they are scarce; there are not enough to go around. Another kind of forgoing treatment, which is not done for purposes of rationing, is based on the emerging consensus described in chapters 13 through 17. This consensus is based, first, on a recognition that not all treatments that prolong biological life are truly beneficial to the patient (in Catholic ethics, this is the distinction between morally ordinary, mandatory treatment and morally extraordinary, optional treatment); second, on the general agreement that there is a moral difference between killing (euthanasia) and allowing to die; and third, on the legal concepts of autonomy, privacy, and liberty to refuse unwanted treatment.

We have already reviewed the distinction between morally ordinary and morally extraordinary medical treatment. We saw that the proportion of burdens and benefits of the treatment was central to the distinction. Although the distinction is not generally used in the context of allocation, it is worth noting that one of the burdens that the Catholic tradition mentions is the burden of cost. It is morally right, says the Catholic tradition, to choose to forgo costly treatments if we have a better purpose for the money. A parent might rightly choose to forgo expensive treatment, even if it would be effective, in order to give the money to children for education. It is true that this tradition was developed long before the advent of third-party payers. Today the burdens and benefits most usually considered are those for the patient.[8] But third-party payers are not always involved, and even when they are, some restrictions for cost containment are justifiable. In any case, the Catholic tradition is clearly open to the possibility that a treatment may rightly be forgone by a patient in order to help others with the resources saved (Boyle 2002, 93–94).

How can the consensus that has emerged be differentiated from the issue of the allocation of scarce resources? It is clear that there is some overlap between the two issues. The more that treatment is forgone as based on the three accepted pillars of the present consensus, the less money is spent on it, and the more resources are available, at least theoretically, for other purposes. And it is possible that patients, families, and health care providers may have the scarce-resource question in the backs of their minds when making some decisions to forgo treatment.

However, despite instances of overlap (times when resource allocation is a factor—usually a hidden or implicit one—in decisions to forgo) there is an easy way to distinguish decisions to forgo treatment when they are made on the basis of the three pillars already discussed from decisions to forgo treatment based on allocation of resources. The former decisions, the ones we make all the time in hospitals, are ones we ought to make even if resources were infinite. The reason we do not treat pneumonia in a patient with terminal metastatic cancer is that the patient does not want this morally extraordinary treatment, and therefore we must not treat. The reason we are morally and ethically justified in removing ventilator and nutritional support from a patient in a persistent vegetative state is that this treatment is not in that person's best interests (as decided by the patient before lapsing into unconsciousness, or as decided by the surrogate who expresses the patient's intent). We would be ethically justified in forgoing the treatment despite any scarcity of resources. Thus, although the areas overlap, they are not the same.

Should Doctors Allocate at the Bedside?

This distinction enables us now to look at the very difficult question of whether physicians should ever refuse treatment to individual patients based on the need for cost containment and allocation within the society. Although in theory it seems the answer is clear—they should not—in practice, at least in some cases, that answer may not be adequate in today's health care environment.

An example of this dilemma might be a case in which a physician knows that a certain treatment, such as monoclonal antibodies, which are very expensive, adds only a 1 or 2 percent likelihood that a patient's life will be saved from acute sepsis (infection). The usual cheaper drug is almost as good, but in some cases the more expensive drug saves a life that the less expensive medicine will not. The doctor cannot know ahead of time what will happen in this case. Can the physician refuse to use the better drug?

The answer is no. We have seen why in chapter 20, on medical futility. In the present example, the more expensive drug is not medically futile. We can rightly expect a chance of a better result with the more expensive treatment. So, unless the hospital or other agency has a public and well-known policy of not using the drug, a policy made on the ethical basis of the need for better allocation of health care resources, families and patients should decide, not physicians. Ethically and legally there seems little doubt: the drug must be given if it is the medical standard of care for this kind of sepsis. Physicians and hospitals should not reject it in individual clinical situations for reasons of cost containment or allocation. They can do so as part of a general and public policy, but hospitals are very unlikely to have these kinds of policies in our competitive health care market. The medical standard of care is to use the drug. Doctors should not allocate at the bedside.

Why not? Because there are simply too many possible conflicts of interest. In today's financial climate, where managed care contracts are so prevalent, hospitals directly and doctors directly, indirectly, or both are compensated more for spending less. Do we really think that physicians and hospital administrators, if given the authority to make this kind of decision on a case-by-case basis, would not be tempted to treat the rich corporate executive who has a living will that insists on everything (with six lawyers in tow to make sure he got it) more readily than to treat the medically identical indigent minority woman from the local housing project? This kind of decision should not be made by providers on a case-by-case basis. Admittedly, this conclusion is not universally supported. It is supported, however, by many and probably by most ethicists (Pellegrino and Thomasma 1988, 185–89; Boyle 2002, 93; Ethics Committee of the Society of Critical Care Medicine 1997). Even such a thoroughgoing utilitarian as Peter Singer, known for his insistence that resources be distributed globally so that they might do the most good, argues that "the physician should not also be the person who decides which forms of health care are sufficiently cost-effective to be offered to her or his patient. Leaving this decision to the physician may clash too violently with the principle that physicians should further the best interests of their patients" (Ratiu and Singer 2001, 48).

As we saw in chapter 20, however, this rejection of bedside allocation does not mean that it is wrong to make such decisions on a policy basis. Medicare can rightly decide not to use the expensive drug for persons for whom it will do little or no human good—for example, for patients with other illnesses who will probably die soon regardless of the outcome of the sepsis. Indeed, Medicare might justly decide that the drug is too expensive to cover for any patient, regardless of condition. And this policy could be made explicitly on the basis of cost. Societies have limited resources and are permitted to choose how to spend them. But these are social policies, subject to public debate and open to examination. Physicians should not make individual decisions for individual patients based on the need for cost containment.

But this answer works better in theory than in some actual contexts, and thus is opposed, or at least criticized, by some (Morreim 1995, 58–63; Baily 2003, 39–40). In a system increasingly dominated by managed care organizations (MCO), physicians find themselves increasingly caught between advocating for their patients and defending their own jobs. MCOs threaten to expel physicians whose treatments exceed certain anticipated costs. Physicians are usually obliged to tell patients if there are better treatments available that their MCO insurance will not pay for, although the risk of lawsuits might mitigate that obligation (Morreim 1995, 112–15). But doctors are not always obliged to give the treatment and absorb the cost themselves, or take the risk of being fired by the MCO (Morreim 1995, 69–102). In a sense, this conclusion is at odds with what has been said in the preceding paragraphs, that physicians should not ration at the bedside. In another sense it is not because the decision has already been made by another agency, in this case by the MCO, so the physician is not making a bedside decision. Physicians cannot easily resolve this kind of conflict. Doctors should not in general make bedside allocation decisions. They are too dangerous. But physicians cannot be obliged to jeopardize their livelihoods when the cause of the injustice is outside their control. Perhaps the principle of cooperation that we saw in chapter 12 can help here. Physicians are obliged to try to change the unjust system but may in some cases materially cooperate with it when opposition would only cause more harm than good. These difficult issues are part of the systemic problem we are examining, and, as long as the unjust system remains, these questions may well be unresolvable.[9]

The Problem with Allocation Arguments

Allocation decisions inevitably mean that at some point we are going to spend less on one worthy project and more on another. Arguments such as this seldom convince us. This is partly due to our resistance to the idea that we cannot, as free individuals, have it all and have it all right now. Our resistance is due to greed—each of us wants access to everything and few of us want our taxes to go up so that others can have it, too. And our resistance is due to our delight with technology.

In addition to this resistance, there are problems with allocation arguments themselves. These problems are not always taken seriously by those who argue for a better national health system with a more equitable allocation of resources. The next chapter treats these difficulties in greater theoretical detail, but some brief overview is helpful here.

A first problem is why we should cut back on this surgery or on that ICU bed instead of on this school or on that bomber. Or why should we not outlaw television or opera or medical schools or houses that costs more than two hundred thousand dollars or vacations to Europe and spend the resources saved on housing the poor and feeding the third world? Does the moral obligation to share mean that just about any expense on personal or family pleasure or comfort is morally wrong? Sometimes moralists give us that impression, and we rightly resist it. Ultimately, such questions cannot be answered in an entirely satisfactory way; despite this, they do need to be raised and thought about.

A second problem is the difficulty we all have, and ought to have, in deciding to let one named person die in order to free up resources for larger unnamed groups. Some have claimed that this was a reason for the federal government's decision to pay for all kidney dialysis and transplants; named individuals were dying for lack of treatment (Beauchamp and Childress 2001, 208). This child will die in the well, or from kidney failure, unless we spend millions. Yet the millions of dollars could save thousands of children if we bought them food. Another aspect of this problem is the issue of family relationships. We do have obligations to our families that we do not have to strangers. Yet this cannot mean that we have no responsibilities to share resources beyond our families.

We often hear in this context that a human life—by which we usually mean the life of this or that named individual—is "priceless" or "of infinite value." Implied in this is the idea that we ought to spend whatever it takes to save that one life. But we forget that what we ought to mean when we say that human life is priceless or of infinite value is not that it is worth an infinitely high price or an infinite number of dollars but that it cannot be measured by price in dollars, few or many. The intrinsic value of human life, upheld in earlier chapters, is transcendental (Sulmasy 2011, 188–89); it transcends measurement. And we also forget that measuring a named individual life in this way means that we may well undervalue many other human lives.

A third problem is the complexity of economics. Things are seldom as simple as spending on this person or on those persons. Money saved here may go there, or it may not. Monetary systems, supply and demand, incentives, taxes, and other similar complex matters are all part of allocation decisions. They are difficult issues to deal with, so we avoid them as long as we can.

In the context of these dilemmas, there is at least one way to make allocation arguments better, that is, to make them more convincing. We ought to be able to argue with some strength that those medical procedures that are very expensive and that are at best of questionable benefit to those who get them should not get public funding except as limited experimental research. This seems reasonable, but it is hard to convince people that this means there should be little or no public funding for certain health care measures, such as artificial heart implants as bridges to human heart transplants. Once the application is made to this or that health care expenditure, those representing certain patients or research projects are quick to insist on the need of the patients and the worthiness of the projects.

Competing Visions of Who People Are

There are two competing visions about who people are as we relate in society. One vision says that we are basically isolated individuals, and the only reason we care about each other, at least in large groups beyond the family, is that we have to keep others from hurting us. This vision of humankind tends to think that we do not owe anyone anything except what we actually contract to give them. It denies the existence of positive rights and insists that no one has the right to be helped; we merely have the right to be left alone. Certain libertarian and contractarian theories of justice tend in this direction.[10] Justice thus becomes something we decide on rather than something we discover to be true and try to embody. Metaethically, this is the "rational positivism" we spoke of in the endnote to chapter 9. Allocation systems are just, according to this first vision, if reasonable and free individuals agree to them. Whatever social contract we agree to set up becomes right by the very fact that we agree to it.

But this ignores the real social situation of real people. The second vision proposes that we are social beings, and that we thrive only in society. This vision proposes that we do owe others real help, that nations do have a moral obligation to spend resources on the poor, that systems that allocate without recognizing these obligations are unjust. Now there is no doubt that many who subscribe to this second vision, as do the authors of this book, are all too often ready to propose unworkable allocation solutions. They are too likely to advocate centralized planning and to think they can eliminate sin, just as many Marxists thought they could eliminate nationalism. But this vision does challenge us with something that approaches the notion of civic virtue. We cannot simply posit a system of allocation and call it fair. We have to discover what is just. Metaethically, this supposes some kind of natural law theory, or at least some foundation for ethics. It is true that there is not only one fair solution. And there is no perfect solution. But we must do better than we are doing now.

Rationing on the Basis of Age

Perhaps the most engaging attempt to propose allocation of health care resources by a limitation of life-prolonging measures based on age is that made by Daniel Callahan, cofounder and former director of The Hastings Center, in his book *Setting Limits: Medical Goals in an Aging Society* (1987). His proposal, startling as it may be at first reading or first hearing, deserves serious study.

Callahan argues his proposal from two perspectives. The first is the problem we have already noted of increased health care costs. In an appendix to his book, Callahan cites statistics showing that US pension and health care costs for the aged alone would, by the year 2040, be 60 percent of the entire federal budget (ibid., 227). This is due both to increased costs of health care and to the increased number of elderly among us, especially of the very old, that is, those over eighty-five or so.

Callahan's argument is not mainly one of statistics, however. His major argument depends on our understanding of the meaning of life. He wants us to see life as biography and not just as biology. He points out that our concept of medicine has shifted from one primarily of caring to one of caring and curing. We actually can cure illnesses, something we used not to be able to do. This advance has led to a change in our understanding of health, from an understanding connected with fate and luck to one open to active medical intervention. Sometimes it seems as if we might medically conquer death and never die.[11]

In such a context, says Callahan, we need to discover again that the goal of aging is not to defer dying as such but to live old age well. The goal of aging is not individualistic disengagement from the lives of others and from social responsibility but is rather active transmission to the young of the lessons learned through a long life. A social system that sets a goal of indefinitely extending life acts to erode the social sense that there is meaning to old age. It would be better for the old, says Callahan, if such a system were not available. Then old age might better understand itself as a valid stage in the living process rather than as a time when science will at some point fail to win a victory over the defeat that is death. He thus makes his proposal: "I want to argue that medicine should not be used for the further extension of the life of the aged, but only for the full achievement of a natural and fitting life span and thereafter for the relief of suffering" (Callahan 1987, 53).

Callahan describes a "tolerable death": "My definition of a tolerable death is this: the individual event of death in a life span when (a) one's life possibilities have on the whole been accomplished; (b) one's moral obligations to those for whom one has had responsibility have been discharged; and (c) one's death will not seem to others an offense to sense and sensibility, or tempt others to despair and rage at the finitude of human existence."

"Note," he goes on to say, "the most obvious feature of this definition: it is a biographical, not a biological definition" (ibid., 66). Thus we see the two bases of Callahan's argument: first, the fact of limited resources, and second, a biographical understanding of life and of a tolerable death. Although the two bases of Callahan's argument work together, he implies that the argument from the meaning of life as biography would be sufficient by itself, even if resources were not limited, to support his proposal that treatment funding for the elderly be limited (ibid., 53).

As a philosopher, Callahan wants to see our society reinstate what he calls a "thick" as opposed to a "thin" theory of the good. It would mean a society in which we agree that the meaning he proposes for old age and for a tolerable death would be the anthropology acceptable to all of us, so that we actually support the idea of medicine ceasing its attempts to extend our life span beyond the biographical optimum, and so that we would continue to support this even if resources were unlimited. Our agreement on this would thus be similar to our general agreement to forgo treatments that are of great burden or of little benefit. We would recognize that old age as such is a sufficient criterion from the social perspective to make it burdensome and of little benefit to extend life further.

But people differ about what life means and about what makes it worth living. Although we have generally agreed that some treatments for some patients in some conditions are of little or no human benefit, we have not done this widely enough to resolve the "medical futility" issue (see chapter 20), and we certainly have not agreed that age by itself makes this the case. In this context, we tend to have a "thin" theory of the good: we tend to believe, at the worst, that the good is what individuals claim it to be, or, at best, that the federal government cannot be in the business of imposing one notion of what old age should mean on others who disagree.

It is not likely that Callahan's "thick" theory will take hold in the United States, with its high emphasis on individual freedom, and it is not clear that it ought to. It is true that the individualism in our society of which Callahan speaks is often pernicious. But it also has important positive ethical implications (Kelly 1988). It serves to counterbalance a move toward absorption of the individual in some sort of state-imposed or society-imposed soup. Yet it must also be admitted that it is this same "thin" theory that is one of the reasons for the ennui or alienation that so many old people experience. We simply do not know what old age means, and so we go on trying to extend it indefinitely in the hope that it is important that it be extended.

As important as Callahan's insistence on life as biography is, it will probably never by itself be able to persuade society to deny funding for life-extending treatment for the very old. Too many of us might disagree that the meaning of old age requires that medicine stop despite the fact that it can extend our lives and let us live what we as individuals and what those around us might think to be a meaningful and fulfilling life. Most of us would surely insist that we do not want to live forever, but this may well be due mainly to our not wanting to be biologically alive but severely handicapped, perhaps bedridden and dependent on machines. That is what we probably mean when we say we do not want to live forever. It is not at all certain that we would refuse if we were offered a treatment that would promise us eternal earthly life with healthy bodies and the potential for growing wisdom and greater experience. As long as we think medicine might someday bring us this gift, it is unlikely that this part of Callahan's argument will persuade.

But even if we never agree on a "thick" theory of the good, even if we never agree on what old age ought to mean, or that it ought to mean we should stop trying to extend longevity, we will still have to deal with the other basis of Callahan's argument, the limited-resource problem that faces us. Insisting on extending our own lives means inevitably that we have fewer resources left to enhance the lives of those younger than we are. At some point, we simply must let go and give others a chance at living.

What are we to think, then, about the moral rightness or wrongness of restricting health care expenditures on the basis of age? Can we make an argument that age is a morally irrelevant factor and that it is simply wrong to discriminate this way, as it would be wrong (and here a consensus has emerged) to discriminate on the basis of race or sex or on the basis of social contribution? We have agreed, generally at least, in issues of immediate microallocation (who of three people gets the organ or the bed) that race, sex, religion, and even past or future social contribution are factors that must not be included. Only medical need, benefit, and random choice are valid factors. The person medically most in need and most likely to benefit is chosen; if there are more than one, flip a coin, or first come, first served. Can we rule out age?

The answer is no. Age can be shown to be unlike morally irrelevant factors such as race, gender, religion, or national origin. Age is a factor that does not exclude any living person. We all have a chance of growing old. The authors of this book will never be black, or women, or Asian. To restrict treatment on bases such as these would allow us to escape the restriction; it would discriminate against others while leaving us untouched. That is the reason behind the heinousness of race and sex discrimination. The discriminators gain while the oppressed lose. The oppressors need not worry that the restrictions they enact will restrict their own access to what they want.

But age does not necessarily entail this kind of injustice. Of course that does not mean that age should be used as a basis for just any kind of restriction. It means that age may rightly be used as a basis for those restrictions where it can reasonably be shown that it is morally relevant. Age can reasonably be shown to be morally relevant when it comes to flying commercial airplanes. Those under twenty-one and those over seventy or so should not be allowed to do it. We do not recoil morally from such restrictions.

Callahan and a number of others are therefore proposing that age is a morally relevant basis for restriction not of life-enhancing treatments but of life-extending treatments. Since resources are better spent elsewhere; since there is no way of increasing these resources to the point where the problem of allocation would disappear; since this is not the same kind of invidious discrimination as that based on race, sex, and similar criteria; and since there is at least a plausible argument that the meaning of old age is not enhanced by life-extending treatment, such restriction is morally justified, at least in theory (Beauchamp and Childress 2001, 259–62).

Callahan's proposal has, needless to say, come under considerable criticism.[12] According to some, it is never right to deny resources to the neediest among us; they must get priority. Surely the very old, especially those who are sick, are among our neediest. Restricting resources allocated to their health care is thus unjust. For others, however, age-based rationing is not necessarily wrong. Robert Veatch, while disagreeing with Callahan on certain matters of philosophical theory, agrees with his basic conclusion that age may be used as a basis for restriction (Veatch 1988). Veatch suggests a way to answer the criticism that the old are the most in need. He says that while this is true from a "slice-of-time" perspective—those old persons who are sick are, right now, very much in need—it is not true from an "over-a-life-time" perspective. Over our lifetimes, those who get very old are actually quite well off. They are among the least needy when compared with others who have been less fortunate. Veatch thus concludes, like Callahan, that while it would be immoral to refuse to care for the old, to relieve suffering, to include them—and this means us when we get there—in meaningful social relationship, it may well be right to exclude them—and this also means us when we get there—from expensive life-extending technologies. Norman Daniels makes a sophisticated book-length philosophical argument for a similar position (Daniels 1988).[13]

Even though age as a criterion for allocation cannot be ruled out a priori, serious political and ethical obstacles to its practical implementation remain. Many authors argue that age cannot be used as a basis for allocation until we have a more just health care system than we now have in the United States (Beauchamp and Childress 2001, 262). This seems a compelling claim; we must establish universal access before we start trimming medical treatment for the old. We may well decide not to use age as a criterion, at least not explicitly. But we will have to decide on some criteria, and we are morally obliged to make sure that these criteria are indeed just, or at least that they do indeed approach justice.

Toward a Better Health Care System

There is no consensus about the question of how to allocate resources, but there is a growing convergence toward the acceptance of some basic parameters. This last section points out features of such a system based on an approach suggested by Charles Dougherty (1988).

First, our health care system must have some form of national health insurance, paid for by tax dollars, that guarantees all of us, regardless of wealth or employment, access to primary care. This would include care for those whose disease process is such that no cure is possible. We should try as much as possible to eliminate the cost containment that now occurs by rationing against this access to basic care. That means a system like Canada's or England's, or it at least means a system like Germany's, where private insurance for the needy is supplemented from tax dollars. Doctor visits and procedures such as check-ups, inoculations, basic health education, and the drugs and medicines needed for primary care should be available to all. This includes access to basic mental health care.[14] Some minimal deductible or copayment might be acceptable as a hedge against misuse, but even this should be waived for the poor. In addition, and still on the level of primary care, we must allocate more dollars to educational attempts at prevention of illness. Prenatal and well-baby programs are morally obligatory and may also be cost-effective.

Second, the same health insurance program should cover most medical procedures that are reasonably likely to return patients to health. This is consistent with the argument made earlier that we should not spend resources on procedures that are unlikely to benefit those who get them. This second requirement is also consistent with the argument of Callahan and others that age may rightly serve as a criterion for denying public funding for life-extending technologies. A national health insurance program should cover most medical procedures that offer a decent likelihood of returning patients to a reasonably healthy state.[15] There may well be exceptions. Some procedures may be so expensive that we will simply decide not to pay for them for anyone. This will be hard to do, but it is not unjust. What is unjust is to go about our business as usual, rationing in hidden ways against the most defenseless. The first and second levels imply as well that we should continue to pay for basic medical research.

Third, we ought to continue to allow the wealthy to get any treatment they desire, and to allow people to buy supplemental health insurance from private insurance companies to cover procedures that the governmental program does not cover. It can be argued that an individual might, in some cases, act wrongly when requesting such treatment, but it is better to allow this freedom to individuals. Such a free market will maintain an incentive for creation of new procedures, and will enable us to keep a share of the health care system somewhat free of government regulation. This means a two-or-more-tier system, a compromise that may well be acceptable to those who support different conceptions of justice (Beauchamp and Childress 2001, 244–47).

Such an approach would be far from perfect. These are its barest outlines. But, as Beauchamp and Childress say, "These issues are too complex for ethical theory to resolve" (ibid., 247). Whether the United States will gather the political will to try to approach justice in health care is still uncertain. There was momentum in the early 1990s that was halted by the failure of the Clinton plan, which was probably misconceived and in any case politically moribund from the start, and by the accompanying victory of the insurance companies and the Republicans in the 1994 election (Ashley and O'Rourke 1997, 109–10). There was additional momentum with the passage during the Bush administration of a controversial Medicare program that provides some minimal support for the purchase of prescription drugs. And a major attempt at including more Americans in health insurance has now been enacted in the Obama administration with the passage of the PPACA. At least we can claim that in the past twenty years or so we have begun to take a look at what is and will continue to be the most important issue in health care ethics.

Conclusion

Ethicists such as Callahan insist—and in this they are quite right—that we are already rationing our health care dollars. But this "soft" or "covert" rationing, as Callahan calls it (2011, 27), is less explicit than "hard" rationing, where legislators and voters actually decide where and how to allocate resources. We simply do not want to engage in hard rationing. It is easy to see why. Those excluded or restricted will fight back. Yet soft rationing clearly results in the reduction of resources to those who are not organized, to those who have little or no voice, to the poor for whom access to health care is so often limited. And poverty cannot justly be a basis for exclusion when health care is distributed.

Scarce resource arguments are notoriously hard to make. They usually leave us unconvinced, and for good reason. We do not want to face them. Yet our society is already rationing its medical care. We must look at how we do it and try to do it better.

Notes

1. Some authors distinguish these two terms. Allocation means deciding on the basis of disease or other medical criteria; rationing means deciding which person or persons of equal need get a limited resource, or deciding on the basis of age or other criteria not considered to be strictly medical. Although the distinction is helpful, it is not clear that the two can be completely distinct, or that, as some argue, we ought to allocate but never ration.

2. The problem stems from a claimed difference in what counts as a live birth as opposed to a miscarriage among the nations compared. It seems that American statistics count as live births premature fetuses who cannot survive and who are considered miscarriages in other nations. Different American states may compile their data differently. This would affect not only infant mortality figures but life-expectancy figures as well. It is uncertain how much this kind of discrepancy affects the final rankings, or even how much discrepancy exists. The final figures are quoted in the literature with no explanation of whether the data on which they are based are comparable. It is unlikely that the incomparability of the data base, to the extent it does exist, would be enough to put the United States at the top or even near the top of the infant mortality list. But issues like this do make it clear that comparative statistics are only as good as the figures on which they are based.

3. See also Churchill 1987, 10, who cites figures from 1983 of twenty-five million at any one time, and thirty-four million at some period during a year. The thirty-seven million figure is from Waldman, Lachman, and Bradburn 1990, 47.

4. It seems that only some preventive measures actually save money in the long run, despite the often-made claim to the contrary. Preventing smoking, for example, while admirable in reducing illness, results in longer lives for those who do not smoke, with the added health care costs those longer lives require (Menzel 2011b, 17).

5. One of the strongest bases of support for universal health insurance provided either by a single-payer tax-funded system or by a universal insurance mandate coupled with government

subsidy for those unable to afford the premiums is found in the fact that in the United States there is already a law mandating emergency room care for all persons regardless of ability to pay or even, in some cases, willingness to pay (Menzel 2011a, 84–90). This has been the case since 1989, when the Emergency Medical Treatment and Labor Act (EMTALA) was enacted in Washington. Since emergency room care is already mandated, and since it is terribly inefficient to treat nonemergent care in emergency rooms, efficiency alone indicates the need to make sure all persons carry health insurance. Otherwise those who are insured carry the burden of those who are not. The alternative would be to repeal EMTALA. This would result in the deaths of persons whose lives could otherwise be saved, which would be immoral, but it would be consistent with the free-market individualism that opposes universal insurance. As it stands, the health care system in the United States is both unjust and inefficient.

Most opposition to the PPACA came from those who oppose government involvement in health care, reject the idea of universal health insurance and the right to health care, and oppose further government spending and increased taxes. But opposition also came from the American Catholic bishops despite their consistent and well-known support for health care rights. The bishops feared that the steps taken to prohibit public funding for abortion were insufficiently strong despite President Obama's executive order against it, and also rejected a requirement that insurance companies include coverage for contraception, even to workers in some Catholic organizations (see chapter 24 for a detailed analysis of this issue in the context of the principle of cooperation). On the other hand, the Catholic Health Association supported the bill (Furton 2011b, 419; see also Saunders 2010, 653–56).

6. Political opposition to even the remotest possibility of rationing health care has been strong in the United States during the debate about the PPACA. Even conversations between doctors and patients about the possible forgoing of treatment have been called "death panels" by Sarah Palin and other Republican opponents of what they call "Obamacare," as we note at the end of chapter 17 (Callahan 2011, 23). This "blatant and unethical mischaracterization" led to the removal of the provision to pay physicians to listen to their patients about these matters (Walter and Goold 2011). Democrats no less than Republicans have opposed any significant form of rationing (Callahan 2011, 25).

This kind of opposition has not been limited to the United States. In England, the National Institute for Clinical Excellence (NICE) has recently come under fire for its decisions not to pay for certain very expensive cancer drugs that offered only marginally greater benefit than much cheaper alternatives (Callahan 2011, 24–26; Latham 2011). Pharmaceutical companies in England, along with the British tabloid press, convinced the public that NICE was killing people to save money, and the future of NICE with its ability to ration treatment is uncertain. During the 2010 debate on health care reform in the United States, Republican opponents warned that the new bill might result in something like NICE for the United States, calling NICE "a real-life, socialist, bureaucratic 'death panel'" (Latham 2011, 53). As a result of this, Congress amended the PPACA to forbid any recommendations that Medicare not pay for certain treatments if the recommendations were based on a comparison of cost to expected benefit (Latham 2011).

It is important to understand what the issue is here. Research and experience suggest that some treatments are marginally more effective than others. The drug Erbitux, for example, extends the life of the average cancer sufferer that takes it by 1.2 months over the standard treatment. The cost for this gain, measured in life-years, is $800,000 per year of life gained (Menzel 2011a, 97). Similarly Cetuximab, a drug for non–small cell lung cancer, when added to traditional therapy, extends patients lives by an average of about five weeks at a cost of $80,000. To treat the sixty thousand patients with this disease in the United States, increasing their lives by an average of five weeks each would cost $4.8 billion dollars annually (Largent and Pearson 2012, 32–33). Another example is Provenge, a drug for terminal prostate cancer advertised as reducing the risk of death by 24 percent. But this does not mean that 24 percent of the patients do not die. It means patients live an average of four months longer than they would on the standard treatment, and then they die. The drug costs $93,000 or about $300,000 per year of life gained. The number of drugs like these is increasing rapidly and will increase only more rapidly with the development of "personalized medicine," drugs aimed at specific subgroups of patients based on their individual genetic makeup. Drug companies will be able to sell each of these drugs only to small groups of patients, and the resulting high cost of each drug coupled with the huge increase in their number will overwhelm both public and private insurance providers (ibid., 28).

These are the kinds of treatments that Medicare should rightly refuse to pay for in order that monies available from the savings could be used for other, clearly more important purposes. Individuals would still be free to pay for these treatments themselves or to pay for private insurance that would cover it. Yet opposition to any form of rationing, loudly proclaimed by politicians of both parties for their own purposes, has resulted in the legal prohibition for Medicare to consider costs in making decisions about which treatments to cover. As long as a drug provides any comparative advantage at all, it must be paid for, even at a cost of hundreds of thousands of dollars for minimal life gained. Individual patients have no incentive to decline the treatment, since they do not pay anything for it. In a nation that continues to refuse to provide basic health care for its citizens, and that claims that this refusal is based on cost, this policy is patently unjust.

The result of all of this is a refusal to make the difficult decisions openly and an inevitable continuation of the "soft rationing" Callahan so rightly decries. Ironically, perhaps even perversely, a deficit-reduction proposal passed by the Republican-controlled House of Representatives in 2011 would essentially eliminate Medicare altogether rather than face difficult allocation decisions. Somehow it is better to have no health care at all, except presumably for the wealthy, than to face up to the need for the ethical control of health care costs.

7. In addition to political opposition to needed ethical and transparent rationing, other factors also contribute to the difficulty the United States faces in reforming its health care system. One of these is the trend toward the lowering of diagnostic thresholds (Welch 2011). Over the years the numbers that designate "abnormal" test results have changed, so that a test that once would have been considered normal is now said to indicate a condition that requires treatment. "High normal" becomes "abnormal," "normal" becomes "high normal," and so on. This has happened with cholesterol numbers, blood pressure numbers, prostate tests, other cancer tests, osteoporosis numbers, diabetes numbers, and so on. The treatments cost money and often carry risks. In theory, setting the break point between normal and abnormal (the diagnostic threshold) ought to be done by independent research, but even when this is the case, there is usually no clear reason to draw a line at one point rather than at another slightly different point. So other factors intervene. Physicians and their malpractice insurance companies recognize that juries are likely to award large settlements if it can be shown that a physician did not order a treatment for a test result that many consider normal but that some claim to be abnormal. Thus, doctors—fearing lawsuits—are more likely to overtreat than to undertreat. Pharmaceutical corporations want people to use their drugs, so they encourage physicians to prescribe them for marginal conditions. And much of the research on which the diagnostic thresholds are supposed to be based is funded by and controlled by these same corporations, who have a significant incentive to lower the thresholds to sell more drugs.

8. A counter position has been proposed, which argues that the interests of the family ought to be given equal weight to those of the patient, even when decisions are made by surrogates (Hardwig 1990). According to this position, the criteria of patient autonomy and patient best interests should be rejected or radically changed. While it is true that the Catholic tradition has

insisted on the moral rightness of a patient deciding for him- or herself to forgo treatment in order to help others, this criterion is far more problematic when the decision is made by surrogates and is based on their own interests. Possibly some reconciliation between the generally accepted "best interests of the patient" standard and Hardwig's insistence that the best interests of the family be given equal weight would result from recalling the flexibility of the "ordinary-extraordinary" distinction and its moral nature. Doubtless much treatment that would be rejected "in the best interests of the family" would also be rejected if the "best interests of the patient" were given primacy but were interpreted humanly, not biologically or medically. But Hardwig's proposal is fraught with danger if it means that families could override the patient's interests in favor of their own. The *Cruzan* decision worries about the precise kind of danger Hardwig's proposal seems to risk. We dealt with these issues at length in chapter 16.

9. For a succinct and particularly evocative analysis of this issue from both bioethical and economic-ethical perspectives, see Baily 2003. Baily points out that although earlier bioethicists adopted the position that physicians should not ration at the bedside, this opinion is changing in the context of managed care (39–40). She argues for establishing a national minimal standard of care as the only way to move toward a resolution of the problem (40–41).

10. For lengthy development of these issues, see Dougherty 1988. See also Beauchamp and Childress 2001, 230–35.

11. Recent developments in biogerontology have suggested to some the possibility of a mean life expectancy of 112 years and a maximum of 140 years. Proponents claim that this life would be one of "compressed morbidity," meaning that the ills usually associated with old age would not occur until very shortly before death. Virtual immortality is even considered possible by some (Juengst et al. 2003, 25–27). Callahan continues to oppose this, supporting what he calls the "traditionalist view of the life cycle" and arguing that such an approach harms not only society as a whole but even the individuals whose lives are extended (Callahan 2003). David Gems, on the other hand, argues that society would indeed be harmed but that longer-living individuals would be given a chance at a richer life (Gems 2003).

12. For one rejection of the entire position, and for citations of many authors on both sides, see Kilner 1988.

13. Daniels makes his argument from the basis of what he calls a "prudential life-span account." All persons have a right to an "age-relative normal opportunity range." Working from a contractarian approach where prudent deliberators must choose a just system for their society, Daniels argues that this just system may rightly include restrictions on life-extending technology to the old. This is not a question of discriminating among birth cohorts (between different people born in different years) but of discriminating among age groups (among the same people at different times in their lives). Prudent deliberators will choose to postpone some expenses in order to save for old age, but they need not postpone enough to enable them to extend their lives beyond a "prudential lifespan" (Daniels 1988).

14. For detail on the complex issues of rationing mental health care, see J. L. Nelson 2003.

15. Inevitably, people have different ideas of what "reasonable health" means. But this phrase is preferable to the one used by Charles Dougherty, who wants national health insurance to provide funding for treatments "likely to preserve or restore functioning typical for a normal member of the species" (Dougherty 1988, 189). It is clear from his book that Dougherty does not intend it, but this might mean no funding for any treatment whatsoever for anyone less than "normal," mentally or physically. We should rightly avoid the extreme of vitalism, which insists, for example, on treating all handicapped newborns regardless of severity of illness or of quality of outcome. But we surely ought to continue to fund the kinds of simple surgery that allow infants born with Down syndrome to live. Similarly, nursing home care and personal care services needed by many partly disabled elderly ought to be funded even though "normal" functioning might not be possible (Daniels 1988, 79, 103–16).

CHAPTER 29

THE USE AND MISUSE OF THE ALLOCATION ARGUMENT

ALLOCATION-OF-RESOURCE ARGUMENTS can take many forms, and there are a number of important systemic questions involved in the larger context of such arguments. In theory, they demand for their solution a complete system of justice, but even then there are difficulties, since such systems seldom solve specific issues. In any case, no such attempt can be made here. Those attempts that have been made—for example, that of John Rawls ([1971] 1999)—have met with mixed reviews and leave open the specific kind of question we want to explore in this chapter.[1] While the applications here will be limited to medical ethics, the methodological questions have implications for other areas of social ethics as well.

This chapter deals with the allocation-of-scarce-resource argument as that argument occurs explicitly or implicitly in the following form: it is morally wrong to spend X money on A while situation B exists, on which the X money ought to be spent instead. This form of the allocation argument distinguishes it from another, easier question, one usually considered an issue of "microallocation." This other question concerns who, of a limited number of named potential recipients, should receive the organ, the machine, or the hospital bed. These issues have not been completely resolved either, but there is agreement concerning some of the factors that may rightly be included (medical factors, time on the list, randomization) as well as those that should not usually be considered (race, gender, social worth).[2]

In the first and second sections of this chapter, we suggest reasons why the allocation argument in the form "X money should not be spent on A as long as situation B exists, on which the money should be spent instead" is so often unpersuasive. In the third section, we advance a suggestion for making it more persuasive by arguing that it can take on a more directly normative quality—that is, it can more persuasively lead to the conclusion that spending the money on A really is wrong—if it is combined with an argument about the benefits or lack of benefits of doing A in the first place. The chapter concludes with an application of this "combination argument" to the current procedure in medicine of using artificial hearts as bridge devices to human heart transplants.

Resistance to Allocation Arguments

Why is it that the allocation argument—"It is wrong to spend X money on A while situation B exists, on which the money ought to be spent instead"—sounds valid at first reading or first hearing but so often fails to be persuasive? We recognize its importance, we know that it urges us to attend to the gross inequalities of our world, and we accept it, even proclaim it as a countervailing exhortation to materialism, consumerism, and selfishness. But when it comes to a normative application of this form of the allocation argument, so that we might really accept the idea that we "ought" to stop spending money on *A* and spend it on *B* instead, the argument often fails to convince. For example, while it seems correct to urge that more health care dollars and energies should be allocated to prevention, and fewer resources, relatively speaking, should be allocated to cure, when it actually comes down to choosing which cures will no longer be available, the allocation argument leaves us unconvinced.

We do ration our health care dollars, as noted in the last chapter. But, to use Daniel Callahan's term, we do it "softly." And "soft" rationing is usually unjust because it tends to follow the path of least resistance, which means that those who have the greatest moral claim on resources are the ones least likely to get them because they have the least powerful voice. Yet "hard" rationing—such as the attempts in Oregon to prioritize treatments for funding and to reduce state funding for transplant surgery in order to make funds available for other purposes—while theoretically a better way to make these kinds of decisions is itself fraught with difficulties (Beauchamp and Childress 2001, 254–57). It is simply very hard to be convinced that some named individual person will have to die ("monies should not be spent on *A*") in order that some other goal may be achieved ("while situation B exists, on which the money should be spent instead"). Why does this form of the allocation argument so often fail to lead to concrete normative conclusions that people are willing to carry out?

There are a number of reasons. Some of these are problematic aspects of the argument itself. Others are resistances that the argument is intended to address and that it urges us to overcome. These latter are surely powerful. The first set of resistances can be summarized as the human resistance to the good, which is a part of the theological doctrine of original sin. We do not allocate our resources more justly because we do not want to. We like to spend our money as we do. Selfishness, greed, and lust for money and power all play a role.

A second set of these resistances is our reliance on technology, our hope that technological answers to the allocation questions will be found by eliminating the scarcity of resources that makes allocation necessary. This is the hope, for example, in cold fusion, which might mean an end to the need to conserve energy. We would prefer not to face the allocation issue that might require us to make hard choices. And surely technology can and does, in many instances, alleviate scarcity and thus reduce the need for allocation. Rejecting technology is not the answer. Physicians and nurses should not want to reject CT scans and heart monitors any more than authors should want to reject computerized word processing.

However, this reliance on technology often increases the scarcity we hope to reduce. So much is spent on high-tech procedures that less is left for other purposes. It is true that the original microallocation question of who gets the dialysis machine was "solved" by eliminating the scarcity through federal funding. The technology has been literally a lifesaver for many persons. But the "solution" has meant that these monies are not available for other purposes. Reliance on technology tends to exacerbate the problem of scarcity at least as much as it alleviates it.

Problems with the Allocation Argument

Greed, selfishness, and a too-eager reliance on technology are powerful forces contributing to our reluctance to accept specific normative conclusions from the allocation argument. But there are problematic aspects to the argument itself. Even if we overcome our selfishness and agree to rely less on technology, problems would remain. When faced with determining exactly which expenses we should not make, or how much wealth is indeed greedy, we find ourselves often without firm norms.

Catholic moral theology is a case in point. Whereas it has been quick (too quick, in our judgment) to make absolute normative applications in areas of sexual ethics and in those areas of medical ethics that deal with reproduction or that otherwise can be "solved" by the physicalist analysis of the traditional principle of double effect, the Catholic tradition has not, at least not usually, attempted to make similar applications in the area of allocating resources. Is it morally wrong to get a heart transplant? What about a second one? Official Catholic teaching prohibits direct sterilization, but there is no norm against expensive neonatology, no insistence that the money be spent instead on prenatal care. No general consensus has emerged in Catholic ethics to conclude that it is wrong to drive a six- or an eight-cylinder car, to take a European vacation, or to buy a DVD player to play movies on a large-screen TV, although it might be implied from many more general statements about consumerism and the unequal distribution of resources that such conclusions would follow.

Why are such conclusions not more often derived from the allocation argument, and why do they seem so unpersuasive? We think it is because the allocation argument itself is problematic in at least five ways. First, the argument is too open-ended. Purpose *A* (the purpose for which spending money is said to be wrong because purpose *B* should get it instead) can be virtually anything that can be seen to be of less importance than purpose *B*. The general argument that we ought to redress the imbalance in our health care policies where too much is spent on expensive cures for the few and too little on prevention for the many is one to which we subscribe. We think this is clear, for example, when one compares the monies spent on expensive peri- and neonatology with those spent on prenatal preventive care, especially for the poor. But how is the argument convincing that it is the neonatal monies that should go to prenatal prevention and not the funds spent on eight-cylinder cars, European vacations, and DVD players? While most of us would agree that we should spend more on prevention of illness than we do, it is very hard to provide adequate justification for the source of the funds. It is easy to identify situation *B*. It is far harder to provide warrants for identifying *A*.[3]

Since *A* can be almost anything, the allocation argument in the form we are examining makes it wrong to do almost anything! Analogously, *A* can be almost if not quite any human activity. Surely food for the starving is more important than teaching Shakespeare. Does this make literature classes and summer Shakespeare festivals morally wrong uses of monies? Of course not. But it is hard to begin with the allocation argument and show *why* not. Even if we were to accept the idea that other expenses more properly fit into category *A* than Shakespeare festivals (the monies spent on gambling, for example), how could we justify going to Niagara-on-the-Lake for Shakespeare just because others go to Las Vegas for the slots? They should spend the money on the poor instead of on the tables, we might say, but just because they do not would not relieve us of the presumed obligation to give up Shakespeare.

Second, there is the question of guilt.[4] The allocation argument, because of its relative inability to exclude almost any resource-expending pleasurable human activity from category *A*, threatens to create false feelings of guilt. If it is indeed morally wrong to take a vacation while monies are needed for food, then we should not do it. If we do, we are guilty of a wrong action and possibly of a sin. But this, it would seem, must be extended to any human action that might fit category *A*. After we have eliminated European vacations, eight-cylinder cars, and DVD players, what next? It would seem there is no end.

The traditional distinction between the so-called positive and negative norms of the natural law, where the former were said to oblige but not to oblige continuously while the latter were said to oblige always, has been correctly criticized by moral theologians as minimalist and often physicalist. Yet the distinction had the advantage of allowing that the positive norms came to an end somewhere. It may be difficult to avoid all deliberate sexual stimulation of thought, word, and deed until married, but at least the obligation is located and limited. If *A* is as widely extended as it would seem to be, then the scrupulous person—indeed, on the presumption that the allocation argument and its implied normative conclusions are correct, the good, virtuous person—is caught in an ethical bind from which there might seem to be no escape save severe poverty or even death. If so many human activities are judged to be wrong uses of resources, then moral uprightness becomes equated with an almost extreme asceticism. Those of us who have counseled people who are tortured with scrupulous consciences in the area of sex ought to be slow to develop other devices of inflicting similar pain.

Anne Patrick points out the dangers of inflicting guilt, using images with which many of us can identify:

> Moral theology, we must admit, is not everyone's favorite subject. The knowing laugh that humorist Garrison Keillor evokes when he refers to . . . "Our Lady of Perpetual Responsibility" says much about moral theology. . . . Moral theology has provided more than one generation with sweaty brows and clammy palms as they examined their consciences and worked up the courage to confess hard-to-name sins in dark confessional boxes around the country. Moral theology, in short, has supplied the peculiarly Catholic variety of guilt so prominent in the literature of parochial school nostalgia. . . . The phrase "moral burnout" is not too strong to describe a syndrome suffered by devout persons who identified all the opinions published in official Catholic books or uttered by religious authority figures as clearly and certainly God's opinion too, and then tried to live in their God-given bodies in the real world. (Patrick 1989, 3)

At this point a counterargument is often made. The allocation argument, it is claimed, is not intended to apply to individual expenses such as vacations, cars, and heart transplants. It is intended to point to structural flaws within the national and international economy, flaws we ought to work to eliminate. In the meantime, even though it is true that spending monies on *A* means that *B* is not funded, it is morally right to do so since individuals cannot be required to give up *A*. We are not exactly sure what to do with this. We agree entirely that the basic intent of allocation arguments, and of redistributive justice generally, is to enact structural change. But we are not sure how the argument, if it is accepted in the form we are examining, can exempt individuals from being bound to stop spending on A simply because the perfect economic system has not yet arrived.

Third, the argument as it stands can be criticized for failing to attend to the more complex aspects of world economics. It is at least possible, and often likely, that doing away with A will not make more funds available for B. This problem is more apparent when one deals with social policy than with individual decision. If an individual decides not to buy a car but to buy food for a poor neighbor instead, that person can be relatively certain where the money goes. But if Medicare were to cut down on reimbursement for certain surgeries, politics might dictate that the savings go to tax cuts for the wealthy instead of to preventive care for the poor. And the complexities of economics get in the way of drawing normative conclusions from the allocation argument. Redistribution is not possible without continuing productivity. Continuing productivity requires at least some restriction on the breadth and the quantity of egalitarian distribution. These issues are too vast for further pursuit here. They necessarily involve the debate between capitalism and socialism with the possibility of some third alternative that might reduce the evils of both. It is enough here to say that the economy as it is poses problems for the allocation argument—problems that the argument cannot transcend, and that make normative conclusions drawn from it less persuasive than they would otherwise be.

A fourth problem has been pointed out in feminist ethics, although in a much different context from the one we are working in here. It concerns the issue of relationships. Carol Gilligan argues that Lawrence Kohlberg's (1981) stages of ethical development are inadequate, and one of her reasons is that they give too little weight to relationships. They are too abstract, too universal, she argues, and women in Kohlberg's scheme are seen too often to be fixated at a lower, less mature level of moral development (the third stage in Kohlberg's six stages) because women's moral reasoning tends to emphasize personal relationships more than abstract concepts such as equality based on justice and human rights (Gilligan 1982, 18).[5] Women, says Gilligan, emphasize care and connectedness, stressing attachment and seeing individual autonomy and separation as an "illusory and dangerous quest" (ibid., 48). Women's patterns of moral decision making reach judgments that are not universalizable in the traditional sense but that nonetheless offer insights and validity often missed in the more logical male emphases on abstract principles of utility and justice as fairness.

We will not try to develop here the relationship between this approach to ethics and the more usual insistence on universalizability. Some universalizable rules surely apply within family groups, and the principle of universalizability properly requires that some degree of specificity of morally relevant circumstances be included in norms and rules. But it is clear that feminist ethics has something to say about the inadequacy of the allocation argument stated in the form we have suggested. The allocation argument in this form is precisely the kind of abstract argument from justice that some feminist ethicists criticize. It may well be that it *is* morally right to spend money on A even though, in the abstract, situation B is more worthy than A. It is difficult, if not impossible, to give a thoroughly convincing justification for two quite correct moral judgments: first, that it is morally wrong for a physician or a scholar to attend a medical or an academic conference while his or her own child is at home without food; but second, that it is morally right to attend that convention, despite the expense, while thousands die of hunger in our world. Relationship, or "nearness" (Daniels 2012, 40–42), does count toward responsibility. Allocation rules that ignore this are, for that reason, often unconvincing.

A fifth and final problem with the allocation argument is similar to the problem of relationship and has received some attention in ethical scholarship (Daniels 2012; Largent and Pearson 2012). It is the problem of how to decide concerning the moral relevance of the distinction between identified individuals and more vague and unnamed groups. In the allocation argument, *A* may be an identified named person while situation *B* is wider but less easily identified. Should identified children be left in wells to die so that the energy and expense of saving them can be transferred to larger populations who are likewise in desperate need, but whose names are not known?

In medical ethics, the traditional physician–patient relationship establishes a bond of obligation between a doctor and the patients he or she happens to accept. But it leaves far less easily determined the obligations the physician has to sick people whom he or she has *not* accepted as patients.[6] Thus, it has become an acceptable practice—indeed, it is often seen by transplant surgeons to be obligatory—that a second, third, and subsequent organ be transplanted in cases of organ rejection even though other candidates are equally in need and may even have greater potential to benefit. This practice seems to be in conflict with both utilitarian and fairness approaches to justice, at least theoretically, and may well be wrong when proposed as an absolute. Yet it would doubtless be humanly difficult, if not impossible, for transplant teams to abandon patients after the first rejected transplant.

This fifth factor, like the other four, is a complex issue and is not easily open to rational "solution." But it is one more reason why we are reluctant to find the allocation argument convincing when we try to apply it to specific cases so that we might draw from it concrete norms for our conduct.

Before turning to our own suggestion for strengthening the allocation argument, we want to use as an example one attempt to apply the argument directly in medical ethics that we think fails. Donald DeMarco argues that in vitro fertilization (IVF) is immoral because it is "a violation of distributive justice. . . . The extraordinary cost incurred in operating fertility centers which offer a relatively small number of people a relatively small chance of having their own children is inconsistent with society's more general obligation to provide all its citizens with basic health care" (DeMarco 1988, 1).

Now there is much reason to worry concerning fertility centers and IVF. Many centers fail to inform couples of the often very low likelihood of success. There are a number of ethical questions that urge hesitancy. Indeed, if it can be shown that the population served by IVF is not truly benefited by the procedure, then the allocation argument would become the "combination argument" that we propose shortly, and would justify the judgment that IVF should not be done, or at least that it should not receive public funding. But DeMarco's argument as it stands is inadequate, and this becomes even more apparent later in his brief essay when he states:

> Society has a duty to respond to people's health needs, since people have a right to have these needs met. Basic needs are universal and as such are appropriately discussed in the framework of rights. Wants, on the other hand, are private rather than universal.

An individual may have any number of wants which are peculiar to him. These wants, no matter how intensely he experiences them, are not the same as needs and consequently are not the subject of rights. An individual may want a high income, pleasurable vacations, and a second car. [Why not a first car—is it only a second one that is a want while the first is a need? If so, why is a pleasurable vacation a want and not a need?] He may also want contraception, sterilization, and access to an in vitro fertilization program. At best, these are privileges rather than rights. But when society allows the medical profession to deprive some people of their basic rights to health care in order to try to satisfy the wants of others, the issue of social justice is brought into sharp focus. Social justice demands that rights be met before wants are satisfied. (DeMarco 1988, 2–3)

The problematic nature of this argument should be clear from what we have already said. DeMarco puts contraception, sterilization, and in vitro fertilization into his category *A*, along with pleasurable vacations and a second car. He calls them privileges, but then, especially for IVF but at least implicitly for the others, he argues that they are immoral because the resources spent on them ought to go instead to true health care needs. It is clear that his choice of the medical procedures to be rejected is influenced by the fact that they are condemned by physicalist Catholic medical ethics. And his distinction between "wants" and "needs" lacks criteria. This kind of application of the allocation argument will convince only those searching for further support of an ethical judgment already made on other grounds—grounds that proscribe the procedures in question as morally wrong apart from any problem of allocation. In the absence of such grounds, the allocation argument advanced here fails to convince for the reasons we have already proposed.

Improving the Allocation Argument

Is the allocation argument then utterly useless? The first answer to this would probably be no, and we think this answer is intuitively correct. Most obviously, it has merit as exhortation. Even if it is hard to apply convincingly to individual cases—that is, even if it is hard to identify *A*—the allocation argument properly urges us to worry about distributive justice. It *is* a scandal that there is in our world both great wealth and great poverty. Although the allocation argument may not be conclusive in concrete instances, it does make us pause. It points out to us the necessity of at least imagining a better way. If it is optimistic, even utopian in the common meaning of that term, the society urged upon us by the argument for a just allocation is nonetheless a society toward which struggle—prudent and cautious perhaps, but struggle nonetheless—ought to be exerted.

In this the allocation argument is not unlike other principles often derived from theology that are seen to be important in medical ethics. As was note in chapter 5, these theological principles—for example, the principle of God's dominion over human life—are often misused in medical ethics when it is implied that they can solve medical ethical issues. But these principles act more as hermeneutic themes than as norms and rules. They give us hints. They make us pause and think. The allocation argument does these things well, and for this reason alone it should not be abandoned. It reminds us that we are not isolated individuals, that we have obligations to others, even to unnamed others in vague faraway groups, that we do not have absolute rights to private property, that wants and needs, even if not easily distinguished, are not identical. As exhortation, as hint, as caution, the allocation argument is of significant importance.

But there may be even more. Perhaps the allocation argument can be helpful in leading to normative conclusions. Our proposal here might allow us, in some cases, to combine the allocation argument as such with another claim that, while not of itself conclusive, might, in combination with the allocation argument, provide moral warrant for judging that spending the money on A is morally wrong. We suggest that the allocation argument, when combined with the empirical claim that A is at best of dubious benefit for those on whom the money is spent, properly serves as a basis for the moral judgment that the funds ought to be spent elsewhere instead. Although the combination argument is not directly helpful in identifying B, and although it does not answer problems three, four, and five enumerated earlier, it can help in identifying A, and this opening toward an answer to problems one and two might enable us, tentatively at least, to derive normative judgments on the basis of the demand for allocation.

Artificial Heart Implants

The best way to develop what we mean by this "combination argument" is to apply it to a specific issue in medical ethics: the use of the artificial human heart. There are two uses proposed. Artificial hearts can be used as permanent implants and as temporary devices intended to keep people alive until a human heart is available for transplant. We find it harder to arrive at a moral judgment about permanent artificial implants than about transitional implants because it is more difficult to be sure about the benefits of permanent devices.

Moral judgment about permanent artificial hearts is complex. Theoretically, the artificial heart would seem to be an ethical as well as a technological advance over cadaver transplants. A permanent artificial heart would eliminate that portion of organ scarcity that results from too few donors. It is likely that the costs would decrease if more hearts were made. The problem of rejection, and thus the cost and dangers of immunosuppressant drugs, would seem to be less than with human or animal hearts. It might be easier to "fix" and to "do maintenance on" a human-made heart than an organic one.

Thus far, however, there has been little widespread success with the permanent artificial heart. This is true in the early stages of most medical techniques, and some are of the opinion that despite the present difficulties, there is sufficient hope of benefit to patients to permit the procedure as a therapy of last resort. But is there such a hope? Our moral judgment, in the combination argument we propose, must depend in part on whether the hope of benefit is proportionate to the risk of harm. At present, it seems that there may be little likelihood of real benefit to the recipient of a permanent artificial heart. Some of the machines radically inhibit mobility. Some patients suffer from periods of physical and mental incapacity. As long as there is little or no hope of real human benefit, experimentation with permanent artificial hearts must be strictly limited. If there are patients whose hearts offer them no hope of survival, and for whom human heart transplants are and will remain impossible, limited experimentation with permanent artificial hearts would seem to be ethical, provided all the requirements of informed consent are adhered to strictly, provided there is indeed no other way to gain the needed knowledge, and provided the experimental protocol is properly designed and approved. If these experiments are of little or no real benefit to recipients, then when it is determined that they are not advancing vital knowledge, no more should be attempted.

On the other hand, if these experiments show promise (and recent developments suggest that advances are being made), then we do not see a way to forbid them by the allocation argument. For all the reasons we have noted, it seems impossible to forbid permanent artificial hearts just because the monies might better be spent on other purposes. Our society may make a reasonable political decision not to fund them with public monies, and such a decision would, in principle, be just. But we can find no reason why society must make this decision if permanent artificial hearts show promise of helping those who need them. Thus, the final judgment about permanent artificial hearts rests on their results. If they are of little or no human benefit to those who get them, then they should not be funded except for limited experimentation, and even that should be shut off when no more knowledge can be gained. But if they bring real benefits, then we do not see how the allocation argument can forbid them.

But what about the temporary artificial heart? Here major ethical problems arise. Instead of costs being reduced, as might be true for permanent artificial hearts, costs are increased because a second expensive procedure is added. The scarcity of organs is not alleviated. Indeed, since more patients are alive to need them, the scarcity problem is increased. Thus, temporary artificial hearts as a therapy for end-stage heart disease should not be attempted. As long as there are too few cadaver hearts, the temporary use of artificial hearts only adds to the list of those needing them without adding to the list of donors. This would change if enough human hearts should become available, but that seems unlikely, and for now the procedure is of no benefit to end-stage heart patients as a whole. Potential recipients without artificial hearts are passed over in favor of those with them, who would otherwise already have died. Since this is done at great cost, and since it merely shifts the outcome of who will live and who will die from one group to another within the population of those needing heart transplants, it does seem to be a morally wrong procedure.

Ethically, then, it seems that as long as there is a shortage of human hearts for transplant, temporary artificial implants should be limited to a restricted number of experimental procedures intended to gain knowledge that might help in designing permanent implants. The reason for this conclusion is a combination of general criteria for the just allocation of resources together with the claim that there is a lack of any real benefit to the population of potential recipients of the temporary devices. Although individuals are helped, there is no benefit to the population of those needing transplants.

Note that there is a difference here between saying that temporary artificial hearts *must not* be used because of the combination argument we are making here, and saying that they *need not* be used because they are morally extraordinary. Morally extraordinary treatment is optional, not ethically wrong. Patients have the moral option of deciding whether they want the treatment. In the present case, we are saying that transitional artificial hearts *must not* be used (except in strictly limited experimental protocols) as long as they offer no benefit to the population of heart patients who need transplants.

A difficult problem remains. Who is obliged to reject this expense? On whom does the obligation for a better allocation rest? Theoretically, it rests on all of us. The medical profession should not use temporary artificial heart implants as a standard treatment modality for patients with end-stage heart disease. Public funding should not support it. And dying patients should not consent to it. Given the inherent difficulties with allocation arguments, however, it is perhaps arrogant and overreaching to conclude that individuals are obliged to refuse to accept temporary artificial hearts. Theoretically that conclusion may be justified. But practically it will be better for our society to work toward a better system of health care delivery, one where such expenditures are not publicly funded, and one where all citizens are aware of the social nature of medicine and of its costs.

Conclusion

Despite the difficulty we often encounter in coming to precise conclusions about how we should allocate our resources, we do need to trouble ourselves about this issue. If we believe that humans are one in God's creative love, then we need to be concerned about all humans, not just about the ones in our own hospitals or offices. And this concern must be one of the reasons why we will reject procedures that are not only expensive but also of dubious benefit to the few whom they are supposed to help.

Notes

1. This last point is noted briefly by Kaufmann 1973, 91. General systems of justice often leave specific questions unanswered. For a system of justice similar to Rawls's but differing in some details and critical of Rawls on some counts, see Sterba 1980, esp. 29–62. Sterba argues for a "basic needs minimum," which he says is less demanding than that required by Rawls's maximin principle. But Sterba points out the requirement that persons contribute to the basic needs of future generations and distant peoples. Although he applies his system to a rejection of abortion on demand, and states that his system requires considerable sacrifice (151), he does not explicitly state the kinds of expenses that must be forgone or the amount of wealth that is immorally high. Another approach to distributive justice is suggested by Alan Gewirth, who derives it from his "principle of generic consistency" (Gewirth 1978). On Rawls, see Rawls (1971, 1999; Daniels 1974; Wolff 1977).

2. One aspect of this "easier" issue that is probably impervious to an acceptable solution is the question of how many "American" organs should be made available for "foreigners." One figure often used is 10 percent. This seems to many to be an acceptable compromise between the strange notion that only Americans are worthy of getting American organs and the danger of making so many organs available to the wealthy from foreign countries who are able to come to the United States that many Americans are in effect shut out. But why 10 percent? Why not 20 percent, as suggested by the National Task Force on Organ Transplantation (Jonasson 1986)? The American Society of Transplant Surgeons proposed a maximum of 5 percent (ibid.). The 10 percent figure is supported by Kleinig (1986). Why is any limitation just? No theoretically acceptable solution is apparent. In this, the problem is similar to the one explored in this chapter.

3. We think this is true even if *A* is identified as military spending, which it very often is. Unless it can be argued persuasively that military spending is in itself either unnecessary or otherwise morally wrong, the problem occurs even when *A* is military expense. We must, of course, strive for the kinds of international structural changes that would reduce our reliance and the reliance of other nations on the military. It is true that military expenses are morally wrong when they are not necessary. But we cannot accept the argument that all of the defense budget is in this category. And, as has been noted, even the elimination of the entire military budget, which would be immoral, would not ultimately solve the problem of scarce resources. Nations that spend far less on their defense than the United States also spend less on health care. An exploration of this question depends, of course, on a complex series of analyses that are impossible here.

4. See Kaufmann 1973, esp. 66–96, 112–37. Kaufmann tends at times to reject altogether the notion of justice in order to get rid of guilt (e.g., 112), a proposal we do not accept. Still, he makes excellent points not easily answered.

5. The third stage, says Kohlberg, emphasizes "trying hard," "pleasing others," and relationships, and does not yet demonstrate the universality of principles of justice found in stages five and six. For a development of these stages, see Duska and Whelan 1975, 46, 58–64, 87–88. For another feminist approach to relational ethics, see Noddings 2003.

6. This area has been examined in the context of a physician's duty to care for AIDS patients (Freedman 1988; Arras 1988; Annas 1988).

CHAPTER 30

GLOBAL BIOETHICS

MEDICINE AND ETHICS have been associated with each other from the beginning. Hippocrates (ca. 460–370 BC) is known as "the father of medicine." He was a contemporary of the famous Greek philosophers Socrates and Plato. He argued in his works that medicine should be emancipated from mythical and magical thinking since medical interventions are based on experience and reasoning (see chapter 1). He explains that one can no longer assume that diseases have a supernatural cause but one should make accurate observations and experiments to identify what pathological processes are going on and how they can be remediated. For Hippocrates, this scientific methodology of observation and analysis is not separated from religion and should be combined with an ethical approach. A good physician is not only competent but also responsible; he will follow certain ethical rules. These rules are formulated in the Hippocratic Oath (Carrick 1985, 60). Greek medicine was not unique. Healing activities are as old as humankind. Ancient Mesopotamia was famous for its medicine. Hammurabi, king of Babylon in the eighteenth century BC, promulgated one of the first law codes in history, written on clay tablets. In the ancient Indian medicine of Ayurveda, the physician Charaka (third century BC) produced a code of conduct that emphasized compassion as the basic ideal in medicine (Francis 1996). He built on an older tradition in which Hindu physicians took the so-called vaidya's oath, which obligated them to give absolute priority to the care for their patients (Young 2009).

Although the term "medical ethics" was used for the first time in the nineteenth century, consideration of ethical questions in connection to health, disease, and health care is not new (Baker and McCullough 2009). But the focus of ethics had not been the same. For a long time the emphasis of medical ethics was on the person of the doctor, on conduct according to professional rules, or on professional duties. The importance of the virtuous conduct of physicians was transformed when, in the nineteenth century, medical associations emerged and when social changes such as health insurance and health care systems developed. The rise of medicine as a profession made it clear that individual virtues were insufficient; professional rules and standards needed to be defined and exemplified as codes of conduct. What has remained consistent during these changes is that medical professionals themselves continued to determine what were the standards for good conduct as well as the criteria for the virtuous doctor.

Other significant changes took place in the second half of the twentieth century. The growth of medical science and technology as well as social changes, such as the civil rights movement, necessitated two changes in medical ethics. First, the ethics discussion was no longer focused on the behavior of health care professionals. Many ethical issues went beyond the usual orientation on good conduct, professional ethics, and professional virtues. New ethical problems have emerged related to death and dying, continuing or foregoing treatment, and allocation of scarce resources. The scope of medical ethics therefore has enlarged. Second, the ethical debate is no longer in the hands of medical professionals. The media, policymakers, and health administrators were originally involved, but increasingly all citizens became aware of the significance of ethical issues in the field of health, disease, and care. These changes became visible in different terminology: "medical ethics" was regarded as too narrow; "health care ethics" and "bioethics" became more popular.

Bioethics

The first person to use and elaborate the term "bioethics" in print was the US cancer researcher Van Rensselaer Potter (1911–2001). He became interested in ethical issues precisely because of his research. Cancer is a complex problem that requires interdisciplinary cooperation. A focus on individual and medical perspectives is insufficient since many cancers are related to lifestyle and individual behavior—smoking, for example—but also to environmental pollution with carcinogenic substances. Medical research will bring some limited progress at the individual level, for example, with new chemotherapies that can alleviate suffering and prolong life expectancy, or with new surgical interventions. But much more progress can be accomplished at the level of populations with preventive programs educating people to live more healthily. His long years of cancer research convinced Potter that a broader approach beyond the individual medical perspective was necessary. At the same time he regretted that his long-term preoccupation with cancer had prevented him from addressing more important issues. Potter summarized these priority problems of our time as the six P's: population, peace, pollution, poverty, politics, and progress (Potter 1971, 150).

For Potter, it is clear that an innovative approach in ethics is necessary. To be able to deal with the priority problems of humankind, we need a new discipline that combines the science of living systems, or biological knowledge ("bio"), with the knowledge of human value systems and philosophy ("ethics"). This new discipline of "bioethics" introduces a broader perspective than the usual medical ethics approach.

Bioethics Is Different—in Theory

The first characteristic of bioethics is that it is oriented toward the future. This orientation is prominent in the title of Potter's first book: *Bioethics—Bridge to the Future*. Bioethics should be a bridge between the present and the future because the survival of humankind requires a focus on long-term interests and goals. For Potter, the overarching concern of bioethics is long-term global human survival. This goal can only be reached by forging compromises between individual interest and social good, and between the quality of the environment and the "sanctity of the dollar" (Potter 2001, 20).

Second, bioethics is an interdisciplinary enterprise. It indicates the need to bridge science and philosophy. The basic problems of humankind are multidimensional. To address them it is necessary to combine all categories of knowledge, in particular biological knowledge and ethics. We cannot proceed with experts working only in their own specialties. What should be created, according to Potter, is "a new breed of scholars," persons who combine a knowledge of new science with old wisdom (Potter 1964, 1022). Also urgently needed are new methods and approaches. The fundamental problems of humankind can only be addressed with a mix of basic biology, social sciences, and the humanities. Interdisciplinary groups should be established that exchange new ideas and examine old ideas in the light of scientific knowledge. These new approaches can provide the wisdom that is fundamental for the overarching long-term goal of human survival. We do not merely need more technology, specialized knowledge, or philosophical reflection. What is required in the first place is "knowledge of how to use knowledge," which Potter called "wisdom" (Potter 1971, 1).

The third characteristic of bioethics is that human beings are part of nature. We cannot continue to degrade and destroy the environment. Bioethics should widen its scope and focus on the question of how to preserve, in Potter's words, "the fragile web of nonhuman life that sustains human society" (Potter 1970, 243). Ethics should be extended from individual and social issues to environmental concerns. Bioethics therefore has a wide scope.

Bioethics Is Not So Different—in Practice

Since it was introduced in the scholarly literature in 1970, the term "bioethics" became popular and widely used. One of the early centers in this field, the Kennedy Institute at Georgetown University, established in 1971, included "bioethics" in its original name. Already in 1978 more than 1,500 colleges in the United States offered courses in bioethics (Potter 1987). The new name was assumed to highlight the broadening of scope of medical ethics. But Potter believes this was misleading. His new idea was misused because "bioethics" in practice continued to focus on medical issues. It was simply an "outgrowth of medical ethics" (Potter 1988, 1). It was concerned with the perspective of the individual patient: how can individual lives be enhanced, maintained, and prolonged through the application of medical technologies? And it was exclusively interested in the short-term consequences of medical and technological interventions. Although Potter concedes that medical bioethics has a broader approach than traditional medical ethics, it is still too narrow to address what are, in his view, the basic and urgent ethical problems of humankind that are threatening the human survival. To adequately address these problems, according to Potter, a new science of survival is necessary. It was for this purpose he had proposed a new discipline called "bioethics." Because contemporary bioethics is not generating new perspectives and new syntheses, Potter wants to reemphasize the concern for the future of the human species by qualifying the terminology. What we currently have is medical bioethics. It needs to be combined with ecological bioethics. Both approaches in bioethics should be merged in a new synthetic approach called "global bioethics."

Global Bioethics

In Potter's vision (1988) global bioethics unites two meanings of the word "global." First, it is a system of ethics that is worldwide in scope. Second, it is unified and comprehensive.

The fact that bioethics today is a worldwide ethics can also have two meanings: international or planetary. Bioethical issues and concerns transcend national boundaries. But global bioethics is more than international bioethics; it is not merely a matter of crossing borders; it concerns the planet as a whole. Bioethics today is relevant to all countries and takes into account the concerns of all human beings wherever they are. Although bioethics emerged in Western countries, it has expanded globally. There is now a new social space, not simply a collection of countries, regions, and continents, that engages bioethical discourse. This new space has emerged because ethical problems today are planetary. An important source of inspiration for Potter was the work of Pierre Teilhard de Chardin (1881–1955), French philosopher, geologist, and Jesuit (ten Have 2012). Potter referred frequently to Teilhard. Writing in the 1940s and 1950s, Teilhard anticipated what we now call "globalization." Humanity will develop into a global community. Due to the processes of "planetary compression" (intensified communication, travel, exchanges through economic networks) and "psychic interpenetration" (increased interconnectedness and a growing sense of universal solidarity), humankind will be involved in an irresistible process of unification. Human beings are becoming increasingly aware of their interdependency and their common destiny. The world population is growing while the surface of the earth remains the same; therefore, people are obliged to cooperate even more intensely: "We can progress only by uniting" (Teilhard de Chardin 2004, 66). According to Teilhard we are in a process of evolution that will lead to a moral community of citizens of the world. It is this process that he calls "planetization of Mankind" (ibid., 108).

Potter's second meaning of "global" refers to bioethics as more encompassing and comprehensive, combining traditional professional (medical and nursing) ethics with ecological concerns and the larger problems of society. For him, global bioethics is the mainstream into which medical and ecological bioethics eventually must merge. Taking global bioethics seriously will imply a further evolution of ethics: from a focus on relations between individuals, to relations between individuals and society, and ultimately to relations between human beings and their environment. The evolution of ethics in the context of health care reflects this pattern: developing from medical ethics into health care ethics and medical bioethics, we are witnessing today the emergence of global bioethics.

New Issues

Another way of defining the "global" in global bioethics is through issues and problems that are addressed today. Of course, the "traditional" topics continue to be discussed, such as abortion, end-of-life care, reproductive technologies, transplantation medicine, and medical futility. But these concerns are primarily relevant for developed countries, whereas many developing countries cope with issues such as access to medication, traditional medicine, and exploitation. New bioethical problems such as pandemics, organ trade, international clinical trials, climate change, obesity, malnutrition, food production, corruption, bioterrorism, and disasters are global in nature. Global bioethics is characterized by new issues that affect everyone everywhere.

Globalization

In the 1990s drug research rapidly became a global enterprise (see chapter 23). Clinical trials were increasingly outsourced, initially to Eastern Europe and now more often to developing countries, especially India and China. Forty percent of clinical trials were carried out in so-called emerging markets in 2005 (Petryna 2009). This expansion of clinical research into countries without a strong ethical infrastructure (no regulation, no legislation, and few ethics committees or ethics experts) has been associated with many ethical problematic cases. But it has also created new debates, for example, about the use of placebos because standard treatment is not available or too expensive in resource-poor countries (see chapter 23). Health care itself has also increasingly been globalized because it is considered as a global market. This has created a disconcerting brain drain. Health professionals such as nurses are educated in poor countries like the Philippines and then recruited to work in the United Kingdom. Medical tourism is another global phenomenon. For example, patients with chronic diseases such as Parkinson's disease are lured into so-called stem cell clinics in Russia where they pay for futile and unproven treatment. There is also the phenomenon of organ trafficking. People in poor countries such as Pakistan sell their kidneys to rich patients in the United States who don't want to be on a waiting list. Many bioethical problems today are no longer domestic problems. Health care requires global policies and approaches. The 2009 swine flu pandemic originated in Mexico but infected 11–21 percent of the world population. The global response to this pandemic, including the ethical problems engendered, needed international coordination by the World Health Organization.

Global Health and Justice

Broader perspectives in bioethics were advocated since the 1980s with increasing interest in such issues as access to health care, right to health care, prioritizing limited resources, and social determinants of health. This macro focus of bioethical analysis easily leads into a global perspective (Brock 2000; Daniels 2006). Of particular relevance is the issue of global health. Global threats such as pandemics and global warming demonstrate that individuals, communities, and the wider world are deeply connected. Globalizing the concerns of bioethics means that more attention is paid to issues relevant to developing countries, in particular global inequalities in health. Global concerns demonstrate the interdependence of people in the world. If an epidemic disease is breaking out in one country, it will have consequences for other countries. If rich patients want to buy organs, people in poor countries run the risk of being exploited.

Environmental Concerns

Since Potter introduced the notion of bioethics, environmental ethics has developed as a separate discipline in applied ethics. Merging the medical and environmental perspectives was Potter's intention in proposing the new concept of "global bioethics." Both perspectives have different theoretical approaches: individual versus common good, concern for individual patients versus survival of humankind, short-term versus long-term interests, present versus future generations. Recently it has been argued that a clear separation between bioethics and environmental ethics is no longer tenable. It is more important that, in practice and in policy, medical and environmental issues have common causes and grounds. Environmental degradation and loss of biodiversity have serious impact on global health and health care (Mascia and Mariani 2010). Climate change and global warming will change disease patterns and will create new health needs. Recent diseases and epidemics such as mad cow disease, salmonella, and swine flu have threatened human health, demonstrating the interconnections among our food, the way we treat animals, and the environment. The widespread use of antibiotics in animal farms contributes to multidrug resistance while at the same time production of animals for food creates an environmental disaster (as one major source of greenhouse gas emissions). These examples illustrate that concern for individuals is not incompatible with concerns for the biosphere.

Policymaking

Another characteristic of global bioethics is its emphasis on policymaking. The interconnected nature of ethical problems today requires international cooperation and regulation. Now that clinical trials are taking place in many countries around the world, it is necessary to determine the ethical principles and guidelines for the execution of trials in heterogeneous conditions and different social and cultural contexts. Practices such as organ trafficking are almost universally condemned but in practice continue to take place. Eradication of this practice requires legislation and implementation policies not only at the level of each country but also at the international level. Even if some countries legally prohibit it, the practice will move to other countries without a strong international legal framework. This is why professional organizations have taken action. Transplantation of kidneys requires surgeons. Trafficking will be more difficult when the world transplant surgeons unite against illegal and commercialized transplant practices. Because of the need for international cooperation, many international organizations (WHO, UNESCO) are now active in the field of global bioethics.

Universal Ethical Framework

Warren Reich has pointed out that global bioethics utilizes a "comprehensive vision of methods" (Reich 1995, 24). The global perspective of bioethics is not a matter of geographical expansion; rather, it refers to phenomena that have a global dimension—that is, they are no longer dependent on the specifics of a particular culture or society. This is not the same as arguing that global bioethics is a unified field of inquiry in which bioethicists behave in similar ways everywhere in the world, or that there is international agreement on fundamental values. That we have similar bioethical problems in different countries does not imply that we have the same ethical approach everywhere. The global dimension, however, invites us to rethink our usual approaches and ethical frameworks. It makes us aware of the "locality" of our own moral views while encouraging us to search for moral views that are shared globally. In this challenge, bioethics is increasingly connected with international law, particularly human rights law, which has a similar global vision.

The growing importance of global bioethics has reactivated the significance of the notion of moral diversity. The development of global bioethics demands a broader framework of normative interpretation and assessment. Is it justified to apply the principle of informed consent in Nigeria where there is a significantly different culture? Should we respect the Chinese practice of harvesting organs from executed persons? In a global perspective, the ethical systems of different cultures need to be examined and moral values analyzed and applied in specific contexts. This is generally recognized as necessary. It has opened up new and fascinating fields of research. But the next step brings us into the old controversy of universal values and local values. Is there a universal framework of principles and values, or are principles and values different, depending on the local, cultural and religious normative systems?

For some, global bioethics as such is an attempt to universalize a specific set of bioethical principles and to export them to the rest of the world. They claim that the four principles formulated by Beauchamp and Childress (see chapter 8) are typically North American principles that are not valid in other parts of the world. Others maintain that global bioethics necessarily reaches beyond the Western individualist perspective of traditional bioethics. It is true that these principles have been formulated in Western countries, but that does not imply that they have no validity outside of these countries. We should make a distinction between origin and validity. The fact that our numerical notation originated from the Arab culture (and they inherited it from the Hindu culture) does not mean that Arab colleagues can still claim it as theirs or that we can blame them imposing their figures on us. The same is true for ethical principles. Whether or not global bioethics is considered to be "ethical imperialism," it has increased sensitivity regarding the application of basic concepts such as individual autonomy and informed consent across the globe. In many non-Western cultures, the autonomy of individuals is not privileged over communities. Global bioethics, therefore, should recognize that in non-Western countries, responsibilities toward family, community, and society can have more significance than individual rights, but that does not mean that individual rights are insignificant. This was a major issue in the development of the UNESCO Universal Declaration on Bioethics and Human Rights.

The search for global ethical principles focuses on the values that we share as human beings. This will be a futile endeavor for some bioethicists because different and contradictory ethics systems exist. If there is no basis for verification of ethical judgments (we treat this issue in chapter 9), then efforts to formulate ethical principles as universal only mean that the dominating system attempts to impose its principles as the universal ones. But this is a mistaken view. This is demonstrated in the activities of the Parliament of the World's Religions. In 1993 approximately two hundred leaders from more than forty religious and spiritual traditions signed the statement "Towards a Global Ethics." This statement, drafted by German theologian Hans Küng, declares that all traditions share common values such as respect for life, solidarity, tolerance, and equal rights (Küng 1997). The document emphasizes that it is important to show what world religions have in common rather than how they differ.

The 191 member states of UNESCO negotiated for two years to reach a consensus on the text of the declaration, And in 2005 they unanimously adopted the declaration. They agreed on fifteen ethical principles as fundamental for global bioethics. These principles include the four principles of Beauchamp and Childress as well as other principles that play a more significant role in non-Western countries, such as solidarity, social responsibility, and benefit-sharing. One of the principles is that of respect for cultural diversity, but this is the only principle that cannot overrule the other principles. In other words, a health care practice that violates human dignity can never be justified by this principle of respect for cultural diversity. This controversy is clear in the debate about informed consent. Although there is wide consensus that informed consent is a fundamental principle, it is also argued that in other cultures the emphasis is different. In African countries, a communitarian approach underlines the importance of the group or tribe. In health care and research decisions, the group discusses the issue and the community leader is the one taking the lead in decision making. In Arab countries the head of the family is crucial, and the husband makes decisions rather than the wife. Nonetheless, the principle requires that in the end the concerned individual needs to provide informed consent. Such different approaches to implementation of principles are common, but they do not affect the validity of the principles. Informed consent in North America requires a great deal of bureaucracy, and patients are required to sign extensive documentation. In many other countries, however, one's word is one's bond, and asking for a signature is a sign of distrust.

The emergence of global bioethics has stimulated interest in perspectives wider than those that focus on the individual and has expanded the idea of the moral community. This is demonstrated in debates on the new principle of protecting future generations and on intergenerational justice. The UNESCO Declaration on the Responsibilities of the Present Generations towards Future Generations (UNESCO 1997) connects our responsibilities to posterity with the need to ensure the continued existence of humankind. These are the same concerns advocated in Potter's conception of global bioethics. Furthermore, the notion of the global moral community is introduced in global bioethics through the principle of benefit sharing. This novel principle is important in the context of bioprospecting, that is, the search for and collection of natural substances for possible development of new medications. Those natural resources are abundantly available in developing countries with rich biodiversity such as Brazil and Indonesia. In many developing countries, traditional medicine is based on such natural resources. These resources and the traditional knowledge of indigenous populations have been appropriated ("biopiracy") by Western companies to fabricate new profitable drugs without any compensation to the indigenous communities. These new debates in fact refer to a more fundamental discourse on "global community" or "world moral community," which regards humanity itself as a moral community. In this discourse two interrelated arguments are used (Agius 2005). One argument is that the global community includes not only human beings but all of nature. The concept of community is broadened to include more than humans; nonhuman species need to be considered members of our community since we all share dependency and vulnerability. In fact, this is Potter's view. He argues that ethics should extend the idea of community from human community to a community that includes soil, water, plants, and animals. Humankind coexists with ecosystems; together they constitute the "entire biological community" (Potter 1988, 78). The second argument is that the earth is not the possession of one particular generation; each generation inherits it and should not bequeath it in an irreversibly damaged state to future generations. Because of the interdependence of human life and the fragility of our planet, we need a new vision of human community that encompasses past, present, and future generations. The future of the human species can only be guaranteed if humanity itself is regarded as a collectivity or a "global community."

The idea that humanity as a global community should be the real focus of bioethics has become morally relevant because it no longer refers merely to extent (a worldwide scope involving "citizens of the world" who are increasingly connected and related due to processes of globalization) but also to content (the identification of global values and responsibilities as well as the establishment of global traditions and institutions). This development is related to the concept of the "common heritage of humankind." Introduced in international law in the late 1960s to regulate common material resources, such as the ocean bed and outer space, the concept was expanded in the 1970s to include culture and cultural heritage. This has led to the construction of a new global geography of symbols indicating that humanity itself can be regarded as a community. Cultural heritage is no longer only representative of a particular culture but of human culture in general. The temples in Abu Simbel in Egypt were entirely relocated in 1968 to avoid their destruction after the construction of the Aswan Dam in the Nile River. This relocation showed that the international community regarded the temples not merely as a product of the Egyptian civilization from the thirteenth century BC. Although built by Pharaoh Ramses, they were the common property of humankind and needed to be preserved. Labeling some cultural products as a world heritage produces a global grammar in which diverse and local phenomena receive a universal significance and require global management. These cultural treasures are expressions of human identity at a global level, they are part of the quest of citizens of the world, and they become indicators of world culture. Regarding and categorizing cultural property as world heritage implies a global civilization project that seeks to create a new global community representing humanity as a whole, enable the identification of world citizens, and evoke a sense of global solidarity and responsibility.

This process of creating the global community as a moral community was further promoted through the application of the concept of "common heritage" in global bioethics, first in the late 1990s in the field of genetics and promoted by genetic researchers themselves, followed in the 2000s by the adoption of a global framework of ethical principles by almost all countries in the world (ten Have and Jean 2009). With such a universal framework, global bioethics can now claim to represent a global geography of moral values that enables humanity itself to be regarded as a moral community. It implies that citizens of high-income countries can no longer be indifferent to clinical research practices or organ trade in low-income countries since the same moral values and standards apply within the global community, although the application is always modified according to local circumstances and local communities. Membership in the global community furthermore draws on a growing number of global institutions and movements (e.g., Doctors without Borders, Bioethics beyond Borders, Oxfam, fair trade, UNESCO). In other words, there is no longer a necessary conflict between individualism and communitarianism. There is a global community of shared values.

These values are the product of intensive and continuous negotiation, deliberation, and dialogue. They are reflected in a universal framework that overrides the diversity of principles and values in different parts of the world and in various religions and cultural traditions. But this framework proceeds without the articulation of absolute principles and values since there is not one supreme principle that trumps the others. Bioethics will continue to proceed with rational deliberation through interpreting, weighing, and applying multiple ethical principles at the same time.

Conclusion

Now that the original notion of bioethics initiated by Potter is revived as "global bioethics," many new issues are on the agenda—systemic corruption, conflicts of interests, and protection of future generations as well as ecological problems such as climate change. These issues require analysis, research and, more important, international action and policies. Bioethical discourse can no longer focus only on the quandaries of rich countries but must also focus on the problems of developing countries. This revival of global bioethics underlines the fact that bioethics is no longer solely an academic discipline but is also public discourse and political concern.

Glossary

Advance directives: Declarations (usually written) made by competent persons stating which treatments they would want (treatment directives or living wills) and which surrogates they would wish to make the decisions (proxy directives) if they are later incapable of doing so themselves.

Allowing to die: Contrasted with killing; the forgoing of life-sustaining treatment such that the patient is allowed to die of the underlying condition. Includes both withholding treatment and withdrawing treatment. *See also* pain control.

Autonomy: Self-rule; the principle or value of making decisions for oneself. One of the four "basic principles" of bioethics.

Beneficence: The principle or value of doing good, of benefitting others (including primarily, though not solely, the patient). One of the four "basic principles" of bioethics.

Best-interests standard: Legally supported standard whereby decisions are made by a surrogate for an incompetent patient based on what is known to be or thought to be in the patient's interests. *See also* substituted judgment standard.

Competency: Condition of a person whereby he or she is ethically or legally able to make decisions. Strictly, "competency" is determined by courts and thus the proper term is "decisional capacity," but "competency" is usually used. Most ethicists hold for a sliding scale of competency whereby persons who reject beneficial and nonburdensome life-sustaining treatments must be clearly competent to do so whereas minor decisions may be made by marginally competent persons. Determining competency is usually quite simple but can be very difficult.

Confidentiality: The requirement that information gained in the therapeutic relationship not be given to those who have no right to it.

Consequentialism: The theory that ethical judgments are made on the basis of reasonably foreseeable effects. *See also* deontology.

Consult: *See* ethics consult.

Cooperation principle: Principle determining the rightness or wrongness of actions done that help other actions that are judged to be wrong. Formal cooperation: cooperation where the cooperating agent identifies with or intends the evil of the primary action; this is always wrong. Material cooperation: cooperation where the cooperating agent does not identify with or intend the evil of the primary action; this may be right or wrong depending on the proximity of the cooperation to the primary action (hence proximate and remote material cooperation) and on whether serious scandal is risked.

Cumulative legislation: A statutory law that is not intended to change or restrict existing rights or previous laws.

Deontology: Wider sense: the requirement that factors must be included in making ethical judgments other than immediate and quantifiable consequences; insistence on including, for example, patient autonomy and not just what will make the patient physically better or result in longer life. Stricter sense: the theory that ethical judgments are made on the basis of innate characteristics in the action itself, thus eliminating consequences altogether in some cases; thus all abortion, all active euthanasia, all lying, all mechanical birth control, for example, are always wrong regardless of situation or consequences. *See also* consequentialism.

Direct/indirect euthanasia (or active/passive euthanasia): Older and confusing usage whereby forgoing treatment is included as euthanasia, and euthanasia includes not only killing but also allowing to die. Direct or active euthanasia means killing. Indirect or passive euthanasia means allowing to die, including in certain cases of pain control. Distinction is often made according to the principle of double effect.

Double effect principle: Principle with four conditions claiming to determine when actions with both good and bad effects are morally right or wrong; includes both deontological and consequentialist conditions.

Durable power of attorney: Legal directive whereby a person appoints another person to be attorney in fact with power to do certain functions when the person becomes unable to do so, which may include admission to hospitals, consent to treatment, and consent to forgo treatment. It is a form of proxy advance directive, sometimes used when states do not have an adequate advance directive law that provides for appointment of a health care proxy.

Emotivism: The ethical epistemological (metaethical) theory that there is no basis for ethical judgment; it is all a matter of emotion.

Ethics consult: Consult initiated by someone connected with a clinical case for getting advice concerning ethical issues; usually done by a team of members from the institutional ethics committee.

Euthanasia: Wider sense: "good death," "dying well"; more usual narrower sense: killing a terminally ill patient. *See also* voluntary/nonvoluntary/involuntary euthanasia and direct/indirect euthanasia.

Extraordinary means (of preserving life): Procedures whose burdens outweigh the benefits so that a patient has no moral obligation to accept them; morally optional treatment.

Forgoing treatment: Withholding treatment and withdrawing treatment.

Formal norm: Norm in which the moral quality attributed to the action is already implied in the term used for the action, as in "Murder is wrong." *See also* material norm.

Informed consent: The process of giving necessary information to the patient or surrogate to enable that person to consent to or refuse to consent to treatment, and the process of obtaining the consent.

Informed consent form: The actual piece of paper that the patient signs; not a legal substitute for informed consent.

Justice: The principle or value of rendering to each person his or her due, of acting fairly, and including social distribution and allocation issues; one of the four "basic principles" of bioethics.

Killing: Actually doing something that kills or hastens death and is intended to do precisely that.

Living will: *See* advance directive.

Material norm: Norm in which the moral quality attributed to the action is not already implied in the term used for the action, as in "Killing is wrong." *See* also formal norm.

Metaethics: The epistemology of ethics, asking whether ethics makes any sense. *See* positivism, relativism, emotivism, and natural law theory.

Natural law theory: The ethical epistemological (metaethical) theory that there is a basis for ethical judgment found in the patterns of human personhood and society as these patterns are discovered by reason and life experience. Also (and unfortunately) the normative theory

that certain actions are intrinsically wrong because they are "against nature," hence physicalism. *See* also deontology.

Noncognitivism: The ethical epistemological (metaethical) theory that there is no basis for
ethical judgment; ethics has no meaning. *See* emotivism.

Nonmaleficence: The principle or value of doing no harm, traditional in medical ethics; one of
the four "basic principles" of bioethics.

Ordinary means (of preserving life): Procedures whose benefits outweigh the burdens to the
extent that a patient has a moral obligation to accept them; morally obligatory treatment.

Pain control: Relief of pain, usually by pharmacological agent. Ethically and legally pain may,
and—if the proper decision maker agrees—must be eliminated in a dying patient even if this
contributes causally to the hastening of death, provided no one intends (wants as an end to
be chosen for its own sake) that the patient die and provided the amount and means of
delivery of the agent are such that they are proper for the elimination of pain.

Palliative support: Treatment aimed at relief of pain and suffering rather than at sustaining the
patient's life.

Palliative support care orders form: Form used by physicians to order palliative support and
to order the forgoing of certain life-sustaining treatments, based on the informed consent
of patient or surrogate.

Paternalism (or parentalism): Choosing (treatment) for others on the basis of their good
whether or not they want it; opposed to autonomy.

Patient Self-Determination Act (PSDA): Federal law requiring that admitted patients be
informed about hospital policy and state law concerning forgoing treatment, that they be
asked about their advance directives, and that these be recorded if they are available.

Persistent vegetative state (PVS): Condition of a person, usually caused by oxygen deprivation
to the cerebral cortex (higher brain), resulting in total and irreversible inability to perform
internal or external conscious acts. PVS patients undergo sleep–wake cycles (eyes open and
close) and other movements directed by the brain stem but are unaware of these movements
or of themselves or anything around them.

Physicalism: Roman Catholic approach that determines right and wrong by emphasizing the
physical and biological aspects of actions and agents.

Physician-assisted suicide: Patient-chosen and patient-accomplished suicide with the direct
and formal help of the physician, usually by prescribing drugs and informing the patient
how much to take to accomplish the suicide. Illegal in most states; Oregon and Washington
laws permitting it implicitly found constitutional by Supreme Court; circuit court decisions
concluding that laws forbidding it are unconstitutional later reversed by Supreme Court.

Positivism: The ethical epistemological (metaethical) theory that all ethical principles and
norms are merely imposed or posited and have no rational or ontological basis. Divine
positivism: God imposes arbitrarily. Ecclesiastical positivism: the Church imposes. Biblical
positivism: the Bible imposes. Rational positivism: reasonable people impose (similar in
theory to relativism and emotivism, though very different in practice).

Principle of cooperation: *See* cooperation principle.

Principle of double effect: *See* double effect principle.

Principle of totality: *See* totality principle.

Proxy directive: *See* advance directive.

Relativism: The ethical epistemological (metaethical) theory that there is no basis for ethical
judgment; it is all a matter of personal opinion or taste.

Substituted judgment standard: Legally supported standard whereby decisions are made by a
surrogate for a now-incompetent patient based on what the patient is known to have
wanted. *See also* best-interests standard.

Surrogate: Proper decision maker for incompetent patient; usually members of the family, sometimes proxy appointed by advance directive; least often a court appointed guardian.

Terminal illness or condition: Stricter sense, usually incorporated into advance directive laws: a condition from which a person will, in the reasonable judgment of physicians, almost certainly die in a short time even if aggressive medical interventions are done. In this sense, PVS, for example, is not a terminal condition since nutrition can prolong physical life. Larger sense, usually preferred by philosophers and theologians: a condition from which a person will almost certainly die, prescinding from the question of medical intervention. In this sense, PVS is a terminal condition. The difference is often important in distinguishing between killing and allowing to die and in interpreting advance directive laws.

Totality principle: Stricter and more usual sense: Roman Catholic principle that a part of the body may be sacrificed for the sake of the whole body, applied primarily to nonsterilizing "mutilating" procedures such as amputations. Wider and less common sense: the principle that orders human values when they conflict.

Utilitarianism: Wider sense: moral method basing judgment of right or wrong on reasonably foreseeable consequences. Stricter sense: moral method basing judgment on presumably quantifiable calculus of utility for the greatest good of the greatest number.

Voluntary/nonvoluntary/involuntary euthanasia: *See* euthanasia. Distinguished according to whether the patient actually asks to be killed, the patient cannot ask but is killed by surrogate decision, or the patient asks not to be killed but is killed anyway.

Withdrawing treatment: Deciding to stop treatment that has been begun; ethically and legally the same as withholding if all other factors are equal.

Withholding treatment: Deciding not to begin treatment.

Cases Cited

Baxter v. Montana, 521 U.S. 702 (2007)

Brophy v. New Eng. Sinai Hosp., Inc., 497 N.E.2d 626 (Mass. 1986)

Bush v. Schiavo, 885 So. 2d 321 (Fla. 2004)

Compassion in Dying v. Washington, 79 F.3d 790 (9th Cir. 1996)

Cruzan v. Director, 497 U.S. 261 (1990)

Doe v. Bolton, 410 U.S. 179 (1973)

Gilgunn v. Massachusetts General Hospital, No. SUC 92–4820 (Super. Ct. Suffolk County, Mass., April 22, 1995)

Griswold v. Connecticut, 381 US 479 (1965)

In re Conroy, 98 N.J. 321, 486 A.2d 1209 (N.J. 1985)

In re Doe, 45 Pa. D. & C.3d 371 (C.P. Phila. County 1987)

In re Eichner, 423 N.Y.S.2d 580 (Sup. Ct. Nassau County 1979)

In re Fiori, 673 A.2d 905 (Pa. 1996)

In re Guardianship of Schiavo, 851 So. 2d 182 (Fla. 2d Dist. Ct. App. 2003)

In re Jobes, 529 A.2d 434 (N.J. 1987)

In re Quinlan, 335 A.2d 647 (N.J. 1976)

In re Wanglie, No. PX-9I-283 (Minn. 4th Dist. Ct. Hennepin County, July 1, 1991)

Martin v. Martin, 538 N.W.2d 399 (Mich. 1995)

McConnell v. Beverly Enters., Conn., Inc., 533 A.2d 596 (Conn. 1989)

Planned Parenthood v. Casey, 505 U.S. 833 (1992)

Quill v. Vacco, 80 F.3d 716 (2d Cir. 1996)

Roe v. Wade, 410 U.S. 113 (1973)

Schiavo ex rel. Schindler v. Schiavo, No. 8:05-CV-530-T-27TBM (M.D. Fla. Mar. 22, 2005)

Superintendent of Belchertown State Sch. v. Saikewicz, 370 N.E.2d 417 (Mass. 1977)

Vacco v. Quill, 117 S. Ct. 2293 (1997)

Washington v. Glucksberg, 117 S. Ct. 2258 (1997)

Webster v. Reproductive Health Services, 492 U.S. 490 (1989)

Wendland v. Wendland, 110 Cal.Rptr.2d 412 (2001)

References

Ackerman, Terrence F., and Carson Strong. 1989. *A Casebook of Medical Ethics.* New York: Oxford University Press.

Agar, N. 2004. *Liberal Eugenics: In Defence of Human Enhancement.* Hoboken, NJ: Wiley-Blackwell.

Agich, George J., and Stuart J. Youngner. 1991. "For Experts Only? Access to Hospital Ethics Committees." *Hastings Center Report* 21, no. 5 (September–October): 17–25.

Agius, Emmanuel. 2005. "Environmental Ethics: Towards an Intergenerational Perspective." In *Environmental Ethics and International Policy,* edited by Henk A. M. J. ten Have, 89–115. Paris: UNESCO Publishing.

Agnew, Leslie Robert Corbert. 1967. "Medicine (History of)." In *New Catholic Encyclopedia.* Vol. 9. New York: McGraw-Hill.

Ahmann, John. 2001. "Therapeutic Cloning and Stem Cell Therapy." *National Catholic Bioethics Quarterly* 1, no. 2 (Summer): 145–50.

Alter, Jonathan. 2003. "A Genuinely Healthy Debate." *Newsweek,* May 5, 48.

American Academy of Neurology. 1989. "Position of the American Academy of Neurology on Certain Aspects of the Care and Management of the Persistent Vegetative State Patient." *Neurology* 39 (January): 125–26.

American College of Medical Genetics. 2006. "Newborn Screening: Towards a Uniform Screening Panel and System." *Genetics in Medicine* 8 (Supplement 1): 1–252S.

American College of Physicians. 1990. "Life, Death, and the American College of Physicians: The *Cruzan* Case." *Annals of Internal Medicine* 112:802–4.

American Medical Association. 1986. *Current Opinions.* Chicago: American Medical Association.

American Society for Bioethics and Humanities. 1998. *Core Competencies for Health Care Ethics Consultation.* Glenview, IL: American Society for Bioethics and Humanities.

———. 2010. *Core Competencies for Health Care Ethics Consultation.* 2nd ed. Glenview, IL: American Society for Bioethics and Humanities.

Andereck, W. S. 1992. "Development of a Hospital Ethics Committee: Lessons from Five Years of Case Consultation." *Cambridge Quarterly of Healthcare Ethics* 1, no. 1 (Winter): 41–50.

Anderson, Marie A., Robert L. Fastiggi, David E. Hargroder, Joseph C. Howard, and C. Ward Kischer. 2011. "Ectopic Pregnancy and Catholic Morality: A Response to Recent Arguments in Favor of Salpingostomy and Methotrexate." *National Catholic Bioethics Quarterly* 11, no. 1 (Spring): 65–82.

Annas, George J. 1986. "Do Feeding Tubes Have More Rights Than Patients?" *Hastings Center Report* 16, no. 1 (February): 26–28.

———. 1988. "Legal Risks and Responsibilities of Physicians in the AIDS Epidemic." *Hastings Center Report* 18, no. 3 (April–May): suppl., 26–32.

———. 1996. "The Promised End: Constitutional Aspects of Physician-Assisted Suicide." *Legal Issues in Medicine* 335, no. 9 (August 29): 683–87.

———. 2005. "Culture of Life: Politics at the Bedside-the Case of Terri Schiavo." *New England Journal of Medicine* 352, no. 16 (April 21): 1710–15.

———. 2009. "Globalized Clinical Trials and Informed Consent." *New England Journal of Medicine* 360, no. 20: 2050–53.

Appel, Jacob M. 2007. "A Suicide Right for the Mentally Ill? A Swiss Case Opens a New Debate." *Hastings Center Report* 37, no. 3 (May–June): 21–23.

Aristotle. 1962. *Nicomachean Ethics*. Translated by Martin Ostwald. Englewood Cliffs, NJ: Prentice Hall.

Arkes, H., N. P. Astraiaco, T. Berg, E. C. Brugger, N. M. Cameron, J. Capizzi, M. L. Condic, S. B. Condic, K. T. FitzGerald, K. Flannery, et al. 2005. "Production of Pluripotent Stem Cells by Oocyte-Assisted Reprogramming: Joint Statement with Signatories." *National Catholic Bioethics Quarterly* 5, no. 3 (Autumn): 579–83.

Arras, John D. 1988. "The Fragile Web of Responsibility: AIDS and the Duty to Treat." *Hastings Center Report* 18, no. 3 (April–May): suppl., 10–20.

Arribas-Ayllon, Michael, Srikant Sarangi, and Angus Clark. 2011. *Genetic Testing: Accounts of Autonomy, Responsibility and Blame*. New York: Routledge.

Ashley, Benedict M. 1988. "Reactions of Various Scholars and Their Comments on the Working Paper, No. 1." In *A Report to the Congregation for the Faith "Feeding and Hydrating the Permanently Unconscious and Other Vulnerable Persons,"* 34–36. Braintree, MA: Pope John XXIII Medical-Moral Research and Education Center.

Ashley, Benedict M., Jean K. deBlois, and Kevin D. O'Rourke. 2006. *Health Care Ethics: A Theological Analysis*. 5th ed. Washington, DC: Georgetown University Press.

Ashley, Benedict M., and Albert S. Moraczewski. 2001. "Cloning, Aquinas, and the Embryonic Person." *Kennedy Institute of Ethics Journal* 11, no. 3 (September): 189–201.

Ashley, Benedict M., and Kevin D. O'Rourke. 1997. *Health Care Ethics: A Theological Analysis*. 4th ed. Washington, DC: Georgetown University Press.

———. 2002. *Ethics of Health Care: An Introductory Textbook*. 3rd ed. Washington, DC: Georgetown University Press.

Augustine. 1887a. "Against Two Letters of the Pelagians (*Contra duas epistolas pelagianorum*)." Translated by Peter Holmes, Robert Wallis and Benjamin Warfield. In *A Select Library of the Nicene and Post-Nicene Fathers of the Christian Church*. Vol. 5, *Saint Augustin: Anti Pelagian Writings*, edited by Philip Schaff, 375–434. Boston: Rand Avery.

———. 1887b. "On Grace and Free Will (*De gratia et libero arbitrio*)." Translated by Peter Holmes, Robert Wallis, and Benjamin Warfield. In *A Select Library of the Nicene and Post-Nicene Fathers of the Christian Church*. Vol. 5, *Saint Augustin: Anti Pelagian Writings*, edited by Philip Schaff, 437–65. Boston: Rand Avery.

———. 1887c. "On Marriage and Concupiscence (*De nuptiis et concupiscentia*)." Translated by Peter Holmes, Robert Wallis, and Benjamin Warfield. In *A Select Library of the Nicene and Post-Nicene Fathers of the Christian Church*. Vol. 5, *Saint Augustin: Anti Pelagian Writings*, edited by Philip Schaff, 258–308. Boston: Rand Avery.

———. 1887d. "On Original Sin (*De peccato originale*)." Translated by Peter Holmes, Robert Wallis, and Benjamin Warfield. In *A Select Library of the Nicene and Post-Nicene Fathers of the Christian Church*. Vol. 5, *Saint Augustin: Anti Pelagian Writings*, edited by Philip Schaff, 237–55. Boston: Rand Avery.

———. 1887e. "On the Gifts of Perseverance (*De Dono Perseverantiae*)." Translated by Peter Holmes, Robert Wallis and Benjamin Warfield. In *A Select Library of the Nicene and Post-Nicene Fathers of the Christian Church*. Vol. 5, *Saint Augustin: Anti Pelagian Writings*, edited by Philip Schaff, 521–52. Boston: Rand Avery.

———. 1887f. "On the Predestination of the Saints (*De praedestinatione sanctorum*)." Translated by Peter Holmes, Robert Wallis and Benjamin Warfield. In *A Select Library of the Nicene and Post-Nicene Fathers of the Christian Church*. Vol. 5, *Saint Augustin: Anti Pelagian Writings*, edited by Philip Schaff, 493–519. Boston: Rand Avery.

———. 1901. "On the Morals of the Manichaeans (*De moribus manichaeorum*)." Translated by Richard Stothert. In *A Select Library of the Nicene and Post-Nicene Fathers of the Christian Church*. Vol. 4, *Saint Augustin: The Writings against the Manichaeans, and Against the Donatists*, edited by Philip Schaff, 69–89. New York: Charles Scribner's Sons.

———. 1903. "The City of God (*De civitate dei*)." Translated by Marcus Dods. In *A Select Library of the Nicene and Post-Nicene Fathers of the Christian Church*. Vol. 2, *Saint Augustin's City of God and Christian Doctrine*, edited by Philip Schaff, 1–511. New York: Charles Scribner's Sons.

———. 1998. "Answer to Julian (*Contra Julianum*)." Translated by Roland J. Teske. In *The Works of Saint Augustine: A Translation for the 21st Century*. Vol. 1, 24, *Answer to the Pelagians, II*, edited by John Rotelle, 225–536. Hyde Park, NY: New City Press.

Austriaco, Nicanor Pier Giorgio. 2002a. "Notes on Bioethics: Science." *National Catholic Bioethics Quarterly* 2, no. 3 (Autumn): 509–12.

———. 2002b. "On Static Eggs and Dynamic Embryos: A System Perspective." *National Catholic Bioethics Quarterly* 2, no. 4 (Winter): 659–83.

———. 2003a. "Notes on Bioethics: Science." *National Catholic Bioethics Quarterly* 3, no. 1 (Spring): 179–82.

———. 2003b. "Notes on Bioethics: Science." *National Catholic Bioethics Quarterly* 3, no. 3 (Autumn): 573–86.

———. 2003c. "Notes on Bioethics: Science." *National Catholic Bioethics Quarterly* 3, no. 4 (Winter): 789–91.

———. 2008. "Notes and Abstracts: Science." *National Catholic Bioethics Quarterly* 8, no. 2 (Summer): 343–47.

———. 2010. "Notes and Abstracts: Science." *National Catholic Bioethics Quarterly* 10, no. 4 (Winter): 775–78.

———. 2011a. "Notes and Abstracts: Science." *National Catholic Bioethics Quarterly* 11, no. 2 (Summer): 347–53.

———. 2011b. "Abortion in the Case of Pulmonary Arterial Hypertension: A Test Case for Two Rival Theories of Human Action." *National Catholic Bioethics Quarterly* 11, no. 3 (Autumn): 503–18.

Baily, Mary Ann. 2003. "Managed Care Organizations and the Rationing Problem." *Hastings Center Report* 33, no. 1 (January–February): 34–42.

Baily, Mary Ann, and Thomas H, Murray. 2009. *Ethics and Newborn Screening: New Technologies, New Challenges*. Baltimore: Johns Hopkins University Press.

Baker, Robert B., and Lawrence B. McCullough, eds. 2009. *The Cambridge World History of Medical Ethics*. New York: Cambridge University Press.

Baron, Charles H. 2006. "Not DEA'd Yet: *Gonzales v. Oregon*." *Hastings Center Report* 36, no. 2 (March–April): 8.

Bashford, A., and P. Levine. 2010. *The Oxford Handbook of the History of Eugenics*. Oxford: Oxford University Press.

Battin, Margaret P. 2008. "Terminal Sedation: Pulling the Sheet over Our Eyes." *Hastings Center Report* 38, no. 5 (September–October): 27–30.

Beauchamp, Tom L. 2003. "A Defense of the Common Morality." *Kennedy Institute of Ethics Journal* 13, no. 3 (September): 259–74.

Beauchamp, Tom L., and James F. Childress. 2001. *Principles of Biomedical Ethics*. 5th ed. Oxford: Oxford University Press.

———. 2009. *Principles of Biomedical Ethics*. 6th ed. New York: Oxford University Press.

Becker, Richard P. 2011. "Hypodermoclysis and Proctoclysis as Basic Care: Avoiding Unnecessary Terminal Dehydration." *National Catholic Bioethics Quarterly* 11, no. 4 (Winter): 649–59.

Bedau, Mark A, and Emily C. Parke, eds. 2009. *The Ethics of Protocells: Moral and Social Implications of Creating Life in the Laboratory*. Cambridge, MA: MIT Press.

Bell, Nora K. 1993. "Ethics Committees: Providing Moral Guidance in the Hospital." *Trustee* (April): 6–8.

Bellah, Robert N., Richard Madsen, William M. Sullivan, Ann Swidler, and Steven M. Tipton. 1986. *Habits of the Heart: Individualism and Commitment in American Life*. New York: Harper & Row.

Berger, Jeffrey T. 2010. "Rethinking Guidelines for the Use of Palliative Sedation." *Hastings Center Report* 40, no. 3 (May–June): 32–38.

Bernard of Clairvaux. 1953. *The Letters of St. Bernard of Clairvaux*. Translated by Bruno Scott James. Chicago: Henry Regnery.

Bernard, Claude. 1957. *An Introduction to the Study of Experimental Medicine*. New York: Dover Publications.

Berteaux, John A. 2002. "Is the Racial Divide in Health Care the Result of Racism?" *Sensabilities* 6, no. 1 (Fall): 13–15.

Betta, M. 2010. *The Moral, Social, and Commercial Imperatives of Genetic Testing and Screening: The Australian Case*. Dordrecht: Springer.

Billings, J. Andrew. 1985. "Comfort Measures for the Terminally Ill: Is Dehydration Painful?" *Journal of the American Geriatrics Society* 33, no. 11: 808–10.

Billings, J. Andrew, Larry R. Churchill, and Richard Payne. 2010. "Severe Brain Injury and the Subjective Life." *Hastings Center Report* 40, no. 3 (May–June): 17–21.

Black, Lisa Gasbarre. 2011. "Double Effect and US Supreme Court Reasoning." *National Catholic Bioethics Quarterly* 11, no. 1 (Spring): 41–48.

Blackhall, Leslie J. 1987. "Must We Always Use CPR?" *New England Journal of Medicine* 317, no. 20 (November 12): 1281–85.

Bonah, Christian, Etienne Lepicard, and Volker Roelcke, eds. 2003. *La medicine expérimental au tribunal. Implications éthiques de quelques procès médicaux du XX siècle européen.* Paris: Éditions des Archives Contemporaires.

Bone, Roger C., Eric Rachow, John Weg, and members of the ACCP/SCCM Consensus Panel. 1990. "Ethical and Moral Guidelines for the Initiation, Continuation, and Withdrawal of Intensive Care." *Chest* 97:952–53, 955.

Bouscaren, Timothy Lincoln. 1933. *Ethics of Ectopic Operations.* Chicago: Loyola University Press.

Boyle, Joseph. 2002. "Limiting Access to Health Care: A Traditional Roman Catholic Analysis." In *Allocating Scarce Medical Resources,* edited by H. Tristram Engelhardt Jr. and Mark J. Cherry, 77–95. Washington, DC: Georgetown University Press.

Boyle, Philip J. 1988. "DNR and the Elderly." *Issues in Health Care* (a publication of the St. Louis Univ. Medical Center for Health Care Ethics), December.

Boyle, Philip J., Edwin R. DuBose, Stephen J. Ellingson, David E. Guinnn, and David B. McCurdy. 2001. *Organizational Ethics in Health Care.* San Francisco: Jossey Bass.

Brand-Ballard, Jeffrey. 2003. "Consistency, Common Morality, and Reflective Equilibrium." *Kennedy Institute of Ethics Journal* 13, no. 3 (September): 231–58.

Brandt, Richard B. 1961. *Value and Obligation: Systematic Readings in Ethics.* New York: Harcourt, Brace & World.

Brennan, Troyen A. 1988. "Incompetent Patients with Limited Care in the Absence of Family Consent." *Annals of Internal Medicine* 109 (November 15): 819–25.

Bresnahan, James F., and James F. Drane. 1986. "A Challenge to Examine the Meaning of Living and Dying." *Health Progress* 67, no. 10 (December): 32–37, 98.

Briggle, Adam. 2010. *A Rich Bioethics. Public Policy, Biotechnology, and the Kass Council.* Notre Dame, IN: University of Notre Dame Press.

Broad, C. D. 1959. *Five Types of Ethical Theory.* Patterson, NJ: Littlefield, Adams and Co.

Brock, Brian. 2010. *Christian Ethics in a Technological Age.* Grand Rapids, MI: Eerdmans.

Brock, Dan W. 2000. "Broadening the Bioethics Agenda." *Kennedy Institute of Ethics Journal* 10, no. 1: 21–28.

Browne, Thomas (1642) 1963. *Religio Medici.* Edited by James Winny. Reprint, Cambridge: Cambridge University Press.

Brugger, E. Christian. 2005. "ANT-OAR: A Morally Acceptable Means for Deriving Pluripotent Stem Cells. A Reply to Criticisms." *Communio* 32, no. 4 (Winter): 753–69.

Buchanan, A. E. 2011a. *Beyond Humanity? The Ethics of Biomedical Enhancement.* Oxford: Oxford University Press.

———. 2011b. *Better than Human: The Promise and Perils of Enhancing Ourselves.* Oxford: Oxford University Press.

Buchanan, A. E., D. W. Brock, N. Daniels, and D. Wikler. 2000. *From Chance to Choice: Genetics and Justice.* Cambridge: Cambridge University Press.

Burke, Greg. 2001a. "Reply to 'A Necessary Tension.'" *Ethics & Medics* 26, no. 8 (August): 2–3.

———. 2001b. "Tube Feeding and Advanced Dementia." *Ethics & Medics* 26, no. 3 (March).

———. 2011. "Notes and Abstracts: Medicine." *National Catholic Bioethics Quarterly* 11, no. 3 (Autumn): 563–69.

Burke, Raymond L. 2005. "The Evil of So-Called Euthanasia." Bishop's Statement.

Burt, Robert A. 1996. "Constitutionalizing Physician-Assisted Suicide: Will Lightening Strike Thrice?" *Duquesne Law Review* 35, no. 1 (Fall): 159–81.

Byrnes, W. Malcolm. 2005. "Why Human 'Altered Nuclear Transfer' Is Unethical." *National Catholic Bioethics Quarterly* 5, no. 2 (Summer): 271–79.

———. 2008. "Direct Reprogramming and Ethics in Stem Cell Research." *National Catholic Bioethics Quarterly* 8, no. 2 (Summer): 277–90.

Cahill, Lisa Sowle. 1970. *Sex, Gender and Christian Ethics*. Philadelphia, PA: Fortress Press.

———. 1990. "Can Theology Have a Role in 'Public' Bioethical Discourse?" *Hastings Center Report* 20, no. 4 (July–August): 10–14.

———. 2003. "Biotech and Justice: Catching Up with the Real World Order." *Hastings Center Report* 33, no. 5 (September–October): 34–44.

Callahan, Daniel. 1970. *Abortion: Law, Choice and Morality*. New York: Macmillan.

———. 1987. *Setting Limits: Medical Goals in an Aging Society*. New York: Simon and Schuster.

———. 1991. "Medical Futility, Medical Necessity: The-Problem-Without-a-Name." *Hastings Center Report* 21, no. 4 (July–August): 30–35.

———. 2003. "A New Debate on an Old Topic." *Hastings Center Report* 33, no. 4 (July–August): 3.

———. 2008. "Organized Obfuscation: Advocacy for Physician-Assisted Suicide." *Hastings Center Report* 38, no. 5 (September–October): 30–32.

———. 2011. "Rationing: Theory, Politics, and Passions." *Hastings Center Report* 41, no. 2 (March–April): 23–27.

Callahan, Sidney. 1999. "A New Synthesis: Alternative Medicine's Challenge to Mainstream Medicine and Traditional Christianity." *Second Opinion*, no 1 (September): 57–78.

Campbell, Courtney S. 2004. "Harvesting the Living?: Separating 'Brain Death' and Organ Transplantation." *Kennedy Institute of Ethics Journal* 14, no. 3 (September): 301–18.

Caplan, Arthur L. 1996. "Odds and Ends: Trust and the Debate over Medical Futility." *Annals of Internal Medicine* 125 (October 15): 688–89.

Caplan, Arthur L., and Glenn McGee. 2001. "Fetal Cell Implants: What We Learned." *Hastings Center Report* 31, no. 3 (May–June): 6.

Capron, Alexander Morgan. 1995. "Abandoning a Waning Life." *Hastings Center Report* 25, no. 4 (July–August): 24–26.

Carrick, Paul. 1985. *Medical Ethics in Antiquity*. Dordrecht: D. Reidel Publishing Company.

Carson, Ronald A. 1989. "The Symbolic Significance of Giving to Eat and Drink." In *By No Extraordinary Means: The Choice to Forgo Life-Sustaining Food and Water*, edited by Joanne Kynn. Bloomington: Indiana University Press.

Cataldo, Peter J. 2004. "Compliance with Contraceptive Insurance Mandates: Licit or Illicit Cooperation in Evil?" *National Catholic Bioethics Quarterly* 4, no. 1 (Spring): 103–30.

Catechism of the Catholic Church. 1994. Mahwah, NJ: Paulist Press.

Catholic Health Association. 2004. "Statement on the March 20, 2004, Papal Allocution." Available at www.chausa.org.

Catholic Health Association of Wisconsin. 1989. *Nutrition and Hydration Guidelines*. Madison: Catholic Health Association of Wisconsin (March).

Catholic Organization for Life and Family, and Catholic Health Association of Canada. 2002. "Giving Something of Ourselves." *Ethics & Medics* 27, no. 8 (August): 1–4.

Cavanaugh, Thomas A. 2011. "Double-Effect Reasoning, Craniotomy, and Vital Conflicts: A Case of Contemporary Catholic Casuistry." *National Catholic Bioethics Quarterly* 11, no. 3 (Autumn): 453–63.

Chapman, Audrey R. 1999. *Unprecedented Choices: Religious Ethics at the Frontiers of Genetic Science*. Minneapolis, MN: Fortress Press.

Chauvet, Louis-Marie. 1977. "Marriage, a Sacrament Unlike the Others." *Theology Digest* 25, no. 3: 240–45.

Chernew, Michael E., Richard A. Hirth, and David M. Cutler. 2009. "Increased Spending on Health Care: Long-Term Implications for the Nation." *Health Affairs* 28, no. 5 (September–October): 1253–55.

Cherry, Mark J. 2002. "Facing the Challenges of High-Technology Medicine: Taking the Tradition Seriously." In *Allocating Scarce Medical Resources*, edited by H. Tristram Engelhardt Jr. and Mark J. Cherry, 19–31. Washington, DC: Georgetown University Press.

Chiong, Winston. 2005. "Brain Death without Definitions." *Hastings Center Report* 35, no. 6 (November–December): 20–30.

Churchill, Larry R. 1987. *Rationing Health Care in America: Perceptions and Principles of Justice*. Notre Dame, IN: University of Notre Dame Press.

Clarke, Adele E., Laura Mamo, Jennifer Ruth Fosket, Jennifer R. Fishman, and Janet K. Shim, eds. 2010. *Biomedicalization: Technoscience, Health, and Illness in the US*. Durham, NC: Duke University Press Books.

Cohen, Cynthia B. 1988a. "Ethics Committees." *Hastings Center Report* 18, no. 1 (February–March): 11.

———. 1988b. "Is Case Consultation in Retreat?" *Hastings Center Report* 118, no. 4 (August–September): 23.

———, ed. 1988c. *Casebook on the Termination of Life-sustaining Treatment and the Care of the Dying*. Bloomington: Indiana University Press.

———. 2004. "Stem Cell Research in the US after the President's Speech of August 2001." *Kennedy Institute of Ethics Journal* 14, no. 1 (March): 97–114.

———. 2007. *Renewing the Stuff of Life: Stem Cells, Ethics, and Public Policy*. New York: Oxford University Press.

Cole-Turner, Ronald, ed. 1997. *Human Cloning*. Louisville, KY: Westminster Press.

———. 2008. *Design and Destiny. Jewish and Christian Perspectives on Human Germline Modification*. Cambridge, MA: MIT Press.

———. 2011. *Transhumanism and Transcendence: Christian Hope in an Age of Technological Enhancement*. Washington, DC: Georgetown University Press.

Cole-Turner, Ronald, and Brent Waters, eds. 2003. *God and the Embryo: Religious Voices on Stem Cells and Cloning*. Washington, DC: Georgetown University Press.

Collins, Francis. 2010. *The Language of Life*. New York: Harper Collins Publishers.

Congregation for the Doctrine of the Faith (CDF). (1974) 1999. "Declaration on Procured Abortion." In *Medical Ethics: Sources of Catholic Teaching*. 3rd ed., edited by Kevin D. O'Rourke and Philip J. Boyle, 36–38. Washington, DC: Georgetown University Press.

———. 1976. "Reply of the Sacred Congregation for the Doctrine of the Faith on Sterilization in Catholic Hospitals (*Quaecumque Sterilizatio*)." *Origins* 6 (March 13): 33–35.

———. (1980) 1998. "Declaration on Euthanasia." In *On Moral Medicine: Theological Perspectives in Medical Ethics*. 2nd ed., edited by Stephen E. Lammers and Allen D. Verhey, 650–55. Grand Rapids, MI: Eerdmans.

———. 1987. "Instruction on Respect for Human Life in Its Origins and on the Dignity of Procreation (*Donum vitae*)." *Origins* 16, no. 40 (March 19): 697–711.

———. 2007. "Responses to Certain Questions of the United States Conference of Catholic Bishops Concerning Artificial Nutrition and Hydration" (August 1).

———. 2008. "Instruction *Dignitatis Personae*: Bioethical Questions and the Dignity of the Human Person." *Origins* 38, no. 28 (December 18): 437–49.

Conner, Paul. 2002. "The Indignity of Human Cloning." *National Catholic Bioethics Quarterly* 2, no. 4 (Winter): 635–58.

Council on Ethical and Judicial Affairs of the American Medical Association. 1999. "Medical Futility in End-of-Life Care." *Journal of the American Medical Association* 281:937–41.

"Courting the Issues: Decisions in Minnesota and Missouri." 1991. *Hospital Ethics* 7, no. 2 (March–April): 1–5.

Cowen, Chad A., Irina Klimanskaya, Jill McMahon, Jocelyn Atienza, Jeannine Witmyer, Jacob P. Zucker, Shunping Wang, Cynthia C. Morton, Andrew P. McMahon, Doug Powers, and Douglas A. Melton. 2004. "Derivation of Embryonic Stem-Cell Lines from Human Blastocysts." *New England Journal of Medicine* 350:1353–56.

Cowley, Geoffrey. 2003a. "Pay More, Get Less?" *Newsweek*, May 19, 11.

———. 2003b. "Ratings: Not Mother's Day." *Newsweek*, May 12, 8.

Crigger, Bette-Jane, ed. 1998. *Cases in Bioethics: Selections from the Hastings Center Report*. 3rd ed. New York: St. Martin's Press.

Cronin, Daniel A. 1958. *The Moral Law in Regard to the Ordinary and Extraordinary Means of Conserving Life*. Rome: Pontifical Gregorian University.

Crowley-Matoka, Megan, and Robert M. Arnold. 2004. "The Dead Donor Rule: How Much Does and Public Care and How Much Should *We* Care?" *Kennedy Institute of Ethics Journal* 14, no. 3 (September): 318–32.

Crozier, G. K. D., and Christopher Hajzler. 2010. "Market Stimulus and Genomic Justice: Evaluating the Effects of Marker Access to Germ-Line Enhancement." *Kennedy Institute of Ethics Journal* 20, no. 2 (June): 161–79.

Cunningham, Bert Joseph. 1944. *The Morality of Organic Transplantation*. Catholic University of America Studies in Sacred Theology, vol. 86. Washington, DC: Catholic University of America Press.

Curran, Charles E. 1964. "Christian Marriage and Family Planning." *Jubilee* (August).

———. 1968. "Absolute Norms and Medical Ethics." In *Absolutes in Moral Theology?*, edited by Charles E. Curran, 108–53. Washington, DC: Corpus Press.

———. 1970a. "Absolute Norms in Moral Theology." In *A New Look at Christian Morality*, 73–123. Notre Dame, IN: Fides Press.

———. 1970b. *Medicine and Morals*. Washington, DC: Corpus Press.

———. 1970c. "Natural Law and Contemporary Moral Theology." In *Contemporary Problems in Moral Theology*, 97–158. Notre Dame, IN: Fides Press.

———. (1973) 1996. "Abortion: Its Moral Aspects." In *Abortion: A Reader*, edited by Lloyd Steffen, 245–59. Cleveland: Pilgrim Press.

———. 1977. "Utilitarianism and Contemporary Moral Theology: Situating the Debate." *Louvain Studies* 6:239–55.

———. 1999. *The Catholic Moral Tradition Today: A Synthesis*. Washington, DC: Georgetown University Press.

Daar, J. F. 1995. "Medical Futility and Implications for Physician Autonomy." *American Journal of Law and Medicine* 21: 221–40.

Daniels, Norman, ed. 1974. *Reading Rawls: Critical Studies of "A Theory of Justice."* New York: Basic Books.

———. 1988. *Am I My Parents' Keeper? An Essay on Justice between the Young and the Old*. New York: Oxford University Press.

———. 2006. "Equity and Population Health: Toward a Broader Bioethics Agenda." *Hastings Center Report* 36, no. 4: 22–35.

———. 2012. "Reasonable Disagreement about Identified vs. Statistical Victims." *Hastings Center Report* 42, no. 1 (January–February): 35–45.

Davis, Henry. 1946. *Moral and Pastoral Theology*. 5th ed. London: Sheed & Ward.

Deane-Drummond, Celia. 2006. *Genetics and Christian Ethics*. New York: Cambridge University Press.

deBlois, Jean, and Kevin D. O'Rourke. 1995. "Issues at the End of Life: The Revised *Ethical and Religious Directives* Discuss Suicide, Euthanasia, and End-of-Life Procedures." *Health Progress* 76, no. 8 (November–December): 24–27.

DeCamp, Matthew, Jennifer K. Walter, and Susan Dorr Goold. 2011. "Conjectural Mixed Motives" (Case Study). *Hastings Center Report* 41, no. 1 (January–February): 11–12.

Declaration of Helsinki. 1964. World Medical Association, revisions in 1975, 1983, 1989, 1996, 2000, 2008. Accessed February 6, 2012. www.wma.net/en/30publications/10policies/b3/index.html.

DeGrazia, David. 2003. "Common Morality, Coherence, and the Principles of Biomedical Ethics." *Kennedy Institute of Ethics Journal* 13, no. 3 (September): 219–30.

DeMarco, Donald T. 1988. "IVF and Social Justice." *Ethics & Medics* 13, no. 7 (July): 1–3.

Derr, Patrick G. 1986. "Why Food and Fluids Can Never Be Denied." *Hastings Center Report* 16, no. 1 (February): 28–30.

Devine, Richard J. 1989. "Save the Body, Lose the Soul." *Health Progress*, June, 68–72.

Diamond, Eugene F. 2002. "Resuscitation and the Operating Room." *Ethics & Medics* 27, no. 5 (May): 3–4.

Doerflinger, Richard M. 1999a. "The Ethics of Funding Embryonic Stem Cell Research: A Catholic Viewpoint." *Kennedy Institute of Ethics Journal* 9, no. 2 (June): 137–45.

———. 1999b. "An Uncertain Future for Assisted Suicide." *Hastings Center Report* 29, no. 1 (January–February): 52.

Dombi, William A. 2005. "Lessons from Schiavo beyond the Legal." *Caring* 24, no. 5 (May): 28–30.

Dorff, Elliot N. 2000a. "End-Stage Medical Care: Halakhic Concepts and Values." In *Life and Death Responsibilities in Jewish Biomedical Ethics*, edited by Aaron L. Mackler, 309–37. New York: Jewish Theological Seminary of America.

———. 2000b. "End-Stage Medical Care: Practical Applications." In *Life and Death Responsibilities in Jewish Biomedical Ethics*, edited by Aaron L. Mackler, 338–58. New York: Jewish Theological Seminary of America.

Dougherty, Charles J. 1988. *American Health Care: Realities, Rights, and Reforms*. New York: Oxford University Press.

Drane, James F. 1988. *Becoming a Good Doctor: The Place of Virtue and Character in Medical Ethics*. Kansas City, MO: Sheed & Ward.

———. 1990. "Methodologies for Clinical Ethics." *Bulletin of the Pan American Health Organization* 24, no. 4: 394–404.

Dreger, Alice. 2010. "Attenuated Thoughts." *Hastings Center Report* 40, no. 6 (November–December): 3.

Dresser, Rebecca. 2002. "The Conscious Incompetent Patient." *Hastings Center Report* 32, no. 3 (May–June): 9–10.

———. 2005. "Schiavo's Legacy: The Need for an Objective Standard." *Hastings Center Report* 35, no. 3 (May–June): 20–22.

———. 2009. "Substituting Authenticity for Autonomy." *Hastings Center Report* 39, no. 2 (March–April): 3.

Driscoll, Thomas J., Jr. 2012. "Organ Donation after Circulatory Determination of Death." *National Catholic Bioethics Quarterly* 12, no. 1 (Spring): 69–84.

DuBose, Edwin R., Ron Hamel, and Laurence J. O'Connell, eds. 1994. *A Matter of Principles: Ferment in US Bioethics*. Valley Forge, PA: Trinity Press International.

Dugdale, Lydia S., and Autumn Alcott Ridenour. 2011. "Making Sense of the Roman Catholic Directive to Extend Life Indefinitely." *Hastings Center Report* 41, no. 2 (March–April): 28–29.

Duska, Ronald, and Mariellen Whelan. 1975. *Moral Development: A Guide to Piaget and Kohlberg*. New York: Paulist Press.

Duwell, M., C. Rehmann-Sutter, and D. Mieth, eds. 2010. *The Contingent Nature of Life: Bioethics and the Limits of Human Existence*. Dordrecht: Springer.

Eberl, Jason T. 2005. "Extraordinary Care and the Spiritual Goal of Life: A Defense of the View of Kevin O'Rourke, OP." *National Catholic Bioethics Quarterly* 5, no. 3 (Autumn): 491–501.

Editorial. 2008. "Trials on Trial. The Food and Drug Administration Should Rethink Its Rejection of the Declaration of Helsinki." *Nature* 453:427–28.

Edmonds, M. 2011. *A Theological Diagnosis: A New Direction of Genetic Therapy, "Disability" and the Ethics of Healing*. London: Jessica Kingsley Publishing.

Edwards, Craig. 2011. "Respect for Other Selves." *Kennedy Institute of Ethics Journal* 21, no. 4 (December): 349–78.

Emanuel, Ezekiel J., David Wendler, and Christine Grady, eds. 2008. "An Ethical Framework for Biomedical Research." In *The Oxford Textbook of Clinical Research Ethics*, edited by Ezekiel Emanuel, Christine Grady, Robert A. Crouch, Reidar K. Lie, Franklin G. Miller, and David Wendler, 123–35. Oxford: Oxford University Press.

Engelhardt, H. Tristram, Jr. 1986. *The Foundations of Bioethics*. New York: Oxford University Press.

Entralgo, Pedro Lain. 1969. *Doctor and Patient*. Translated by Frances Partridge. New York: McGraw-Hill.

Esposito, Mary. 2001. "Adult Stem Cell Research, at Duquesne and Elsewhere, Makes Positive Contribution to Medicine." *Duquesne Times*, October 29, 1.

Ethics Committee of the Society of Critical Care Medicine. 1997. "Consensus Statement of the Society of Critical Care Medicine's Ethics Committee Regarding Futile and Other Possibly Inadvisable Treatments." *Critical Care Medicine* 25, no. 5: 887–91.

"Ethics Committees." 1990. *Medical Ethics Advisor* 6, no. 1 (January): 7–8.

Faden, Ruth R., Liza Dawson, Alison Bateman-House, Dawn Mueller Agnew, Hilary Bok, Dan W. Brock, Aravinda Chakravarti, Xiao-Jiang Gao, Mark Greene, John A. Hansen, et al. 2003. "Public Stem Cell Banks: Considerations of Justice in Stem Cell Research and Therapy." *Hastings Center Report* 33, no. 6 (November–December): 13–27.

Fagerlin, Angela, and Carl E. Schneider. 2004. "Enough: The Failure of the Living Will." *Hastings Center Report* 34, no. 2 (March–April): 30–42.

Fanelli, Daniele. 2009. "How Many Scientists Fabricate and Falsify Research? A Systematic Review and Meta-Analysis of Survey Data." *PLOS One* 4, no. 5: e5738; doi:10.1371/journal.pone.0005738.

Fangerau, Heiner, Jorg M. Fegert, and Thorsten Trapp. 2011. *Implanted Minds: The Neuroethics of Intracerebral Stem Cell Transplantation and Deep Brain Stimulation.* Bielefeld, Germany: Transcript Verlag.

Farah, Martha J., ed. 2010. *Neuroethics.* Cambridge, MA: MIT Press.

Feldman, David F. 1986. *Health and Medicine in the Jewish Tradition.* New York: Crossroad.

Fernandez-Lynch, Holly. 2008. *Conflicts of Conscience in Health Care: An Institutional Compromise.* Cambridge, MA: MIT Press.

Field, Robert I. 2007. *Health Care Regulation in America.* New York: Oxford University Press.

Finney, Patrick A. 1922. *Moral Problems in Hospital Practice: A Practical Handbook.* St. Louis, MO: B. Herder.

Finney, Patrick, and Patrick O'Brien. 1956. *Moral Problems in Hospital Practice: A Practical Handbook.* Rev. ed. St. Louis, MO: B. Herder.

Fins, Joseph J. 2005. "Rethinking Disorders of Consciousness: New Research and Its Implications." *Hastings Center Report* 35, no. 2 (March–April): 22–24.

———. 2006. "Shades of Gray: New Insight into the Vegetative State (In Brief)." *Hastings Center Report* 36, no. 6 (November–December): 8.

Fins, Joseph J., and Nicholas D. Schiff. 2010. "In the Blink of the Mind's Eye." *Hastings Center Report* 40, no. 3 (May–June): 21–23.

Finucane, Thomas E., Colleen Christmas, and Kathy Travis. 1999. "Tube Feeding in Patients with Advanced Dementia: A Review of the Evidence." *Journal of the American Medical Association* 282, no. 14 (October 13): 1365–70.

Fisher, Jill A. 2009. *Medical Research for Hire: The Political Economy of Pharmaceutical Clinical Trials.* New Brunswick, NJ: Rutgers University Press.

Flannery, Kevin L. 2011. "Vital Conflicts and the Catholic Magisterial Tradition." *National Catholic Bioethics Quarterly* 11, no. 4 (Winter): 691–704.

Fleckenstein, Heinz. 1963. "Pastoralmedizin." *Lexikon für Theologie und Kirche* 8.

Fletcher, John C. 1990. "Ethics Consultation Services: An Overview." *Biolaw* 22, no. 34 (January): S339–47.

Fletcher, John C., and Diane E. Hoffmann. 1994. "Ethics Committees: Time to Experiment with Standards." *Annals of Internal Medicine* 120, no. 4 (February 15): 335–38.

Fletcher, Joseph F. 1960. *Morals and Medicine.* Boston: Beacon.

———. 1966. *Situation Ethics: The New Morality.* Philadelphia: Westminster Press.

———. 1975. "Four Indicators of Humanhood: The Enquiry Matures." *Hastings Center Report* 4, no. 6 (December): 4–7.

Florida Catholic Conference. 2005. "Florida Bishops Urge Safer Course for Terri Schiavo." www.flaccb.org/statements/2003/schiavo.pdf.

Flynn, Eileen P. 1990. *Hard Decisions: Forgoing and Withdrawing Artificial Nutrition and Hydration.* Kansas City, MO: Sheed & Ward.

Ford, John C., and Gerald Kelly. 1963. *Marriage Questions.* Contemporary Moral Theology, vol. 2. Cork, Ireland: Mercier Press.

Ford, Norman M. 2001. "The Human Embryo as Person in Catholic Teaching." *Kennedy Institute of Ethics Journal* 11, no. 3 (September): 155–60.

———. 2003. "Using Pluripotent Germ Cells in Regenerative Medicine." *National Catholic Bioethics Quarterly* 3, no. 4 (Winter): 697–705.

———. 2005. "Thoughts on the Papal Address and MANH." *Ethics and Medics* 30, no. 2 (February): 3–4.

Fost, Norman. 2004. "Reconsidering the Dead Donor Rule: Is It Important That Organ Donors Be Dead?" *Kennedy Institute of Ethics Journal* 14, no. 3 (September): 249–60.

Fox, Ellen, and Carol Stocking. 1993. "Ethics Consultants' Recommendations for Life-Prolonging Treatment of Patients in a Persistent Vegetative State." *Journal of the American Medical Association* 270, no. 21 (December 1): 2578–82.

Francis, C. M. 1996. "Medical Ethics in India: Ancient and Modern (I)." *Indian Journal of Medical Ethics* 4, no. 4 (October–December). www.issuesinmedicalethics.org/044ed115.html.

Frankel, Mark S. 2003. "Inheritable Genetic Modification and a Brave New World: Did Huxley Have It Wrong?" *Hastings Center Report* 33, no. 2 (March–April): 31–36.

Freedman, Benjamin. 1981. "One Philosopher's Experience on an Ethics Committee." *Hastings Center Report* 11, no. 2 (April): 20–22.

———. 1988. "Health Professions, Codes, and the Right to Refuse to Treat HIV-Infectious Patients." *Hastings Center Report* 18, no. 2 (April–May): suppl., 20–25.

Freeman, John M., and Kevin McDonnell, eds. 2001. *Tough Decisions: Cases in Medical Ethics.* 2nd ed. Oxford: Oxford University Press.

Friedman M., and G. W. Friedland. 1998. *Medicine's 10 Greatest Discoveries.* New Haven, CT: Yale University Press.

Fukuyama, F. 2002. *Our Posthuman Future: Consequences of the Biotechnology Revolution.* New York: Farrar, Straus and Giroux.

Furton, Edward J. 2004. "Vaccines and the Right of Conscience." *National Catholic Bioethics Quarterly* 4, no. 1 (Spring): 53–62.

———. 2005. "Nutrition and Hydration" (Letter to the Editor). *Hastings Center Report* 35, no. 3 (May–June): 5.

———. 2010. "Embryo Adoption Reconsidered." *National Catholic Bioethics Quarterly* 11, no. 2 (Summer): 329–47.

———. 2011a. "Ethics without Metaphysics: A Review of the Lysaught Analysis." *National Catholic Bioethics Quarterly* 11, no. 1 (Spring): 53–62.

———. 2011b. "In This Issue." *National Catholic Bioethics Quarterly* 11, no. 3 (Autumn): 419–20.

Garrett, Jeremy R., and John D. Lantos. 2011. "Patient Autonomy and the Twenty-First Century Physician." *Hastings Center Report* 41, no. 5 (September–October): 3.

Gaynor, Pamela. 2002. "More Hospitals End Up in the Red." *Pittsburgh Post-Gazette* (April 30): A1, A3.

Gems, David. 2003. "Is More Better? The New Biology of Aging and the Meaning of Life." *Hastings Center Report* 33, no. 4 (July–August): 31–39.

Gerlach, Neil, Sheryl Hamilton, Rebecca Sullivan, and Priscilla Walton. 2011. *Becoming Biosubjects: Bodies. Systems. Technology.* Toronto: University of Toronto Press.

Gert, Heather J. 2002. "Avoiding Surprises: A Model for Informing Patients." *Hastings Center Report* 32, no. 4 (September–October): 23–32.

Gervais, Karen G. 1986. *Redefining Death.* New Haven, CT: Yale University Press.

Gervais, Karen G., Priester Reinhard, Dorothy E. Vawter, Kimberly K. Otte, and Mary M. Solberg, eds. 1999. *Ethical Challenges in Managed Care: A Casebook.* Washington, DC: Georgetown University Press.

Getz, Lorine M. 1982. *Nature and Grace in Flannery O'Connor's Fiction.* New York: Edwin Mellen Press.

Gewirth, Alan. 1978. *Reason and Morality.* Chicago: University of Chicago Press.

Gibson, Joan McIver, and Thomasine Kimbrough Kushner. 1986. "Will the 'Conscience of an Institution' Become Society's Servant?" *Hastings Center Report* 16, no. 3 (June): 9–11.

Gillick, Muriel R. 2000. "Rethinking the Role of Tube Feeding in Patients with Advanced Dementia." *New England Journal of Medicine* 342, no. 3 (January 20): 206–10.

Gilligan, Carol. 1982. *In a Different Voice: Psychological Theory and Women's Development.* Cambridge, MA: Harvard University Press.

Glannon, Walter. 2007. *Bioethics and the Brain.* New York: Oxford University Press.

Glaser, John W., and Ronald B. Miller. 1993. "A Paradigm Shift for Ethics Committees and Case Consultation: A Modest Proposal." *HEC Forum* 5, no. 2: 83–88.

Glover, Jonathan. 2006. *Choosing Children: Genes, Disability, and Design.* New York: Oxford University Press.

Glover, William Kevin. 1948. *Artificial Insemination among Human Beings: Medical, Legal, and Moral Aspects.* Catholic University of America Studies in Sacred Theology. 2nd series, vol. 86. Washington, DC: Catholic University of America Press.

Gold, E. Richard. 1996. *Body Parts: Property Rights and the Ownership of Human Biological Materials.* Washington, DC: Georgetown University Press.

Gómez-Lobo, Alfonso. 2004. "On the Ethical Evaluation of Stem Cell Research: Remarks on a Paper by N. Knoepffler." *Kennedy Institute of Ethics Journal* 4, no. 1 (March): 75–80.

Gordijn, B., and R. Chadwick, eds. 2010. *Medical Enhancement and Posthumanity.* Dordrecht: Springer.

Gordon, John-Stewart. 2011. "Global Ethics and Principlism." *Kennedy Institute of Ethics Journal* 21, no. 3 (September): 251–76.

Gostin, Lawrence O. 2010. "The National Individual Insurance Mandate." *Hastings Center Report* 40, no. 5 (September–October): 8–9.

Grabowski, John S., and Christopher Gross. 2010. "*Dignitas personae* and the Adoption of Frozen Embryos." *National Catholic Bioethics Quarterly* 11, no. 2 (Summer): 307–28.

Green, R. M. 2008. *Babies by Design: The Ethics of Genetic Choice.* Cambridge, MA: Yale University Press.

Griener, Glenn G., and Janet L. Storch. 1994. "The Educational Needs of Ethics Committees." *Cambridge Quarterly of Healthcare Ethics* 3: 467–77.

Grisez, Germain. 1964. *Contraception and the Natural Law.* Milwaukee, WI: Bruce Publishing Company.

———. 1993. *Living a Christian Life.* Quincy, MA: Franciscan Press.

Grisez, Germain, John C. Ford, Joseph Boyle, John Finnis, and William E. May. 1998. *The Teaching of "Humanae vitae": A Defense.* San Francisco, CA: Ignatius Press.

Grisso, Thomas, and Paul S. Applebaum. 1998. *Assessing Competence to Consent to Treatment.* New York: Oxford University Press.

Groll, Daniel. 2011. "What Health Care Providers Know: A Taxonomy of Clinical Disagreements." *Hastings Center Report* 41, no. 5 (September–October): 27–36.

Gruenler, C. 2008. *Quo vadis? Homo sapiens? Ethical Positions concerning Genetic Enhancement of the Human Brain.* Munich: Global Society Press.

Guenin, Louis M. 2008. *The Morality of Embryo Use.* New York: Cambridge University Press.

Guevin, Benedict M. 2007. "The Use of Methotraxate or Salpingostomy in the Treatment of Tubal Ectopic Pregnancies." *National Catholic Bioethics Quarterly* 7, no. 2 (Summer): 249–62.

———. 2007. "Vital Conflicts and Virtue Ethics." *National Catholic Bioethics Quarterly* 11, no. 4 (Winter): 679–88.

———. 2011. "Vital Conflicts and Virtue Ethics." *National Catholic Bioethics Quarterly* 11, no. 4 (Winter): 679–88.

Gummere, Peter J. 2008. *National Catholic Bioethics Quarterly* 8, no. 2 (Summer): 291–305.

Gustafson, James. 1984. *Ethics from a Theocentric Perspective.* Vol. 2, *Ethics and Theology.* Chicago: University of Chicago Press.

Guterl, Fred. 2003. "To Build a Baby." *Newsweek,* June 9, E14–15.

Haas, John M. 2011. "Catholic Teaching Regarding the Legitimacy of Neurological Criteria for the Determination of Death." *National Catholic Bioethics Quarterly* 11, no. 2 (Summer): 279–99.

Habermas, J. 2003. *The Future of Human Nature.* Oxford. Blackwell.

Halevy, Amir. 1999. "Medical Futility in End-of-Life Care." *Journal of the American Medical Association* 282, no. 14 (October 13): 1331–32.

Hall, Robert, T. 2000. *An Introduction to Healthcare Organizational Ethics.* New York: Oxford University Press.

Hamel, Ron. 2003. "Rape and Emergency Contraception." *Ethics & Medics* 28, no. 6 (June): 1–2.

Hamel, Ron, and Thomas Nairn. 2010. "The New Directive 58: What Does It Mean?" *Health Progress* 91, no. 1 (January–February): 70–72.

Hanigan, James P. 1986. *As I Have Loved You: The Challenge of Christian Ethics.* Mahwah, NJ: Paulist Press.

Hanna, Kathi E. 2003. "Senate Passes Genetic Nondiscrimination Bill." *Hastings Center Report* 33, no. 6 (November–December): 8.

Hardwig, John. 1990. "What about the Family?" *Hastings Center Report* 20, no. 2 (March–April): 5–10.

———. 1997. "Is There a Duty to Die?" *Hastings Center Report* 27, no. 2 (March–April): 34–42.

Harris, J. 2010. *Enhancing Evolution: The Ethical Case for Making Better People.* Princeton, NJ: Princeton University Press.

Hartman, Rhonda Gay. 2000. "Adolescent Autonomy: Clarifying an Ageless Conundrum." *Hastings Law Journal* 51, no. 6 (August): 1265–1362.

———. 2001. "Adolescent Decisional Autonomy for Medical Care: Physician Perceptions and Practices." *University of Chicago Law School Roundtable* 8, no. 1: 87–134.

Harvard Medical School, Ad Hoc Committee to Examine the Definition of Brain Death. 1968. "A Definition of Irreversible Coma." *JAMA* 25, no. 6: 337–40.

Hastings Center. 1987. *Guidelines on the Termination of Life-Sustaining Treatments and the Care of the Dying.* Briarcliff Manor, NY: Hastings Center.

Häyry, M. 2010. *Rationality and the Genetic Challenge: Making People Better?* Cambridge: Cambridge University Press.

Health Grades Quality Study. 2004. *Patient Safety in American Hospitals.* Colorado: Health Grades.

Healy, Edwin F. 1956. *Medical Ethics.* Chicago: Loyola University Press.

Helft, Paul R., Mark Siegler, and John Lantos. 2000. "The Rise and Fall of the Futility Movement." *New England Journal of Medicine* 343, no. 4 (July 27): 293–95.

Henderson, D. Scott. 2003. "Deontological and Teleological Misgivings: A Synthetic Alternative for Christian Moral Theology." Course Paper, Duquesne University, Healthcare Ethics Program, April 10.

Hendin, Herbert. 2003. "The Practice of Euthanasia." *Hastings Center Report* 33, no. 4 (July–August): 44–45.

Hendin, Herbert, Chris Rutenfrans, and Zbigniew Zylicz. 1997. "Physician-Assisted Suicide and Euthanasia in the Netherlands." *Journal of the American Medical Association* 277, no. 21 (June 4): 1720–22.

Heng, B. C., C. P. Ye, H. Liu, W. S. Toh, A. J. Rufaihah, and T. Cao. 2006. "Kinetics of Cell Death of Frozen-Thawed Human Embryonic Stem Cell Colonies Is Reversibly Slowed Down by Exposure to Low Temperature." *Zygote* 14, no. 4: 341–48.

Hoffmann, Diane E. 1993. "Evaluating Ethics Committees: A View from the Outside." *Milbank Quarterly* 71, no. 4: 677–700.

Holland, Suzanne. 2001. "Contested Commodification at Both Ends of Life: Buying and Selling Gametes, Embryos, and Body Tissues." *Kennedy Institute of Ethics Journal* 11, no. 3 (September): 264–84.

Hollinger, Paula C. 1989. "Hospital Ethics Committees Required by Law in Maryland." *Hastings Center Report* 19, no. 1 (January–February): 23–24.

Hoose, Bernard. 1987. *Proportionalism: The American Debate and Its European Roots.* Washington, DC: Georgetown University Press.

———. 2001. "Towards the Truth about Hiding the Truth." *Louvain Studies* 6, no. 1 (Spring): 63–84.

Huarte, Joachim, and Antoine Suarez. 2004. "On the Status of Parthenotes: Defining the Developmental Potentiality of a Human Embryo." *National Catholic Bioethics Quarterly* 4, no. 4 (Winter): 755–70.

Hudson, Kathy L. 2006. "Embryo Biopsy for Stem Cells: Trading Old Problems for New." *Hastings Center Report* 36, no. 5 (September–October): 50–51.

Hughes, Marsha Magnusen. 1992. "Reconciling Ethics Differences." *Caring Magazine*, June, 16–20.

Human Fertilisation and Embryology Authority (HFEA). 2002. *Sex Selection: Choice and Responsibility in Human Reproduction.* London: Human Fertilisation and Embryology Authority.

———. 2003. *Sex Selection: Options for Regulation.* London: Human Fertilisation and Embryology Authority.

Hurlbut, William B. 2005. "Altered Nuclear Transfer as a Morally Acceptable Means for the Procurement of Human Embryonic Stem Cells." *National Catholic Bioethics Quarterly* 5, no. 1 (Spring): 145–51.

Hurlbut, William B., Robert P. George, and Markus Grompe. 2006a. "Seeking Consensus: A Clarification and Defense of Altered Nuclear Transfer." *Hastings Center Report* 36, no. 5 (September–October): 42–50.

———. 2006b. "ANT vs. SCNT (Letters Reply)." *Hastings Center Report* 36, no. 6 (November–December): 7.

Hyde, M. J. 2010. *Perfection: Coming to Terms with Being Human.* Waco, TX: Baylor University Press.

Hyun, Insoo. 2002. "Waiver of Informed Consent, Cultural Sensitivity, and the Problem of Unjust Families and Traditions." *Hastings Center Report* 32, no. 5 (September–October): 14–22.

Hyun, Insoo, and Kyu Won Jung. 2006. "Human Research Cloning, Embryos, and Embryo-Like Artifacts." *Hastings Center Report* 36, no. 5 (September–October): 34–41.

Illes, Judy, ed. 2006. *Neuroethics: Defining the Issues in Theory, Practice, and Policy.* New York: Oxford University Press.

Inoue, Yusuke, and Kaori Muto. 2011. "Children and Genetic Identification of Talent." *Hastings Center Report* 41, no. 5 (September–October): 49.

In Re Quinlan. 1982. In *Law and Bioethics: Texts with Commentary on Major US Court Decisions*, edited by Thomas A. Shannon and Jo Ann Manfra, 147–72. New York: Paulist Press.

Institute of Medicine (IOM). 1997. *Non-Heart-Beating Organ Transplantation: Medical and Ethical Issues in Procurement.* Washington, DC: National Academies Press.

———. 2000a. *To Err Is Human: Building a Safer Health System.* Washington, DC: National Academies Press.

———. 2000b. *Non-Heart-Beating Organ Transplantation: Practice and Protocols.* Washington, DC: National Academies Press.

———. 2001. *Crossing the Quality Chasm: A New Health System for the 21st Century.* Washington, DC: National Academies Press.

———. 2002. *Leadership by Example: Coordinating Government Roles in Improving Health Care Quality.* Washington, DC: National Academies Press.

———. 2006. *Organ Donation: Opportunities for Action.* Washington, DC: National Academies Press.

International Association of Catholic Bioethicists. 2008. "Statement on Regenerative Medicine and Stem Cell Research." *National Catholic Bioethics Quarterly* 8, no. 2 (Summer): 323–39.

Ip, K. T., ed. 2009. *The Bioethics of Regenerative Medicine.* Dordrecht: Springer Science & Business Media.

Jamison, Tracy. 2010. "Embryo Adoption and the Design of Human Nature." *National Catholic Bioethics Quarterly* 11, no. 2 (Spring): 111–22.

Janssens, Louis. (1947) 1988. "Time and Space in Morals." Translated by Jan Jans. In *Personalist Morals*, edited by Joseph A. Selling, 9–22. Leuven, Belgium: Leuven University Press.

———. 1963. "Moral Conjugale et Progestogènes." *Ephemerides Theologicae Lovanienses* 24, no. 4: 787–826.

———. 1963–64. "Moral Theology 1963–1964: Conjugal Morality." Student notes transcribed at American College, University of Louvain.

———. 1966. "Moral Problems Involved in Responsible Parenthood." *Louvain Studies* 1, no. 1 (Fall): 3–18.

———. 1972–73. "Ontic Evil and Moral Evil." *Louvain Studies* 4:115–56.

———. 1983. "Transplantations d'organes." *Foi et temps* 4:308–24.

Jasanoff, S. 2011. *Reframing Rights: Bioconstitutionalism in the Genetic Age.* Cambridge, MA: MIT Press.

Jennings, Bruce, Virginia A. Sharpe, Bradford H. Gray, and Alan R. Fleischman, eds. 2004. *The Ethics of Hospital Trustees.* Washington, DC: Georgetown University Press.

John Paul II. 1995. *Evangelium vitae (The Gospel of Life).* March 25. http://www.vatican.va/holy_father/john_paul_ii/encyclicals/documents/hf_jp-ii_enc_25031995_evangelium-vitae_en.html.

———. 2004. "Care for Patients in a 'Permanent Vegetative State.'" *Origins* 33, no. 43 (April 8): 738–40.

Johnson, Mark. 1993. "The Principle of Double Effect and Safe Sex in Marriage: Reflections on a Suggestion." *Linacre Quarterly* 60:82–89.

Joint Commission on Accreditation of Healthcare Organizations. 2004. *Patient Safety: Essentials for Health Care.* 2nd ed. Oakbrook Terrace, IL: Joint Commission Resources.

———. 2008. *Understanding and Preventing Sentinel and Adverse Events in Your Health Care Organization.* Oakbrook Terrace, IL: Joint Commission Resources.

———. 2010. *Root Cause Analysis in Healthcare. Tools and Techniques.* 4th ed. Oakbrook Terrace, IL: Joint Commission Resources.

———. 2011. *Comprehensive Accreditation Manual.* Oakbrook Terrace, IL: Joint Commission Resources.

Jonasson, Olga. 1986. "In Organ Transplants, Americans First? (Case Study)." *Hastings Center Report* 16, no. 5 (October–November): 24.

Jones, David Albert. 2011. "Is There a Logical Slippery Slope from Voluntary to Non-Voluntary Euthanasia?" *Kennedy Institute of Ethics Journal* 21, no. 4 (December): 379–404.

Jotterand, F., ed. 2008. *Emerging Conceptual, Ethical and Policy Issues in Bionanotechnology.* Dordrecht: Springer.

Juengst, Eric T., Robert H. Binstock, Maxwell Mehlman, Stephen G. Post, and Peter Whitehouse. 2003. "Biogerontology, 'Anti-Aging Medicine,' and the Challenge of Human Enhancement." *Hastings Center Report* 33, no. 4 (July–August): 21–30.

Kahlenborn, Chris. 1996. "Seeking Cures from the Dead: Chickenpox Vaccine: A Forced 'Option.'" *Life Advocate* (January): 25–27.

———. 2001. "A Necessary Tension and Tube Feeding." *Ethics & Medics* 26, no. 8 (August): 1–2.

Kalb, Claudia. 2003. "Taking a New Look at Pain." *Newsweek*, May 19, 45–52.

———. 2004. "Brand New Stem Cells." *Newsweek*, March 15, 57.

Kamisar, Yale. 1996. "The 'Right to Die': On Drawing (and Erasing) Lines." *Duquesne Law Review* 35, no. 1 (Fall): 481–521.

Kant, Immanuel. 1981. *Foundations of the Metaphysics of Morals*. Translated by James W. Ellington. Indianapolis: Hackett Publishing Co.

———. 1993. *Grounding for the Metaphysics of Morals; with "On the Supposed Right to Lie because of Philanthropic Concerns."* Translated by James W. Ellington. 3rd. ed. Indianapolis: Hackett Publishing Co.

Kass, L. R., Elizabeth H. Blackburn, Rebecca S. Dresser, Daniel W. Foster, Francis Fukuyama, Michael S. Gazzaniga, Robert P. George, Mary Ann Glendon, Alfonso Gomez-Lobo, William B. Hurlbut, et al. 2003. *Beyond Therapy: Biotechnology and the Pursuit of Happiness*. A Report on the President's Council on Bioethics. Commissioned Report by the President's Council, Washington, DC.

Kaufmann, Walter. 1973. *Without Guilt and Justice: From Decidophobia to Autonomy*. New York: Dell.

Kaveny, M. Cathleen. 1999. "Jurisprudence and Genetics." *Theological Studies* 60, no. 1: 135–47.

———. 2002. "Developing the Doctrine of Distributive Justice: Methods of Distribution, Redistribution, and the Role of Time in Allocating Intensive Care Resources." In *Allocating Scarce Medical Resources*, edited by H. Tristram Engelhardt Jr. and Mark J. Cherry, 177–99. Washington, DC: Georgetown University Press.

Keenan, James F. 1998. "The Case for Physician-Assisted Suicide?" *America*, November 14: 14–19.

———, ed. 2000. *Catholic Ethicists on HIV/AIDS Prevention*. New York: Continuum.

Kelly, David F. 1979. *The Emergence of Roman Catholic Medical Ethics in North America: An Historical–Methodological–Bibliographical Study*. New York: Edwin Mellen Press.

———. 1983. "Sexuality and Concupiscence in Augustine." *Annual of the Society of Christian Ethics*, 81–116.

———. 1988. "Individualism and Corporatism in a Personalist Ethics: An Analysis of Organ Transplants." In *Personalist Morals*, edited by J. Selling, 147–65. Leuven, Belgium: Leuven University Press.

———. 1991. *Critical Care Ethics: Treatment Decisions in American Hospitals*. Kansas City, MO: Sheed & Ward.

———. 1995. "Karl Rahner and Genetic Engineering: The Use of Theological Principles in Moral Analysis." *Philosophy and Theology* 9, no. 1–2: 177–200.

———. 1998. "Methodological and Practical Issues in the *Ethical and Religious Directives for Catholic Health Services*." *Louvain Studies* 23:321–37.

———. 2002. *Critical Care Ethics: Treatment Decisions in American Hospitals*. Eugene, OR: Wipf and Stock.

———. 2006. *Medical Care at the End of Life: A Catholic Perspective*. Washington, DC: Georgetown University Press.

Kelly, Gerald. 1950. "The Duty of Using Artificial Means of Preserving Life." *Theological Studies* 11:203–20.

———. 1958. *Medico-Moral Problems*. St. Louis, MO: Catholic Hospital Association of the United States and Canada.

Kilner, John F. 1988. "The Ethical Legitimacy of Excluding the Elderly When Medical Resources Are Limited." *Annual of the Society of Christian Ethics*, 179–203.

Kimmelman, Jonathan. 2010. *Gene Transfer and the Ethics of First-in-Human Research*. New York: Cambridge University Press.

King, Nancy M. 2003. "Accident and Desire: Inadvertent Germline Effects in Clinical Research." *Hastings Center Report* 33, no. 2 (March–April): 23–30.

King, Patricia A., and Leslie E. Wolf. 1998. "Lessons for Physician-Assisted Suicide from the African-American Experience." In *Physician-Assisted Suicide: Expanding the Debate*, edited by Margaret D. Battin, Rosamond Rhodes, and Anita Silvers, 91–112. New York: Routledge.

Kirschner, Kristi L. 2010. "One City, Two Worlds." *Hastings Center Report* 40, no. 5 (September–October): 6–7.

Kleinig, John. 1986. "In Organ Transplants, Americans First? (Case Study)." *Hastings Center Report* 16, no. 5 (October–November): 25.

Knauer, Peter. (1967) 1979. "The Hermeneutic Function of the Principle of Double Effect." In *Readings in Moral Theology, No. 1*, edited by Charles E. Curran and Richard A. McCormick, 1–39. New York: Paulist Press.

Knoepffler, Nikolaus. 2004. "Stem Cell Research: An Ethical Evaluation of Policy Options." *Kennedy Institute of Ethics Journal* 14, no. 1 (March): 55–74.

Kohlberg, Lawrence. 1981. *The Philosophy of Moral Development: Moral Stages and the Idea of Justice*. San Francisco: Harper and Row.

Korthals, M. 2010. *Genomics, Obesity and the Struggle over Responsibilities*. Dordrecht: Springer.

Kubat, Christopher K. 2002. "TOTS and GIFT Reconsidered." *Ethics & Medics* 27, no. 7 (July): 3.

Küng, Hans. 1997. *Weltethos für Weltpolitik und Weltwirtschaft*. München: Piper Verlag.

Kutz, Christopher. 2000. *Complicity: Ethics and Law for a Collective Age*. New York: Cambridge University Press.

Laffey, Judy. 1996. "Bioethical Principles and Care-Based Ethics in Medical Futility." *Cancer Practice* 4, no. 1 (January–February): 41–46.

Lander, Eric S., Lauren M. Linton, Bruce Birren, Chad Nusbaum, Michael C. Zody, Jennifer Baldwin, Keri Devon, Ken Dewar, Michael Doyle, William FitzHugh, et al. 2001. "Initial Sequencing and Analysis of the Human Genome." *Nature* 409 (February 15): 860–921.

Landry Donald W., and Howard A. Zucker. 2004. "Embryonic Death and the Creation of Human Embryonic Stem Cells." *Journal of Clinical Investigation* 114, no. 9: 1184–86.

Landry Donald W., H. A. Zucker, M. V. Sauer, M. Reznik, and L. Wiebe. 2006. "Hypocellularity and Absence of Compaction as Criteria for Embryonic Death." *Regenerative Medicine* 1, no. 3: 371–75.

Lantos, John D., Peter A. Singer, Robert M. Walker, Gregory P. Gramelspacher, Gary R. Shapiro, Miguel A. Sanchez-Gonzalez, Carol B. Stocking, Steven H. Miles, and Mark Siegler. 1989. "The Illusion of Futility in Clinical Practice." *American Journal of Medicine* 87: 81–84.

Lappetito, Joanne, and Paula Thompson. 1993. "Today's Ethics Committees Face Varied Issues." *Health Progress* 74 (November): 34–39.

LaPuma, John J., Carol B. Stocking, Marc D. Silverstein, Andrea DiMartini, and Mark Siegler. 1988. "An Ethics Consultation Service in a Teaching Hospital: Utilization and Evaluation." *Journal of the American Medical Association* 290, no. 6 (August 12): 808–11.

LaPuma, John J., and David L. Schiedermayer. 1991. "Ethics Consultation: Skills, Roles, and Training." *Annals of Internal Medicine* 114, no. 2 (January 15): 155–60.

LaPuma, John J., and Stephen E. Toulmin. 1989. "Ethics Consultation and Ethics Committees." *Archives of Internal Medicine* 149 (May): 1109–12.

Largent, Emily A., and Steven D. Pearson. 2012. "Which Orphans Will Find a Home? The Rule of Rescue in Resource Allocation for Rare Diseases." *Hastings Center Report* 42, no. 1 (January–February): 27–34.

Larkin, Vincent R. 1960. "St. Thomas Aquinas on the Movement of the Heart." *Journal of the History of Medicine* 15, no. 1 (January): 22–30.

"The Latest Word: Brophy Dies." 1986. *Hastings Center Report* 16, no. 6 (December): 32.

"The Latest Word: In the Courts." 1986. *Hastings Center Report* 16, no. 5 (October): 47.

Latham, Stephen R. 2011. "The 'Real-Life' Death Panel, Reformed." *Hastings Center Report* 41, no. 1 (January–February): 53.

Latkovic, Mark S. 2005. "The Morality of Tube Feeding PVS Patients: Critique of the View of Kevin O'Rourke, OP." *National Catholic Bioethics Quarterly* 5, no. 3 (Autumn): 503–13.

Lauritzen, Paul. 1993. *Pursuing Parenthood: Ethical Issues in Assisted Reproduction*. Bloomington: Indiana University Press.

Lee, Patrick, and Germain Grisez. 2010. "Total Brain Death." *Bioethics*, October 6, 1–10.

Lee, Thomas H., and James J. Mongan. 2009. *Chaos and Organization in Health Care*. Cambridge, MA: MIT Press.

Levine, Carol. 1984. "Questions and (Some Very Tentative) Answers about Hospital Ethics Committees." *Hastings Center Report* 14, no. 3 (June): 9–12.

Liebrecht, John. 1990. "The Nancy Cruzan Case." *Origins* 19, no. 32 (January 11): 525–26.

Lizza, John P. 2006. *Persons, Humanity, and the Definition of Death*. Baltimore: Johns Hopkins University Press.

———, ed. 2009. *Defining the Beginning and End of Life*. Baltimore: Johns Hopkins University Press.

Lo, Bernard. 1987. "Behind Closed Doors: Problems and Pitfalls of Ethics Committees." *New England Journal of Medicine* 317, no. 1 (July 2): 46–50.

Lock, Margaret. 2002. *Twice Dead: Organ Transplants and the Reinvention of Death*. Berkeley: University of California Press.

Lombardo, P. A. 2011. *A Century of Eugenics in America: From the Indiana Experiment to the Human Genome Era*. Bloomington: Indiana University Press.

Lustig, B. A., B. A. Brody, and G. P. McKenny, eds. 2010. *Altering Nature. Vol. 2, Religion, Biotechnology and Public Policy*. Dordrecht: Springer Science & Business Media.

Lynn, Joann. 1993. "Are the Patients Who Become Organ Donors under the Pittsburgh Protocol for 'Non-Heart-Beating Donors' Really Dead?" *Kennedy Institute of Ethics Journal* 3, no. 2 (June): 167–68.

Lysaught, M. Therese. 2011. "Moral Analysis of Procedure at Phoenix Hospital." *Origins* 40, no. 33 (January 27): 537–49.

Mackler, Aaron L., ed. 2000. *Life and Death Responsibilities in Jewish Biomedical Ethics*. New York: Jewish Theological Seminary of America.

———, ed. 2003. *Introduction to Jewish and Catholic Bioethics: A Comparative Analysis*. Washington, DC: Georgetown University Press.

Macklin, Ruth. 1988. "Making Policy by Committee." *Hastings Center Report* 18, no. 4 (August–September): 26.

———. 2004. *Double Standards in Medical Research in Developing Countries*. Cambridge: Cambridge University Press.

Macrina, Francis L. 2012. *Scientific Integrity. Text and Cases in Responsible Conduct of Research*. 4th ed. Washington, DC: ASM Press.

Magill, Gerard. 2002. "The Ethics Weave in Human Genomics, Embryonic Stem Cell Research, and Therapeutic Cloning." *Albany Law Review* 65, no. 3: 701–28.

———. 2006. "Ethical and Policy Issues Related to Medical Error and Patient Safety." In *First Do No Harm. Law, Ethics and Healthcare*, edited by Sheila A. M. McLean, 101–16. Burlington, VT: Ashgate.

———. 2008. "Using Excess IVF Blastocysts for Embryonic Stem Cell Research." *Hofstra Law Review* 37, no. 2 (Winter): 447–85.

———. 2011. "Threat of Imminent Death in Pregnancy: A Role for Double Effect Reasoning." *Theological Studies* 72, no. 4 (December): 848–60.

———. 2012. "A Moral Compass for Cooperation with Wrongdoing." In *Voting and Holiness. Catholic Perspectives on Political Participation*, edited by Nicholas P. Cafardi, 135–57. New York: Paulist Press.

Magill, Gerard, and William B. Neaves. 2009 "Ontological and Ethical Implications of Direct Nuclear Reprogramming." *Kennedy Institute of Ethics Journal* 19, no. 1: 23–32.

Magill, Gerard, and Lawrence D. Prybil. 2004. "Stewardship and Integrity in Health Care: A Role for Organizational Ethics." *Journal of Business Ethics* 50:225–38.

———. 2011. "Board Oversight of Community Benefit: An Ethical Imperative." *Kennedy Institute of Ethics Journal* 21, no. 1: 25–50.

Maguire, Daniel C. 1974. *Death by Choice*. Garden City, NY: Doubleday.

Maguire, Marjorie Reiley. 1983. "Personhood, Covenant, and Abortion." *Annual of the Society of Christian Ethics*, 117–45.

Mahoney, John. 1987. *The Making of Moral Theology: A Study of the Roman Catholic Tradition*. Oxford: Clarendon Press.

———. 2003. "Christian Doctrines, Ethical Issues, and Human Genetics." *Theological Studies* 64, no. 4 (December): 719–49.

Malmqvist, Erik. 2011. "Reprogenetics and the 'Parents Have Always Done It' Argument." *Hastings Center Report* 41, no. 1 (January–February): 43–49.

Mappes, Thomas A. 2003. "Persistent Vegetative State, Prospective Thinking, and Advance Directives." *Kennedy Institute of Ethics Journal* 13, no. 2 (June): 119–39.

Marker, Rita L., and Wesley J. Smith. 1996. "The Art of Verbal Engineering." *Duquesne Law Review* 35, no. 1 (Fall): 81–107.

Marquis, Don. 2010. "Are DCD Donors Dead?" *Hastings Center Report* 40, no. 2 (May-June): 24–31.

Mascia, Matteo, and Lucia Mariani, eds. 2010. *Ethics and Climate Change: Scenarios for Justice and Sustainability.* Padua, Italy: Fondazione Lanza.

May, William E. 1998. "Tube Feeding and the Vegetative State." *Ethics & Medics* 23, no. 12 (December): 1–2.

———. 1999. "Tube Feeding and the Vegetative State." *Ethics & Medics* 24, no. 1 (January): 3–4.

———. 2008. *Catholic Bioethics and the Gift of Human Life.* 2nd ed. Huntington, IN: Our Sunday Visitor.

May, William E., Robert Barry, Orville Griese, Germaine Grisez, Brian Johnstone, Thomas J. Marzen, James T. McHugh, Gilbert Meilaender, Mark Siegler, and William Smith. 1987. "Feeding and Hydrating the Permanently Unconscious and Other Vulnerable Persons." *Issues in Law and Medicine* 3, no. 3: 204–11.

May, William F. 1983. *The Physician's Covenant: Images of the Healer in Medical Ethics.* Philadelphia: Westminster Press.

Mayer, Ryan C. 2011. "Is Embryo Adoption a Form of Surrogacy?" *National Catholic Bioethics Quarterly* 11, no. 2 (Summer), 249–56.

McCartney, James J. 1986. "Catholic Positions on Withholding Sustenance for the Terminally Ill." *Health Progress*, October, 38–40.

———. 1992a. "Ethics in Health Care, Part I: The Process of Ethics Committees." *Clinical Laboratory Management Review* 6, no. 3 (May-June): 222–24.

———. 1992b. "Ethics in Health Care, Part II: The Product of Shared Deliberation, Working within a Pluralistic Culture." *Clinical Laboratory Management Review* 6, no. 4 (July-August): 315–21.

McCormick, Richard A. (1972) 1981. "Genetic Medicine: Notes on the Moral Literature." In *Notes on Moral Theology 1965 through 1980*, 401–22. Lanham, MD: University Press of America.

———. (1989) 1993. "Therapy or Tampering: The Ethics of Reproductive Technology and the Doctrine of Development." In *Bioethics: Basic Writings on the Key Ethical Questions That Surround the Major, Modern Biological Possibilities and Problems.* 4th ed., edited by Thomas A. Shannon, 97–122. Mahwah, NJ: Paulist Press.

———. 1992. "'Moral Considerations' Ill Considered." *America* 166, no. 9 (March 14): 210–14.

———. 1994. *Corrective Vision.* Kansas City, MO: Sheed & Ward.

McCormick, Richard A., and John J. Paris. 1987. "The Catholic Tradition on the Use of Nutrition and Fluids." *America* 156:358.

McDonough, Mary J. 2007. *Can a Health Care Market Be Moral? A Catholic Vision.* Washington, DC: Georgetown University Press.

McFadden, Charles J. 1955. *Medical Ethics.* 3rd ed. Philadelphia, PA: F. A. Davis.

———. 1956. *Medical Ethics.* 4th ed. Philadelphia, PA: F. A. Davis.

———. 1961. *Medical Ethics.* 5th ed. Philadelphia, PA: F. A. Davis.

McHugh, James. 1989. "Artificially Assisted Nutrition and Hydration." *Origins* 19, no. 19 (October 12): 314–16.

McHugh, John A., OP, and Charles J. Callan, OP. 1929. *Moral Theology: A Complete Course.* vol. 1. New York: Joseph F. Wagner.

McIntyre, Alison. 2001. "Doing Away with Double Effect." *Ethics* 111, no. 2 (January): 219–55.

Medical Ethics Advisor. 1993. *Medical Ethics Advisor* 9, no. 5 (May): 57–59.

Meisel, Alan. 1989. *The Right to Die.* New York: John Wiley & Sons.

———. 1995. *The Right to Die*, 2nd ed., 2 vols. New York: John Wiley & Sons.

———. 2003. *The Right to Die*, 2nd Edition 2003 Supplement. New York: Aspen Publishers.

Menzel, Paul T. 2011a. "The Cultural Moral Right to a Basic Minimum of Accessible Health Care." *Kennedy Institute of Ethics Journal* 21, no. 1 (March): 79–119.

———. 2011b. "Dishonesty, Ignorance, or What?" *Hastings Center Report* 41, no. 2 (March-April): 16–17.

Michejda, Maria. 2002. "Spontaneous Miscarriages as Source of Fetal Stem Cells." *National Catholic Bioethics Quarterly* 2, no. 3 (Autumn): 401–11.

Miles, Steven H., and Allison August. 1990. "Courts, Gender and the Right to Die." *Law, Medicine and Health Care* 18, nos. 1–2 (Spring–Summer): 85–95.

Miller, Franklin G., and Diane E. Meier. 1998. "Voluntary Death: A Comparison of Terminal Dehydration and Physician-Assisted Suicide." *Annals of Internal Medicine* 128, no. 7 (April 1): 559–62.

Miller, Franklin G., and Robert D. Truog. 2008. "Rethinking the Ethics of Vital Organ Donations." *Hastings Center Report* 38, no. 6 (November–December): 38–46.

———. 2009. "The Incoherence of Determining Death by Neurological Criteria: A Commentary on *Controversies in the Determination of Death*, A White Paper by the President's Council on Bioethics." *Kennedy Institute of Ethics Journal* 19, no. 2 (June): 185–93.

Miller, Geoffrey. 2007. "Ten Days in Texas." *Hastings Center Report* 37, no. 4 (July–August): 57.

"Minority Papal Commission Report." (1967) 1969. In *The Catholic Case for Contraception*, edited by Daniel Callahan, 174–211. London: Macmillan.

Mirkes, Renée. 2001. "NBAC and Embryo Ethics." *National Catholic Bioethics Quarterly* 1, no. 2 (Summer): 163–87.

Mirowski, Philip, and Esther-Mirjam Sent. 2002. *Science Bought and Sold: Essays in the Economics of Science*. Chicago: Chicago University Press.

Mitchell, C. B., E. D. Pellegrino, and J. Bethke Elshtain. 2007. *Biotechnology and the Human Good*. Washington, DC: Georgetown University Press.

Mitchell, Susan M., and Martha S. Swartz. 1990. "Is There a Place for Lawyers on Ethics Committees? A View from the Inside." *Hastings Center Report* 20, no. 2 (March–April): 32–33.

Modras, Ronald. 1984. "Implications of Rahner's Anthropology for Fundamental Moral Theology." *Horizons* 12:70–90.

Montoya, M. 2011. *Making the Mexican Diabetic: Race, Science, and the Genetics of Inequality*. Berkeley: University of California Press.

Moraczewski, Albert S. 2003. "Stem Cells: Answers to Three Questions." *Ethics & Medics* 28, no. 3 (March): 1–2.

Morlino, Robert C. 2005. "Medical Treatment: Make Decisions Based on Catholic Teaching." Bishop's Statement.

Morreim, E. Haavi. 1995. *Balancing Act: The New Medical Ethics of Medicine's New Economics*. Washington, DC: Georgetown University Press.

———. 2001. *Holding Health Care Accountable: Law and the New Medical Marketplace*. New York: Oxford University Press.

Morris, Julian. 2000. *Rethinking Risk and the Precautionary Principle*. Oxford: Butterworth-Heinemann.

Moskowitz, Ellen. 2003. "The Consensus on Assisted Suicide." *Hastings Center Report* 33, no. 4 (July–August): 46–47.

Mulligan, James J. 2005. "Caring for the Unconscious." *Ethics and Medics* 30, no. 7 (July): 2–4.

Multi-Society Task Force on PVS. 1994. "Medical Aspects of the Persistent Vegetative State." *New England Journal of Medicine* 330, nos. 21 and 22 (May 26 and June 2): 1499–508, 1572–79.

Munsat, Theodore L., William H. Stuart, and Ronald E. Cranford. 1989. "Guidelines on the Vegetative State: Commentary on the American Academy of Neurology Statement." *Neurology* 39: 123–24.

Munson, Ronald. 2002. *Raising the Dead: Organ Transplants, Ethics, and Society*. New York: Oxford University Press.

Munthe, C. 2011. *The Price of Precaution and the Ethics of Risk*. Dordrecht: Springer.

Murphy, Donald J. 1988. "Do-Not-Resuscitate Orders: Time for Reappraisal in Long-Term-Care Institutions." *Journal of the American Medical Association* 260, no. 14 (October 14): 2098–2101.

Murphy, N., and C. C. Knight. 2010. *Human Identity at the Intersection of Science, Technology and Religion*. Surrey, UK: Ashgate.

Murphy, P. 1989. "The Role of the Nurse on Hospital Ethics Committees." *Nursing Clinics of North America* 24, no. 2 (June): 551–56.

Murray, Thomas H. 1988. "Where Are the Ethics in Ethics Committees?" *Hastings Center Report* 18, no. 1 (February–March): 12–13.

Nagy, A., E. Gocza, E. M. Diaz, V. R. Prideaux, E. Iványi, M. Markkula, and J. Rossant. 1990. "Embryonic Stem Cells Alone Are Able to Support Fetal Development in the Mouse." *Development* 110:815–21.

National Bioethics Advisory Commission. 2001. *Ethical and Policy Issues in Research Involving Human Participants*. Bethesda, MD: National Bioethics Advisory Commission.

National Coalition on Health Care, and the Institute for Healthcare Improvement. 2000. *Reducing Medical Error and Improving Patient Safety*. Washington, DC: National Coalition on Health Care.

National Conference of Catholic Bishops. 1995. *Ethical and Religious Directives for Catholic Health Care Services*. Washington, DC: United States Catholic Conference.

National Patient Safety Foundation. 2001. *Patient Safety Initiative 2000. Spotlight on Solutions*. Chicago: National Patient Safety Foundation.

Naumov, Ivan M., James E. Wilberger Jr., and C. Don Keyes. 1991. "Beginning and End of Biological Life." In *New Harvest*, edited by C. Don Keyes and Walter E. Wiest, 31–56. Clifton, NJ: Humana Press.

Nayef, R. F. 2011. *The Politics of Emerging Strategic Technologies: Implications for Geopolitics, Human Enhancement and Human Destiny*. Hampshire, UK: Palgrave Macmillan.

Neher, Jon O. 2004. "Like a River." *Hastings Center Report* 34, no. 2 (March–April): 9–10.

Nelson, Hilde Lindemann. 2002. "What Child Is This?" *Hastings Center Report* 32, no. 6 (November–December): 29–39.

Nelson, James Lindemann, ed. 2003. *Rationing Sanity: Ethical Issues in Managed Health Care*. Washington, DC: Georgetown University Press.

Nelson, Lawrence J. 2003. "Persistent Indeterminate State: Reflections on the Wendland Case." *Issues in Ethics* 14, no. 1 (Winter): 14–17.

Nelson, Lawrence, and Brandon Ashby. 2011. "Rethinking the Ethics of Physician Participation in Lethal Injection Execution." *Hastings Center Report* 41, no. 3 (May–June): 28–37.

New York State Task Force on Life and the Law. 1992. *When Others Must Choose: Deciding for Patients without Capacity*. New York: New York State Task Force on Life and the Law.

———. 1993. *When Others Must Choose: Deciding for Patients without Capacity: Supplement to Report and Legislation*. New York: New York State Task Force on Life and the Law.

———. 1994. *When Death Is Sought: Assisted Suicide and Euthanasia in the Medical Context*. New York: New York State Task Force on Life and the Law.

Newborn Screening Task Force. 2000. "Serving the Family from Birth to the Medical Home." *Pediatrics* 106:383–47.

Niederauer, George. 2012. "Catholic Healthcare West Becomes Dignity Health: What Does It Mean?" *Catholic San Francisco*, February 14. www.catholic-sf.org/news_select.php?newsid=4&id=59532.

Niedermeyer, Albert. 1955. *Allgemeine Pastoralmedizin*. Vienna: Herder.

Noddings, Nel. 2003. *Caring: A Feminine Approach to Ethics and Moral Education*. 2nd ed. Berkeley: University of California Press.

Noonan, John T., Jr. 1967. *Contraception: A History of Its Treatment by the Catholic Theologians and Canonists*. New York: New American Library.

———. (1966) 1969. "Contraception and the Council." In *The Catholic Case for Contraception*, edited by Daniel Callahan, 3–29. London: Macmillan.

"Nurses Bring Holistic View to Ethical Decision Making." 1993. *Medical Ethics Advisor* 9, no. 5 (May): 49–54.

"Nursing Ethics Group: When the Ethics Committee Is Not Enough." 1989. *Hospital Ethics*, January–February: 15–16.

O'Connell, Timothy E. 1978. *Principles for a Catholic Morality*. New York: Seabury Press.

———. 1990. *Principles for a Catholic Morality*. Rev. ed. New York: Harper-Collins.

O'Donnell, Thomas J. 1959. *Morals in Medicine*. 2nd ed. Westminster, MD: Newman Press.

O'Grady, John F. 1975. *Christian Anthropology: A Meaning for Human Life*. New York: Paulist Press.

Olson, Ellen, Eileen Chichin, Frances Brennan, Helene Meyers, and Ellen Schulman. 1994. "Early Experience on an Ethics Consult Team." *Journal of the American Geriatric Society* 42, no. 4 (April): 437–41.

O'Meara, Thomas F. 2003. "Divine Grace and Human Nature as Sources for the Universal Magisterium of Bishops." *Theological Studies* 64, no. 4 (December): 683–706.

Oregon and Washington Bishops. 1991. "Living and Dying Well." *Origins* 21, no. 22 (November 7): 346–52.

"Oregon Death with Dignity Act." 1998. In *Physician-Assisted Suicide: Expanding the Debate*, edited by Margaret D. Battin, Rosamond Rhodes, and Anita Silvers, 443–48. New York: Routledge.

O'Rourke, Kevin D. 1989. "Father Kevin O'Rourke on Hydration and Nutrition: Open Letter to Bishop McHugh." *Origins* 19, no. 21 (October 26): 351–52.

———. 1999a. "On the Care of 'Vegetative' Patients." *Ethics & Medics* 24, no. 4 (April): 3–4.

———. 1999b. "On the Care of 'Vegetative' Patients." *Ethics & Medics* 24, no. 5 (May): 3–4.

———. 2004. "Stem Cell Research: Prospects and Problems." *National Catholic Bioethics Quarterly* 4, no. 2 (Summer): 289–99.

———. 2005. "The Catholic Tradition on Forgoing Life Support." *National Catholic Bioethics Quarterly* 5, no. 3 (Autumn): 537–53.

———. 2008. "When to Withdraw Life Support?" *National Catholic Bioethics Quarterly* 8, no. 4 (Winter): 663–72.

———. 2010. "Catholic Principles and *In-Vitro* Fertilization." *National Catholic Bioethics Quarterly* 10, no. 4 (Winter): 709–22.

O'Rourke, Kevin D., and Jean deBlois. 1992. "Removing Life Support: Motivations, Obligations: An Opinion on NCCB Committee for Pro-Life Activities' Statement on Artificial Hydration and Nutrition." *Health Progress*, July–August, 20–27, 38.

Orr, R. D., and E. Moon. 1993. "Effectiveness of an Ethics Consultation Service." *Journal of Family Practice* 36, no. 1 (January): 49–53.

Otto, Rudolf. (1923) 1950. *The Idea of the Holy.* Translated by John W. Harvey. 2nd ed. New York: Oxford University Press.

Panicola, Michael R., David M. Belde, John Paul Slosar, and Mark F. Repenshek. 2011. *Health Care Ethics: Theological Foundations, Contemporary Issues, and Controversial Cases.* 2nd ed. Winona, MN: Anselm Academic.

Papanikolaou, Evangelos G. 2006. "In Vitro Fertilization with Single Blastocyst-Stage Versus Single Cleavage-Stage Embryos." *New England Journal of Medicine* 354:1130–42.

Parens, E. 1998. *Enhancing Human Traits: Ethical and Social Implications.* Washington, DC: Georgetown University Press.

———. 2004. "Genetic Differences and Human Identities: On Why Talking about Behavioral Genetics Is Important and Difficult." *Hastings Center Report* 34, no. 1 (January–February): S1–S36.

Parens, E., A. Chapman, and N. Press, eds. 2006. *Wrestling with Behavioral Genetics: Science, Ethics, and Public Conversation.* Baltimore: Johns Hopkins University Press.

Parens, Erik, Josephine Johnston, and Jacob Moses. 2009. *Ethical Issues in Synthetic Biology: An Overview of the Debates.* Washington, DC: Woodrow Wilson International Center for Scholars.

Parens, Erik, and Lori P. Knowles. 2003. "Reprogenetics and Public Policy: Reflections and Recommendations." *Hastings Center Report* 33, no. 4 (July–August): S1–S24.

Paris, John J. 1986. "When Burdens of Feeding Outweigh Benefits." *Hastings Center Report* 16, no. 1 (February–March): 30–32.

Paris, John J., Robert K. Crone, and Frank Reardon. 1990. "Physicians' Refusal of Requested Treatment: The Case of Baby L." *New England Journal of Medicine* 322, no. 14 (April 5): 1012–15.

Patrick, Anne E. 1989. "Conscience and Community: Catholic Moral Theology Today." In *Warren Lecture Series in Catholic Studies.* Tulsa, OK: University of Tulsa Press.

Paul VI. 1965. *Gaudium et spes.* Pastoral Constitution on the Church in the Modern World, December 7. www.vatican.va/archive/hist_councils/ii_vatican_council/documents/vat-ii_cons_19651207_gaudium-et-spes_en.html.

———. 1969. "On Human Life." 1968. In *The Catholic Case for Contraception*, edited by Daniel Callahan, 212–38. London: Macmillan.

Pearson, Steven D., James E. Sabin, and Ezekiel J. Emanuel. 2003. *No Margin, No Mission. Health-Care Organizations and the Quest for Ethical Excellence.* New York: Oxford University Press.

Pellegrino, Edmund D. 1979. *Humanism and the Physician.* Knoxville: University of Tennessee Press.

Pellegrino, Edmund D., Adam Schulman, and Thomas W. Merrill, eds. 2009. *Human Dignity and Bioethics*. Notre Dame, IN: University of Notre Dame Press.

Pellegrino, Edmund D., and David C. Thomasma. 1981. *A Philosophical Basis of Medical Practice*. New York: Oxford University Press.

———. 1988. *For the Patient's Good*. New York: Oxford University Press.

———. 1996. *The Christian Virtues in Medical Practice*. Washington, DC: Georgetown University Press.

Pence, Gregory E. 1998. *Who's Afraid of Human Cloning?* Lanham, MD: Rowman & Littlefield.

———. 2000. *Classic Cases in Medical Ethics: Accounts of Cases That Have Shaped Medical Ethics, with Philosophical, Legal, and Historical Backgrounds*. Boston: McGraw-Hill.

Pennsylvania Bishops. 1992. "Nutrition and Hydration: Moral Considerations." *Origins* 21, no. 34 (January 30): 541, 543–53.

Perkins, Henry S., and Bunnie S. Saathoff. 1988. "Impact of Medical Ethics Consultations on Physicians: An Exploratory Study." *American Journal of Medicine* 85, no. 6 (December): 761–65.

Perlin, Terry M. 1992. *Clinical Medical Ethics: Cases in Practice*. Boston: Little, Brown.

Peters, Ted, Karen Lebacqz, and Gaymon Bennet. 2010. *Sacred Cells? Why Christians Should Support Stem Cell Research*. Lanham, MD: Rowman & Littlefield.

Petryna, Adriana. 2009. *When Experiments Travel: Clinical Trials and the Global Search for Human Subjects*. Princeton, NJ: Princeton University Press.

Phillips, Donald F. 1993. "Pastoral Care: Finding a Niche in Ethical Decision Making." *Cambridge Quarterly of Healthcare Ethics* 2:99–106.

Pius XI. 1939. "On Christian Marriage." 1930. In *Five Great Encyclicals*, edited by Gerald C. Treacy, 77–117. New York: Paulist Press.

Pius XII. 1957. "Address on Reanimation." *Acta apostolicae sedis* 49:1027–33.

———. 1958. "The Prolongation of Life: An Address of Pope Pius XII to an International Congress of Anesthesiologists." *The Pope Speaks* 4, no. 4 (Spring): 395–98.

Place, Michael D. 2000. "Letter to Colleagues in the Ministry." Catholic Health Association of the United States, July 25.

Plato. 1991. *The Republic: The Complete and Unabridged Jowett Translation*. Edited and translated by Benjamin Jowett. New York: Vintage Books.

Pollock, David S., and Todd M. Begg. 1990. "The Constitutional Right to Die." Pittsburgh: Pollock and Adams.

Pompey, Heinrich. 1968. *Die Bedeutung der Medizin Für die Kirchliche Seelsorge im Selbstverständnis der Sognannten Pastoralmedizin: Eine Bibliographisch-Historische Untersuchung Bis Zur Mitte Des 19. Jahrhunderts*. Fribourg in Germany: Herder.

Pontifical Commission for the Study of Population Family and Births. (1966) 1978. "The Theological Report of the Papal Commission on Birth Control." In *Official Catholic Teachings: Love and Sexuality*, edited by Odile M. Liebard, 296–320. Wilmington, NC: McGrath Publishing.

Porter, Roy, ed. 2006. *The Cambridge History of Medicine*. New York: Cambridge University Press.

Potter, Van Rensselaer. 1964. "Society and Science: Can Science Aid in the Search for Sophistication in Dealing with Order and Disorder in Human Affairs?" *Science* 146:1018–22.

———. 1970. "Biocybernetics and Survival." *Zygon* 5, no. 3: 229–46.

———. 1971. *Bioethics: Bridge to the Future*. Englewood Cliffs, NJ: Prentice Hall.

———. 1987. "Aldo Leopold's Land Ethics Revisited: Two Kinds of Bioethics." *Perspectives in Biology and Medicine* 30, no. 2: 157–69.

———. 1988. *Global Bioethics: Building on the Leopold Legacy*. East Lansing: Michigan State University Press.

———. 2001. "Moving the Culture toward More Vivid Utopias with Survival as Goal." *Global Bioethics* 14, no. 4: 19–30.

Potts, Michael, P. A. Byrne, and R. G. Nigles. 2000. *Beyond Brain Death: The Case against Brain Based Criteria for Human Death*. Dordrecht: Kluwer Academic Publishers.

Powell, Russell. 2010. "What's the Harm? An Evolutionary Theoretical Critique of the Precautionary Principle." *Kennedy Institute of Ethics Journal* 20, no. 2 (June): 181–206.

Presidential Commission for the Study of Bioethical Issues. 2010. *New Directions: The Ethics of Synthetic Biology and Emerging Technologies*. Washington, DC: Presidential Commission.

President's Commission for the Study of Ethical Problems in Medicine and Biomedical and Behavioral Research. 1981. *Defining Death: Medical, Legal, and Medical Issues in the Determination of Death.* Washington, DC: Government Printing Office.

———. 1982. *Splicing Life: The Social and Ethical Issues of Genetic Engineering with Human Beings.* Washington, DC: Government Printing Office.

———. 1983. *Deciding to Forego Life-Sustaining Treatment.* Washington, DC: Government Printing Office.

President's Council on Bioethics. 2004. *Reproduction and Responsibility: The Regulation of New Biotechnologies.* Washington, DC: Government Printing Office.

———. 2008. *Controversies in the Determination of Death.* Washington, DC: Government Printing Office.

Printz, Louise A. 1989. "Withholding Hydration in the Terminally Ill: Is it Valid?" *Geriatric Medicine,* April, 81–84.

Purtilo, Ruth. 2005. *Ethical Dimensions in the Health Professions.* 4th ed. Philadelphia: Elsevier Saunders.

Quill, Timothy E. 2005. "Terri Schiavo: A Tragedy Compounded." *New England Journal of Medicine* 352, no. 16 (April 21): 1630–31, 1633.

———. 2008. "Physician-Assisted Death in the United States: Are the Existing 'Last Resorts' Enough?" *Hastings Center Report* 38, no. 5 (September–October): 17–22.

Quill, Timothy, Rebecca Dresser, and Dan W. Brock. 1997. "The Rule of Double Effect: A Critique of Its Role in End-of-Life Decision Making." *New England Journal of Medicine* 337, no. 24: 1768–71.

Quindlen, Anna. 2002. "In a Peaceful Frame of Mind." *Newsweek,* February 4, 64.

Racine, Eric. 2010. *Pragmatic Neuroethics: Improving Treatment and Understanding of the Mind-Brain.* Cambridge, MA: MIT Press.

Radin, Margaret Jane. (1987) 1992. "Market-Inalienability." In *The Ethics of Reproductive Technology,* edited by Kenneth D. Alpern, 174–94. New York: Oxford University Press.

Rahner, Karl. (1954) 1961. "Concerning the Relationship between Nature and Grace." In *Theological Investigations,* translated by Cornelius Ernst, vol. 1, 297–317. Baltimore: Helicon.

———. (1959) 1965. "The Concept of Mystery in Catholic Theology." In *Theological Investigations.* Translated by Kevin Smyth, vol. 4, 36–73. Baltimore, MD: Helicon.

———. 1963. *Nature and Grace and Other Essays.* Translated by Dinah Wharton. New York: Sheed & Ward.

———. 1969. *Grace in Freedom.* Translated by Hilda Graef. New York: Herder and Herder.

———. 1972a. "The Experiment with Man: Theological Observations on Man's Self-Manipulation." Translated by Graham Harrison. In *Theological Investigations, vol. 9, Writings of 1965–1967,* 205–24. New York: Herder and Herder.

———. 1972b. "The Problem of Genetic Manipulation." Translated by Graham Harrison. In *Theological Investigations, vol. 9, Writings of 1965–1967,* 225–52. New York: Herder and Herder.

Ramsey, Paul. 1970. *Fabricated Man: The Ethics of Genetic Control.* New Haven, CT: Yale University Press.

Ramsey, W., and K. Frankish, eds. 2010. *The Cambridge Handbook of Artificial Intelligence.* 2nd ed. Cambridge: Cambridge University Press.

Randal, Judith. 1983. "Are Ethics Committees Alive and Well?" *Hastings Center Report* 13, no. 6 (December): 10–12.

Rasmussen, Steen, Mark A. Bedau, Liaohai Chen, David Deamer, David C. Krakauer, Norman H. Packard, and Peter F. Stradler, eds. 2008. *Protocells: Bridging Nonliving and Living Matter.* Cambridge, MA: MIT Press.

Ratiu, Peter, and Peter Singer. 2001. "The Ethics and Economics of Heroic Surgery." *Hastings Center Report* 31, no. 2 (March–April): 47–48.

Ratzinger, Joseph Cardinal. 1997. "Vatican List of Catechism Changes." *Origins* 27, no. 15: 257–62.

———. 2004. "Worthiness to Receive Holy Communion," *Wanderer Press,* 137:29.

Rawls, John. (1971) 1999. *A Theory of Justice.* Rev. ed. Cambridge, MA: Harvard University Press.

Recombinant DNA Advisory Committee (RAC). 1994. "Points to Consider in the Design and Submission of Human Somatic-Cell Gene Therapy Protocols." *Recombinant DNA Tech Bulletin,* 8, no. 4 (December): 181–86.

Reich, Warren T. 1995. "The Word 'Bioethics': The Struggle over Its Earliest Meanings." *Kennedy Institute of Ethics Journal* 5, no. 1: 19–34.

Repenshek, Mark. 2011. "Therapeutic Access to the Embryo: Can Therapeutic IVF Be Justified?" *National Catholic Bioethics Quarterly* 11, no. 4 (Winter): 735–56.

Repenshek, Mark, and John Paul Slosar. 2004. "Medically Assisted Nutrition and Hydration: A Contribution to the Dialogue." *Hastings Center Report* 34, no. 6 (November–December): 13–16.

Rhonheimer, Martin. 2011a. "Reply to Fr. Austriaco." *National Catholic Bioethics Quarterly* 11, no. 1 (Spring): 9–11.

———. 2011b. "Vital Conflicts, Direct Killing, and Justice: A Response to Rev. Benedict Guevin and Other Critics." *National Catholic Bioethics Quarterly* 11, no. 3 (Autumn): 519–40.

Ritchie, Karen. 1989. "When It's Not Really Optional." *Hastings Center Report* 18, no. 4 (August–September): 25–26.

Robinson, John. 2010. "*Baxter* and the Return of Physician-Assisted Suicide." *Hastings Center Report* 40, no. 6 (November–December): 15–17.

Robertson, John A., Jeffrey P. Kahn, and John E. Wagner. 2002. "Conception to Obtain Hematopoietic Stem Cells." *Hastings Center Report* 32, no. 3 (May–June): 34–40.

Rothenberg, Leslie Steven. 1986. "The Dissenting Opinions: Biting the Hands That Won't Feed." *Health Progress*, December: 38–45, 99.

Rothman, David J. 1991. *Strangers at the Bedside. a History of How Law and Bioethics Transformed Medical Decision Making.* New York: Basic Books.

Rubenfeld, S., ed. 2010. *Medicine after the Holocaust: From the Master Race to the Human Genome and Beyond.* Hampshire, UK: Palgrave Macmillan.

Rubin, Susan B. 1998. *When Doctors Say No: The Battleground of Medical Futility.* Bloomington: Indiana University Press.

Rubin, Susan B., and Laurie Zoloth-Dorfman. 1994. "First-Person Plural: Community and Method in Ethics Consultations." *Journal of Clinical Ethics* 5, no. 1 (Spring): 49–54.

Runciman, Bill, Alan Merry, and Merrilyn Walton. 2007. *Safety and Ethics in Healthcare. A Guide to Getting It Right.* Burlington, VT: Ashgate.

Rush, Brittany. 2011. "Where the Money Goes." *Health Care Cost Monitor*, March 3, 1–2.

Saint John's Hospital and Health Center. 1995. "Policy: Ethically Appropriate and Inappropriate Medical Treatment, and Related Matters." Santa Monica, CA: Saint John's Hospital and Health Center.

Sanchez, Gina M. 2012. "Objections to Donation after Cardiac Death." *National Catholic Bioethics Quarterly* 12, no. 1 (Spring): 55–65.

Sandel, M. J. 2007. *The Case against Perfection: Ethics in the Age of Genetic Engineering.* Cambridge, MA: Belknap Press of Harvard University Press.

Sanderson, Katharine. 2011. "Artificial Cells Made to Reproduce Thanks to DNA." *New Scientist* 14 (September 15): 31.

Saunders, William L., Jr. 2010. "Washington Insider." *National Catholic Bioethics Quarterly* 10, no. 4 (Winter): 653–64.

Savulescu, J., and N. Bostrom. 2008. *The Wisdom of Nature: An Evolutionary Heuristic for Human Enhancement.* Oxford: Oxford University Press.

———, eds. 2009. *Human Enhancement.* Oxford: Oxford University Press.

Savulescu, J., R. T. Meulen, and G. Kahane, eds. 2011. *Enhancing Human Capacities.* Oxford: Wiley Blackwell.

Schieve, Laura A. 2006. "The Promise of Single-Embryo Transfer." *New England Journal of Medicine* 354:1190–91.

Schillebeeckx, Edward. 1982. *Interim Report on the Books Jesus & Christ.* Translated by John Bowden. New York: Crossroad.

Schneider, Carl E. 1997. "Making Sausage: The Ninth Circuit's Decision." *Hastings Center Report* 27, no. 1 (January–February): 27–28.

———. 2004. "Benumbed." *Hastings Center Report* 34, no. 1 (January–February): 9–10.

Schneiderman, Lawrence J., Kathy Faber-Langendoen, and Nancy S. Jecker. 1994. "Beyond Futility to an Ethic of Care." *American Journal of Medicine* 92:110.

Schneiderman, Lawrence J., Nancy S. Jecker, and Albert R. Jonsen. 1990. "Medical Futility: Its Meaning and Ethical Implications." *Annals of Internal Medicine* 112, no. 12 (June 15): 949–54.

———. 1996. "Medical Futility: Response to Critiques." *Annals of Internal Medicine* 125 (October 15): 669–74.

Schüller, Bruno. 1986. *Wholly Human: Essays on the Theory and Language of Morality.* Translated by Peter Heinegg. Washington, DC: Georgetown University Press.

Secretary's Advisory Committee on Genetic Testing. 2000. *Enhancing the Oversight of Genetic Testing.* Bethesda, MD: National Institutes of Health.

Selling, Joseph A. 2002. "Proportionate Reasoning and the Concept of Ontic Evil: The Moral Theological Legacy of Louis Janssens." *Louvain Studies* 27:3–28.

———. 2012. "The Recovery of Aquinas's Action Theory: A Reply to William Murphy." *Theological Studies* 73, no. 1 (March): 139–50.

Shalala, Donna. 2001. "Protecting Research Subjects—What Must Be Done." *New England Journal of Medicine* 343 (September 14): 808–10.

Shannon, Thomas A. 1999. "No Restraint." *Catholic Free Press*, April 23, 5.

Shannon, Thomas A., and Lisa Sowle Cahill. 1988. *Religion and Artificial Reproduction. An Inquiry into the Vatican's "Instruction on Respect for Human Life."* New York: Crossroad.

Shannon, Thomas A., and Nicholas J. Kockler. 2009. *An Introduction to Bioethics.* 4th ed. New York: Paulist.

Shannon, Thomas A., and James J. Walter. 1988. "The PVS Patient and the Forgoing/Withdrawing of Medical Nutrition and Hydration." *Theological Studies* 49, no. 4 (December): 623–47.

———. 2004. "Implications of the Papal Allocution on Feeding Tubes." *Hastings Center Report* 34, no. 4 (July–August): 18–20.

———. 2005a. "Assisted Nutrition and Hydration and the Catholic Tradition." *Theological Studies* 66, no. 3 (September): 651–62.

———. 2005b. "Nutrition and Hydration: Shannon and Walter Reply." *Hastings Center Report* 35, no. 3 (May–June): 5.

———. 2005c. "Nutrition and Hydration" (Letter to the Editor). *Hastings Center Report* 35, no. 3 (May–June): 4.

Shannon, Thomas A., and Allan B. Wolter. 1990. "Reflections on the Moral Status of the Pre-Embryo." *Theological Studies* 51, no. 4 (December): 603–25.

Shewmon, D. Alan. 2009. "Brain Death: Can It Be Resuscitated?" *Hastings Center Report* 39, no. 2 (March–April): 18–24.

Shore, David A., ed. 2007. *The Trust Crisis in Healthcare: Causes, Consequences, and Cures.* New York: Oxford University Press.

Shuchman, Miriam. 2007. "Commercializing Clinical Trials: Risks and Benefits of the CRO Boom." *New England Journal of Medicine* 357, no. 14: 1365–68.

Siegler, Mark. 1986. "Ethics Committees: Decisions by Bureaucracy." *Hastings Center Report* 16, no. 3 (June): 22–24.

Siegler, Mark, and Peter Singer. 1988. "Clinical Ethics Consultation: Godsend or 'God Squad?'" *American Journal of Medicine* 85 (December): 759–60.

Singer, Peter. 1992. "From *Animal Liberation.*" In *Today's Moral Issues*, edited by Daniel Bonevac. 4th ed., 81–87. Boston, MA: McGraw-Hill.

———. 1993. *Practical Ethics.* Cambridge: Cambridge University Press.

Sismondo, Sergio, and Mathieu Doucet. 2010. "Publication Ethics and the Ghost Management of Medical Publications." *Bioethics* 24, no. 6: 273–83.

Skene, L., and J. Thompson. 2008. *The Sorting Society: The Ethics of Genetic Screening and Therapy.* Cambridge: Cambridge University Press.

Skinner, B. F. 1971. *Beyond Freedom and Dignity.* New York: Bantam/Vintage.

Sloan, Phillip T., ed. 2000. *Controlling Our Destinies: Historical, Philosophical, Ethical, and Theological Perspectives on the Human Genome Project.* Notre Dame, IN: University of Notre Dame Press.

Slomka, Jacqueline. 1994. "The Ethics Committee: Providing Education for Itself and Others." *HEC Forum* 6, no. 1: 31–38.

Slosar, John Paul, and Daniel O'Brien. 2003. "Rape Protocols and Moral Certitude." *Ethics & Medics* 28, no. 2 (February): 3–4.

Smith, G. P. 2011. *The Christian Religion and Biotechnology: A Search for Principled Decision-Making*. Dordrecht: Springer.

Solomon, Mildred Z. 1993. "How Physicians Talk about Futility: Making Words Mean Too Many Things." *Journal of Law, Medicine & Ethics* 21:231–37.

Sparrow, Robert. 2010. "Better Than Men? Sex and the Therapy/Enhancement Distinction." *Kennedy Institute of Ethics Journal* 20, no. 2 (June): 115–44.

Spath, P. L., ed. *Error Reduction in Health Care: A Systems Approach to Improving Patient Safety*. Washington, DC: AHA Press.

Spencer, Edward M, Ann E. Mills, Mary V. Rorty, Patricia H. Werhane. 2000. *Organization Ethics in Health Care*. New York: Oxford University Press.

SSM Health Care System. 1989. "Continuing or Discontinuing Treatment: Ethical Criteria: Catholic Health-Care System's Brief." *Origins* 19, no. 1 (September 28): 279–86.

Stark, Andrew. 2006. *The Limits of Medicine*. Cambridge: Cambridge University Press.

Sterba, James P. 1980. *The Demands of Justice*. Notre Dame, IN: University of Notre Dame Press.

St. Francis Medical Center. 1995. "Forgoing Treatment Policy." Pittsburgh, PA: St. Francis Medical Center.

Stock, Gregory, and John Campbell, eds. 2000. *Engineering the Human Germline*. New York: Oxford University Press.

Stockwell, B. R. 2011. *The Quest for the Cure: The Science and Stories behind the Next Generation of Medicines*. New York: Columbia University Press.

Stupak, Bart, and Joseph R. Pitts. 2009. "An Amendment to the Affordable Health Care for America Act." US House of Representatives, H.R. 3962.

Suarez, A., and J. Huarte. 2011. *Is This Cell a Human Being? Exploring the Status of Embryos, Stem Cells and Human-Animal Hybrids*. Dordrecht: Springer.

Sugarman, Jeremy. 1994. "Should Hospital Ethics Committees Do Research?" *Journal of Clinical Ethics* 5, no. 2 (Summer): 121–25.

Sulmasy, Daniel P. 1999. "The Rule of Double Effect: Clearing Up the Double Talk." *Archives of Internal Medicine* 159:545–50.

———. 2011. "Speaking of the Value of Life." *Kennedy Institute of Ethics Journal* 21, no. 2 (June): 181–99.

Swift, Francis W. 1966. "An Analysis of the American Theological Reaction to Janssens' Stand on 'the Pill.'" *Louvain Studies* 1, no. 1: 19–53.

Swinton, John, and Brian Brock, eds. 2007. *Theology, Disability and the New Genetics*. London: T & T Clark.

Teilhard de Chardin, Pierre. 2004. *The Future of Man*. New York: Doubleday (original English translation 1964).

Ten Have, Henk A. M. J. 2012. "Potter's Notion of Bioethics." *Kennedy Institute of Bioethics* 22, no. 1 (March): 59–82.

Ten Have, Henk A. M. J., and Michele S. Jean. eds. 2009. *The UNESCO Universal Declaration on Bioethics and Human Rights: Background, Principles, and Application*. Paris: UNESCO Publishing.

Texas Bishops. 1990. "On Withdrawing Artificial Nutrition and Hydration." *Origins* 20, no. 4 (June 7): 53–55.

Thielicke, Helmut. 1966. *Theological Ethics: Foundations*, edited by William H. Lazareth. Grand Rapids, MI: Eerdmans.

———. 1975. *Theological Ethics: Sex*. Translated by John W. Doberstein. Grand Rapids, MI: Eerdmans.

Thomas Aquinas. 1945. *Basic Writings of Saint Thomas Aquinas*. Edited and translated by Anton C. Pegis. New York: Random House.

———. 1948. *Summa theologica: Selections in Introduction to St. Thomas Aquinas*. Edited by Anton C. Pegis. New York: Random House.

———. 1986. *The Division and Methods of the Sciences*. Translated by Armand Maurer. 4th ed. Mediaeval Sources in Translation. Toronto: Pontifical Institute of Mediaeval Studies.

Thomasma, David C. 1991. "Why Philosophers Should Offer Ethics Consultations." *Theoretical Medicine* 12, no. 2 (June): 129–40.

Thurin, Ann, John Hausken, Torbjörn Hillensjö, Barbara Jablonowska, Anja Pinborg, Annika Strandell, and Christina Bergh. 2004. "Elective Single-Embryo Transfer versus Double-Embryo Transfer in In Vitro Fertilization." *New England Journal of Medicine* 351:2392–2401.

Tollefsen, Christopher. 2010. "Divine, Human, and Embryo Adoption." *National Catholic Bioethics Quarterly* 11, no. 2 (Spring): 75–85.

Tomlinson, Tom, and Howard Brody. 1988. "Ethics and Communication in Do-Not-Resuscitate Orders." *New England Journal of Medicine* 318, no. 1 (January 7): 43–46.

Torke, Alexia M., G. Caleb Alexander, and John Lantos. 2008. "Substituted Judgment: The Limitations of Autonomy in Surrogate Decision Making." *Journal of General Internal Medicine* 23, no. 9 (September): 1514–17.

Tracy, David. 1975. *Blessed Rage for Order.* New York: Seabury Press.

Traveline, John M. 2007. "Notes and Abstracts: Medicine." *National Catholic Bioethics Quarterly* 7, no. 4 (Winter): 793–808.

Truog, Robert D., David M. Browning, Judith A. Johnson, and Thomas H. Gallagher. 2011. *Talking with Patients and Families about Medical Error: Guide for Education and Practice.* Baltimore: Johns Hopkins University Press.

Tulskey, James A., and Bernard Lo. 1992. "Ethics Consultation: Time to Focus on Patients." *American Journal of Medicine* 92 (April): 343–45.

Tuohey, John F. 1995. "The Implications of the Ethical and Religious Directives for Catholic Health Care Services on the Clinical Practice of Resolving Ectopic Pregnancies." *Louvain Studies* 20:41–57.

Turda, M. 2010. *Modernism and Eugenics.* Hampshire, UK: Palgrave Macmillan.

Turner, Leigh. 2003. "Zones of Consensus and Zones of Conflict: Questioning the 'Common Morality' Presumption in Bioethics." *Kennedy Institute of Ethics Journal* 13, no. 3 (September): 193–218.

Underwood, Anne. 2003. "Fibromyalgia: Not All in Your Head." *Newsweek,* May 19, 53.

UNESCO. 1997. *Declaration on the Responsibilities of the Present Generations towards Future Generations.* Paris: UNESCO. Accessed December 2, 2011. www.unesco.org/cpp/uk/declarations/generations.pdf.

US Bishops' Pro-Life Committee. 1992. "Nutrition and Hydration: Moral and Pastoral Reflections." *Origins* 21, no. 44 (April 9): 705–12.

United States Catholic Conference (USCC). 1989. "USCC Brief in Nancy Cruzan Case." *Origins* 19, no. 21 (October 26): 345–51.

US Catholic Conference Department of Health Affairs. 1971. *Ethical and Religious Directives for Catholic Health Facilities.* Washington, DC: United States Catholic Conference.

US Conference of Catholic Bishops (USCCB). 1977. "Commentary on the Reply of the Sacred Congregation for the Doctrine of the Faith on Sterilization in Catholic Hospitals." *Origins* 7 (September 15): 399–400.

———. 1981. *Health and Health Care: A Pastoral Letter of the American Catholic Bishops.* Washington, DC: USCCB.

———. 1983. *Commentary on the Reply of the Sacred Congregation for the Doctrine of the Faith on Sterilization in Catholic Hospitals.* Washington, DC: USCCB.

———. 1986. *Economic Justice for All: Pastoral Letter on Catholic Social Teaching and the US Economy.* Washington, DC: USCCB.

———. 1995. *Ethical and Religious Directives for Catholic Health Care Services.* Washington, DC: USCCB.

———. 2001. *Ethical and Religious Directives for Catholic Health Care Services.* 4th ed. Washington, DC: USCCB.

———. 2009a. *Ethical and Religious Directives for Catholic Health Care Services.* 5th ed. Washington, DC: USCCB.

———. 2009b. *Forming Consciences for Faithful Citizenship. A Call to Political Responsibility from the Catholic Bishops of the United States.* Washington, DC: USCCB.

US Government Accountability Office. 2009. *Human Subjects Research: Undercover Tests Show the Institutional Review Board System Is Vulnerable to Unethical Manipulation.* GAO-09-448T, March 2009. Accessed February 10, 2012. www.gao.gov/assets/130/122142.pdf.

Vacek, Edward V. 1988. "Notes on Moral Theology: Vatican Instruction on Reproductive Technology." *Theological Studies* 49, no. 1 (March): 110–31.

Van Allen, Evelyn D., Gay Moldow, and Ronald Cranford. 1989. "Evaluating Ethics Committees." *Hastings Center Report* 19, no. 5 (September–October): 23–24.

van der Heide, Inga G. 1994. "Hospital Ethics Committees in Practice: The Case Review Function of Four HEC's in Connecticut." *HEC Forum* 6, no. 2: 73–84.

Vatican Council II. 1966. "Pastoral Constitution on the Church in the Modern World." Translated by Joseph Gallagher. In *The Documents of Vatican II*, edited by Walter M. Abbott, 199–308. New York: Guild Press.

Vatican Information Service. 2004. "Patients in the Vegetative State Are Always Human," March 22.

Veatch, Robert M. 1973a. "Does Ethics Have an Empirical Basis?" *Hastings Center Studies* 1, no. 1: 50–65.

———. 1973b. "Generalization of Expertise." *Hastings Center Studies* 1, no. 2: 29–40.

———. 1977a. *Case Studies in Medical Ethics*. Cambridge, MA: Harvard University Press.

———. 1977b. "Hospital Ethics Committees: Is There a Role?" *Hastings Center Report* 7, no. 3 (June): 22–25.

———. 1988. "Justice and the Economics of Terminal Illness." *Hastings Center Report* 18, no. 4 (August–September): 34–40.

———. 2000. *Transplantation Ethics*. Washington, DC: Georgetown University Press.

———. 2003. "Is There a Common Morality?" *Kennedy Institute of Ethics Journal* 13, no. 3 (September): 189–92.

———. 2004. "Abandon the Dead Donor Rule or Change the Definition of Death?" *Kennedy Institute of Ethics Journal* 14, no. 3 (September): 261–76.

Venter, J. Craig, Mark D. Adams, Eugene W. Myers, Peter W. Li, Richard J. Mural, Granger G. Sutton, Hamilton O. Smith, Mark Yandell, Cheryl A. Evans, Robert A. Holt, et al. 2001. "The Sequence of the Human Genome." *Science* 291 (February 16): 1304–51.

Verhey, Allen D. 1997. "Playing God." In *Genetic Ethics: Do the Ends Justify the Genes?*, edited by John F. Kilner and Frank E. Young, 60–74. Grand Rapids, MI: Eerdmans.

———. 2010. *Nature and Altering It*. Grand Rapids, MI: Eerdmans.

Vincent, Charles. 2010. *Patient Safety*. 2nd ed. Oxford: Wiley-Blackwell.

Wachter, Robert M. 2008. *Understanding Patient Safety*. New York: McGraw-Hill.

Waldman, Steven, Andrew Lachman, and Elizabeth Bradburn. 1990. "The Insurance Mess." *Newsweek*, April 23.

Walker, Rebecca L., and Nancy M. P. King. 2011. "Biodefense Research and the US Regulatory Structure: Whither Nonhuman Primate Moral Standing?" *Kennedy Institute of Ethics Journal* 21, no. 3 (September): 277–310.

Walter, James J. 2002. "Terminal Sedation: A Catholic Perspective." *Update* 18, no. 2 (September): 6–8.

———. 2011 "Healthcare Reform in the United States: The *Status Quaestionis* of the Ethical Debate." *Louvain Studies* 35, no. 1–2 (Spring–Summer): 117–37.

Walter, Jennifer K., and Susan Dorr Goold. 2011. "Conjectural Mixed Motives (Case Study)." *Hastings Center Report* 41, no. 1 (January–February): 11–13.

Walters, LeRoy B. 2004 "Human Embryonic Stem Cell Research: An International Perspective." *Kennedy Institute of Ethics Journal* 14, no. 1 (March): 3–38.

Walters, LeRoy, and Julie G. Palmer. 1997. *The Ethics of Human Gene Therapy*. New York: Oxford University Press.

Watson, J. D., and F. H. C. Crick. 1953. "Molecular Structure of Nucleic Acids: A Structure for Deoxyribose Nucleic Acid." *Nature* 171:737–38.

Watt, Helen, ed. 2005. *Cooperation, Complicity & Conscience: Problems in Healthcare, Science, Law and Public Policy*. London: Linacre Centre.

Wear, Stephen, Benjamin Phillips, Sally Shimmel, and John Banas. 1995. "Developing and Implementing a Medical Futility Policy: One Hospital's Experience." *Community Ethics* 3, no. 1 (Winter): 2–5.

Weindling, P. J. 2004. *Nazi Medicine and the Nuremberg Trials: From Medical War Crimes to Informed Consent*. London: Palgrave.

Weiss, S. F. 2010. *The Nazi Symbiosis: Human Genetics and Politics in the Third Reich*. Chicago: University of Chicago Press.

Welch, H. Gilbert. 2011. "Low Diagnostic Thresholds Mean Higher Risk of Harmful Treatment." *Island Packet*, May 11, 6A.

West, Mary Beth, and Joan McIver Gibson. 1992. "Facilitating Medical Ethics Case Review: What Ethics Committees Can Learn from Mediation and Facilitation Techniques." *Cambridge Quarterly of Healthcare Ethics* 1:63–74.

White House. 2010. "Executive Order: Ensuring Enforcement and Implementation of Abortion Restrictions in the Patient Protection and Affordable Care Act." March 24. www.whitehouse .gov/the-press-office/executive-order-patient-protection-and-affordable-care-acts-consistency-with-longst.

Wijdicks, Eelco F. M., ed. 2001. *Brain Death*. Philadelphia: Lippincott Williams & Wilkins.

Wilkinson, Stephen. 2010. *Choosing Tomorrow's Children: The Ethics of Selective Reproduction*. Oxford: Clarendon Press.

Wilson, J. M. G., and G. Jungner. 1968. *Principles and Practice of Screening for Disease*. Geneva: World Health Organization.

Wolf, Susan M. 1996. "Physician-Assisted Suicide in the Context of Managed Care." *Duquesne Law Review* 35, no. 1 (Fall): 455–79.

———. 2008. "Confronting Physician-Assisted Suicide and Euthanasia: My Father's Death." *Hastings Center Report* 38, no. 5 (September–October): 23–26.

Wolff, Robert Paul. 1977. *Understanding Rawls: A Reconstruction and Critique of "A Theory of Justice."* Princeton, NJ: Princeton University Press.

Wuerl, Donald W. 2005. "Reflection on Nutrition and Hydration." Bishop's Statement.

Yavarone, Mark. 2004. "Do Anovulants and IUDs Kill Early Human Embryos?" *National Catholic Bioethics Quarterly* 4, no. 1 (Spring): 63–70.

Young, Amos. 2007. *Theology and Down Syndrome. Reimagining Disability in Late Modernity*. Waco, TX: Baylor University Press.

Young, K. K. 2009. "The Discourses of Hindu Medical Ethics." In *The Cambridge World History of Medical Ethics*, edited by Robert B. Baker and Lawrence B. McCullough, 175–84. New York: Cambridge University Press.

Youngner, Stuart J. 1988. "Who Defines Futility?" *Journal of the American Medical Association* 260, no. 14 (October 14) 2094–95.

———. 1994. "Applying Futility: Saying No Is Not Enough." *Journal of the American Geriatrics Society* 42:887–89.

Youngner, Stuart J., Martha W. Anderson, and Renie Shapiro, eds. 2004. *Transplanting Human Tissue: Ethics, Policy, and Practice*. New York: Oxford University Press.

Youngner, Stuart J., Robert M. Arnold, and Renie Shapiro, eds. 1999. *The Definition of Death: Contemporary Controversies*. Baltimore: Johns Hopkins University Press.

Zaner, Richard M. 1988. *Death: Beyond Whole Brain Criteria*. Dordrecht: Kluwer Academic Publishers.

Zoloth, Laurie. 2002. "Reasonable Magic and the Nature of Alchemy: Jewish Reflections on Human Embryonic Stem Cell Research." *Kennedy Institute of Ethics Journal* 12, no. 1 (March): 65–93.

Index

Page numbers followed by *t* indicate tables.